CANNABINOIDS IN HEALTH AND DISEASE

Edited by **Rosaria Meccariello**
and **Rosanna Chianese**

Cannabinoids in Health and Disease
http://dx.doi.org/10.5772/61595
Edited by Rosaria Meccariello and Rosanna Chianese

Contributors

Sophie Layé, Oliver Dewald, Georg Duerr, Abel Santamaria, Gabriela Aguilera, Roberto Coccurello, Teresa Morera-Herreras, Maria Torrecilla, Cristina Miguelez, Asier Aristieta, Jose Angel Ruiz-Ortega, Luisa Ugedo, Thomas Heinbockel, Ze-Jun Wang, Edward Brown, Paul Austin, Elena Kaschina, Katia Befort, Léa Giron, Li Zhang, Rosaria Meccariello

Published by InTech

Janeza Trdine 9, 51000 Rijeka, Croatia

Publishing Process Manager Edi Lipovic
Technical Editor SPi Global
Cover InTech Design team

First published November, 2016
Printed in Croatia

Additional hard copies can be obtained from orders@intechopen.com

Cannabinoids in Health and Disease, Edited by Rosaria Meccariello and Rosanna Chianese
p. cm.
Print ISBN 978-953-51-2429-0
Online ISBN 978-953-51-2430-6

Meet the editors

Dr. Rosaria Meccariello received her degree in biology from the University of Naples Federico II, Italy, and the PhD in comparative endocrinology from the University of Padova, Italy, in 1997 and 2004, respectively. Currently, she is an associate professor of biology at the Department of Movement Sciences and Wellness at Parthenope University of Naples, Italy. She has published over 110 papers in various peer-reviewed international journals, books, proceedings and abstract books. She has a wide experience as a reviewer for international journals, and recently, she has been an editor of a special issue and an e-book. She is an expert in biology of reproduction, spermatogenesis, hypothalamus-pituitary-gonad axis, central and local activity of GnRH, endocannabinoid and kisspeptin systems.

Dr. Rosanna Chianese received her degree in biology from the University of Naples Federico II, Italy, in 2004. In 2006, she carried out a training at the University of Washington, Seattle, USA, during her PhD studies in comparative endocrinology (University of Padova, Italy). For the biennium 2009/2011, she obtained a research fellowship for the project "Mesothelioma and biomarkers" at the Second University of Naples (SUN), Italy. Currently, she is an assistant professor at the Department of Experimental Medicine, SUN. She has experience as reviewer for international journals and since 2005, she has published 25 articles in international journals, 1 book chapter for InTech and 22 abstracts for national and international conferences. Dr. Chianese also teaches face-to-face cellular biology course at SUN.

Contents

Preface

The origin of the therapeutic use of *Cannabis* goes back to time immemorial. One of the most ancient books on medical plants, the *PenT'sao Ching*, recommends its use as a *"poison good"* to improve body energy and to treat rheumatism, malaria, constipation and mental weakness. In the same book, the hallucinogenic effects of the plant were also described. From that moment onwards, evidences of *Cannabis* use were also reported in the Indian holy book Atharvaveda in relation to practices against demons, but also *"as a plant able to give body and mind more perceptive"*. Around 70 AC, Dioscorides, a surgeon in the Roman legions, reported the first representation of the plant in De materia medica, suggesting its use in case of earache, inflammation, oedema and gout. During the nineteenth century, O'Shaughnessy, a British physician and surgeon working in India, described—for the first time—important anticonvulsant and analgesic properties of the *Cannabis*, so that Queen Victoria's doctor prescribed this plant to treat her dysmenorrhea; since then, several European countries tried to identify the active *Cannabis* constituents. Anyway, during the twentieth century, firstly in the USA, then in Europe, some historical-political circumstances induced a reversal of tendency about the enthusiasm that until then followed through *Cannabis* use. In fact, its diffusion for recreational purposes and the introduction of other derivatives of opium as anticonvulsant and analgesic drugs instigated a massive press campaign against *Cannabis* until causing its removal from the United States Pharmacopeia and losing its therapeutic legitimacy. Investigations into the chemistry of *Cannabis* came back to the nineteenth century, when an alkaloid—like most of the active plant constituents, such as morphine and cocaine—was considered the active constituent of *Cannabis*. But only in 1965, a group of Israeli researchers, working on synthetic compounds, suggested that Delta 9-tetrahydrocannabinol (THC) was the most potent among the several active principles of *Cannabis*. From this starting point, different groups tried to isolate numerous components of *Cannabis*, in addition to cannabidiol and THC.

The discovery of *Cannabis* constituents persuaded researchers to understand their mechanisms of action, since the isolation of cannabinoid receptors, the analysis of their pharmacological properties, their binding sites and their distribution in biological systems. As a consequence of specific cannabinoid receptor discovery, the next step in Cannabis history was surely the assumption of the existence of endogenous cannabinoid ligands, defined as *endocannabinoids*. A major challenge in this field was to understand the biological activities of the endocannabinoids in several physiological systems. Anyway, much has been done, but this story is so intriguing that many aspects still need to be elucidated.

The book aims to provide basic concepts in the modulation of endocannabinoid system in both physiological and pathological conditions and integrates data from experimental animal models and clinical observations. Particular attention has been focused on the medical use of cannabinoids and the targeting of endocannabinoid system as a new potential therapeutic strategy for the prevention and treatment of human diseases. In this respect, the book aims to reach basic and clinical scientists, teachers and students interested in the field of cannabinoids.

The book is organized in 10 chapters. The first one provides a general overview on the activity/impairment of endocannabinoid system in human health/disease. Then, four interrelated chapters point out cannabinoid activity in the brain and their potential therapeutic role in the treatment of neurological disorders. In particular, Chapter 2 focuses on the olfactory and limbic system, Chapters 3 and 4 on basal ganglia, and Chapter 5 reveals upcoming experimental evidences concerning cannabinoid activity through glycine receptors. The impact of polyunsaturated fatty acids (PUFAs) on brain health and the links among cannabinoids, diet, food intake and energy balance have been addressed in Chapters 6 and 7, respectively. Furthermore, the next two chapters describe the activity of cannabinoid receptors in the hearth (Chapter 8) and the role of the endocannabinoid system in cardioprotection and myocardial adaptation (Chapter 9). The last chapter of the book focuses on the discussed role of cannabinoids as drug or medication.

We would like to thank all the authors for their valuable contributions and for the constructive interplay throughout the editorial process.

Editor
Rosaria Meccariello
Department of Movement Sciences and Wellness
Parthenope University of Naples, Italy

Co-Editor
Rosanna Chianese
Department of Experimental Medicine
Second University of Naples, Italy

Chapter 1

Introductory Chapter: The Endocannabinoid System in Human Physiology

Rosanna Chianese and Rosaria Meccariello

Additional information is available at the end of the chapter

http://dx.doi.org/10.5772/63818

1. Endocannabinoid system (ECS)

The identification of Δ^9-tetrahydrocannabinol (Δ^9-THC) in 1964 by Gaoni and Mechoulam [1] as the principal biologically active component of *Cannabis sativa* has implicated the indispensable need to unveil the pharmacology of such a molecule and the correlated mechanisms of action. Since then, the subsequent identification of two G-protein-coupled cannabinoid receptors, CB1 [2] and CB2 [3], able to mediate Δ^9-THC effects. The existence of endogenous ligands that share many effects of the Δ^9-THC allows to formulate the attractive hypothesis that an endocannabinoid system (ECS) may play a pivotal role in a variety of centrally and peripherally regulated physiological processes. A plethora of endocannabinoids has been discovered starting from the anandamide [AEA, 4] and 2-arachidonoylglycerol [2-AG, 5] toward; they bind to CB1, CB2, or other cannabinoid receptors. In this regard, a role of GPR119 [6] and GPR55 [7] in endocannabinoid signal transduction has been suggested a long time ago; intriguingly, some endocannabinoids—such as the AEA—also bind to type 1 vanilloid receptor [TRPV1, 8] and to peroxisome proliferator-activated receptor γ [PPARγ, 9], as well as 2-AG binds to specific γ-aminobutyric acid (GABA) receptor (A) subtypes in neuronal cells [10], thus making more intricate the network of the endocannabinoid activated pathways.

Endocannabinoid tone is finely regulated by a highly organized system of biosynthesis and degradation enzymes that are integral part of ECS. The main pathways of AEA biosynthesis and degradation depend on the activity of the N-arachidonoyl-phosphatidylethanolamine phospholipase D (Nape-PLD) [11] and the fatty acid amide hydrolase (FAAH) [12], respectively. Two diacylglycerol lipases (DAGLα and DAGLβ) enzymes are involved in 2-AG biosynthesis [13], whereas monoacylglycerol lipase (MAGL) and to a lesser extend FAAH metabolizes it [14]. The biological activity of endocannabinoids is finely regulated by mechanisms of intracellular uptake. In this respect, many doubts still exist and several hypotheses have been formulated. AEA transport, for instance, may occur by passive and/or facilitated diffusion, this last by an hypothetical endocannabinoid membrane transporter whose chemical identity remains as yet unknown [15], by endocytosis [16], through fatty acid binding protein (FABP) proteins [17] or a FAAH-like AEA transporter protein (FLAT), a cytosolic variant of FAAH that lacks amidase activity, but bounding AEA, facilitates its translocation into cells [18].

2. Endocannabinoid activity in biological systems

Endocannabinoid biosynthesis, uptake, degradation, and activity have been largely reported in the central nervous system (CNS) and in a wide set of peripheral tissues in vertebrates—from fish to mammals, humans included [19]—but also in invertebrates [20]. Thus, this phylogenetically and onthogenetically conserved system is involved in the central and local control of many biological functions.

At cellular level, cell proliferation, differentiation, survival, and apoptotic rate—with different outcomes depending on the molecular targets and cellular context involved—have been reported to be under ECS control in tissues such as gonads, adipose tissues, bone, blood, epithelial cells, and also in the brain [21].

ECS activity is critical in CNS, as elsewhere properly reviewed [22]. In general, physiological functions of ECS in CNS include: pain perception, motor functions, control of tremor, and spasticity, cognitive functions (i.e. learning and memory), thermogenesis, regulation of weak/sleep cycles, axonal pathfinding, synaptic plasticity and adult neurogenesis, emotional behavior, stress response *via* modulation of hypothalamus-pituitary-adrenal gland axis (HPA), feeding and appetite, reproductive functions *via* modulation of hypothalamus-pituitary-gonad axis (HPG) and sex behavior, retinal neurotransmission from the retina to the primary visual cortex [properly reviewed in the following books: 23, 24]. Classically, 2-AG is released in the brain by postsynaptic neurons and acts as rapid retrograde signal to target presynaptic neurons in order to inhibit neurotransmitter release, whereas AEA may function as slow retrograde signal, non-retrograde signal or as TRPV1 agonist [25]. Dopaminergic, glutamatergic, GABA and N-methyl-D-aspartate (NMDA) transmission, and the secretion of neurohormones such as the gonadotropin-releasing hormone (GnRH) are all controlled by endocannabinoids [26, 27]. Direct involvement in the control of pituitary hormone release has also been provided [28].

Besides the brain, endocannabinoid biosynthesis and activity occur in peripheral tissues, such as blood cells, heart, intestine, liver, adipose tissue, muscle, and pancreas, where it seems to be involved in the regulation of inflammation, platelet aggregation, blood pressure, heart rate, vasodilatation, modulation of peristalsis, energy balance *via* lipid and glucose homeostasis and so on [properly reviewed in the following book: 23, 29–32]. However, most studies concern the activity of ECS in the control of reproduction in both sexes, as summarized in **Table 1**. In fact, besides the activity exerted at hypothalamic and pituitary level in order to regulate GnRH release and the discharge of pituitary gonadotropins which in turns sustain sex steroid biosynthesis, direct ECS activity has been reported in both testis and ovary, in male and female reproductive tracts, in gametes and also in reproductive fluids. Functions related to the production of high-quality gametes, fertilization, embryo implantation, embryo growth, and delivery have excellently been reviewed elsewhere, with evidence that the maintenance of gradients of endocannabinoids in reproductive tracts is required to modulate step-by-step several events, from the acquisition of sperm motility to a successful embryo implantation (details and references in **Table 1**).

Female Reproduction	**References**
Folliculogenesis	[35, 36]
Oocyte maturation	[35]
Embryo transport	[37]
Embryo implantation/pregnancy	[38–41]
Endometrial plasticity	[42]
Delivery	[34, 43]
Male reproduction	**References**
Spermatogenesis progression	[44–50]
Sperm motility	[51, 52]
Chromatin remodelling	[53–55]
Sperm fertilizing ability	[34, 56, 57]
Leydig cell functions	[58–60]
Sertoli cell apoptosis	[44, 61]
Sperm capacitation, ZP-induced acrosomal reaction (AR)	[57, 62–64]

Table 1. Main biological activities of ECS in both female and male reproduction.

Thus, the modulation of endocannabinoid tone by FAAH is the main gatekeeper in the control of many physiological functions, from the formation of specialized tissues to neurotransmitter release, neuroprotection of circuit integrity and neuroplasticity, central pain perception, neuroendocrine functions, food intake, energy balance, reproduction, pregnancy, delivery, cardioprotection, inflammatory response, and so on [33].

As a consequence, alterations of ECS activity have been correlated to many diseases such as neurodegenerative disorders and motor dysfunctions, mood disorders as well as psychosis (schizophrenia) and autism, retinopathy, neuroendocrine dysfunctions, obesity, diabetes and metabolic syndrome, cardiovascular disorders and cardiac pathologies, gastrointestinal and urogenital diseases, sepsis, cancer and related inflammation processes, infertility, but also to miscarriage and preterm birth.

Consistently, alteration of the physiological endocannabinoid tone by the occasional use or abuse of phytocannabinoids has been reported to deeply impact human health [34].

3. Conclusions

Due to the above considerations, ECS has emerged as important regulator of both physiological and pathological processes. Considerable attention has been focused on the targeting of the endocannabinoid receptors and of endocannabinoid byosinthetic/hydrolizing enzymes for the treatment of a variety of disorders with high impact on human health. Thus, in the future, the administration of specific cannabinoid receptor agonists/antagonists or the inhibition of endocannabinoid degradation might represent a promising therapeutic strategy for the maintenance/restore of human health and the cure of human diseases such as neurological and cardiovascular diseases, diabetes and obesity, as well as infertility and cancer.

Conflict of interest

The authors declare that there is no conflict of interests regarding the publication of this paper.

Acknowledgements

Work incorporated in this paper was partially supported by Prin MIUR 2010–2011 (Rosaria Meccariello).

The authors apologize for unintended omission of any relevant references.

Author details

Rosanna Chianese[1] and Rosaria Meccariello[2*]

*Address all correspondence to: rosaria.meccariello@uniparthenope.it

1 Dipartimento di Medicina Sperimentale sez "F. Bottazzi", Seconda Università di Napoli, Napoli, Italy

2 Dipartimento di Scienze Motorie e del Benessere, Università di Napoli Parthenope, Napoli, Italy

References

[1] Gaoni Y, Mechoulam R. Isolation, structure and partial synthesis of an active constituent of hashish. J Am Chem Soc 1964;86:1646.

[2] Matsuda LA, Lolait SJ, Brownstein MJ, Young AC, Bonner TI. Structure of a cannabinoid receptor and functional expression of the cloned cDNA. Nature 1990;346:561–564.

[3] Munro S, Thomas KL, Abu-Shaar M. Molecular characterization of a peripheral receptor for cannabinoids. Nature 1993;365:61–65.

[4] Devane WA, Hanus L, Breuer A, Pertwee RG, Stevenson LA, Griffin G, Gibson D, Mandelbaum A, Etinger A, Mechoulam R. Isolation and structure of a brain constituent that binds to the cannabinoid receptor. Science 1992;258:1946–1949.

[5] Mechoulam R, Ben-Shabat S, Hanus L, Ligumsky M, Kaminski NE, Schatz AR, Gopher A, Almog S, Martin BR, Compton DR. Identification of an endogenous 2-monoglyceride, present in canine gut, that binds to cannabinoid receptors. Biochem Pharmacol 1995;50:83–90.

[6] Fredriksson R, Hoglund PJ, Gloriam DE, Lagerstrom MC, Schioth HB. Seven evolutionarily conserved human rhodopsin G protein-coupled receptors lacking close relatives. FEBS Lett 2003;554:381–388.

[7] Lauckner JE, Jensen JB, Chen HY, Lu HC, Hille B, Mackie K. GPR55 is a cannabinoid receptor that increases intracellular calcium and inhibits M current. Proc Natl Acad Sci USA 2008;105:2699–2704.

[8] Starowicz K, Nigam S, Di Marzo V. Biochemistry and pharmacology of endovanilloids. Pharmacol Ther 2007;114:13–33.

[9] Gasperi V, Fezza F, Pasquariello N, Bari M, Oddi S, Agrò AF, Maccarrone M. Endocannabinoids in adipocytes during differentiation and their role in glucose uptake. Cell Mol Life Sci 2007;64:219–229.

[10] Sigel E, Baur R, Rácz I, Marazzi J, Smart TG, Zimmer A, Gertsch J. The major central endocannabinoid directly acts at GABA(A) receptors. Proc Natl Acad Sci USA 2011; 108:18150–18155.

[11] Okamoto Y, Morishita J, Tsuboi K, Tonai T, Ueda N. Molecular characterization of a phospholipase d generating anandamide and its congeners. J Biol Chem 2004;279:5298–5305.

[12] McKinney MK, Cravatt BF. Structure and function of fatty acid amide hydrolase. Annu Rev Biochem 2005;74:411–432.

[13] Stella N, Schweitzer P, Piomelli DA, second endogenous cannabinoid that modulates longterm potentiation. Nature 1997;388:773–778.

[14] Dinh TP, Freund TF, Piomelli D. A role for monoglyceride lipase in 2-arachidonoylglycerol inactivation. Chem Phys Lipids 2002;121:149–158.

[15] Ligresti A, Morera E, van der Stelt M, Monory K, Lutz B, Ortar G, Di Marzo V. Further evidence for the existence of a specific process for the membrane transport of anandamide. Biochem J 2004;380:265–272.

[16] McFarland MJ, Porter AC, Rakhshan FR, Rawat DS, Gibbs RA, Barker EL. A role for caveolae/lipid rafts in the uptake and recycling of the endogenous cannabinoid anandamide. J Biol Chem 2004;279:41991–41997.

[17] Kaczocha M, Glaser ST, Deutsch DG. Identification of intracellular carriers for the endocannabinoid anandamide. Proc Natl Acad Sci USA 2009;106:6375–6380.

[18] Fu J, Bottegoni G, Sasso O, Bertorelli R, Rocchia W, Masetti M, Guijarro A, Lodola A, Armirotti A, Garau G, Bandiera T, Reggiani A, Mor M, Cavalli A, Piomelli D. A catalytically silent FAAH-1 variant drives anandamide transport in neurons. Nat Neurosci 2011;15:64–69.

[19] Cacciola G, Chianese R, Chioccarelli T, Ciaramella V, Fasano S, Pierantoni R, Meccariello R, Cobellis G. Cannabinoids and reproduction: a lasting and intriguing history. Pharmaceuticals 2010;3:3275–3323

[20] Elphick MR, Egertová M. The neurobiology and evolution of cannabinoid signalling. Philos Trans R Soc Lond B Biol Sci. 2001;356:381–408.

[21] Galve-Roperh I, Chiurchiù V, Díaz-Alonso J, Bari M, Guzmán M, Maccarrone M. Cannabinoid receptor signaling in progenitor/stem cell proliferation and differentiation. Prog Lipid Res. 2013;52:633–650.

[22] Mechoulam R, Parker LA. The endocannabinoid system and the brain. Annu Rev Psychol 2013;64:21–47.

[23] Pertwee RG (editor). Endocannabinoids. in Handbook of experimental pharmacology. Springer International Publisher Science, Technology, Medicine, Germany. 2015. 231 p. doi:10.1007/978-3-319-20825-1_2.

[24] Litwack G (editor). Anandamide an endogenous cannabinoid. in Vitamins & Hormones. Elsevier Science Publishing Co Inc, United States (2009). 2009. 81 p. ISBN: 978-0-12-374782-2.

[25] Ohno-Shosaku T, Kano M. Endocannabinoid-mediated retrograde modulation of synaptic transmission. Curr Opin Neurobiol 2014;29:1–8.

[26] van der Stelt M, Di Marzo V. The endocannabinoid system in the basal ganglia and in the mesolimbic reward system: implications for neurological and psychiatric disorders. Eur J Pharmacol 2003;480:133–150.

[27] Meccariello R, Battista N, Bradshaw HB, Wang H. Endocannabinoids and reproduction. Int J Endocrinol 2014;378069.

[28] Battista N, Di Tommaso M, Bari M, Maccarrone M. The endocannabinoid system: an overview. Front Behav Neurosci 2012;6:9.

[29] Watkins BA, Hutchins H, Li Y, Seifert MF. The endocannabinoid signaling system: a marriage of PUFA and musculoskeletal health. J Nutr Biochem 2010;21:1141–1152.

[30] Bab I, Zimmer A. Cannabinoid receptors and the regulation of bone mass. Br J Pharmacol 2008;153:182–188.

[31] Klein TW. Cannabinoid-based drugs as anti-inflammatory therapeutics. Nat Rev Immunol 2005;5:400–411.

[32] Pacher P, Gao B. Endocannabinoids and liver disease. III. Endocannabinoid effects on immune cells: implications for inflammatory liver diseases. Am J Physiol Gastrointest Liver Physiol 2008;294:G850–854.

[33] Katona I, Freund TF. Multiple functions of endocannabinoid signaling in the brain. Annu Rev Neurosci 2012;35:529–558.

[34] Wang H, Xie H, Guo Y, Zhang H, Takahashi T, Kingsley PJ, Marnett LJ, Das SK, Cravatt BF, Dey SK. Fatty acid amide hydrolase deficiency limits early pregnancy events. J Clin Invest 2006;116:2122–2131.

[35] El-Talatini MR, Taylor AH, Elson JC, Brown L, Davidson AC, Konje JC. Localisation and function of the endocannabinoid system in the human ovary. PLoS One 2009;4:e4579.

[36] Cecconi S, Rossi G, Castellucci A, D'Andrea G, Maccarrone M. Endocannabinoid signaling in mammalian ovary. Eur J Obstet Gynecol Reprod Biol 2014;178:6–11.

[37] Maccarrone M. Endocannabinoids: friends and foes of reproduction. Prog Lipid Res 2009;48:344–354.

[38] Sun X, Dey SK. Aspects of endocannabinoid signaling in periimplantation biology. Mol Cell Endocrinol 2008;286:S3–11.

[39] Taylor AH, Ang C, Bell SC, Konje JC. The role of the endocannabinoid system in gametogenesis, implantation and early pregnancy. Hum Reprod Update 2007;13:501–513.

[40] Taylor AH, Amoako AA, Bambang K, Karasu T, Gebeh A, Lam PM, Marzcylo TH, Konje JC. Endocannabinoids and pregnancy. Clin Chim Acta 2010;411:921–930.

[41] Trabucco E, Acone G, Marenna A, Pierantoni R, Cacciola G, Chioccarelli T, Mackie K, Fasano S, Colacurci N, Meccariello R, Cobellis G, Cobellis L. Endocannabinoid system in first trimester placenta: low FAAH and high CB1 expression characterize spontaneous miscarriage. Placenta 2009;30:516–522.

[42] Di Blasio AM, Vignali M, Gentilini D. The endocannabinoid pathway and the female reproductive organs. J Mol Endocrinol 2013;50:R1–9.

[43] Melford SE, Taylor AH, Konje JC. Of mice and (wo)men: factors influencing successful implantation including endocannabinoids. Hum Reprod Update 2014;20:415–428.

[44] Maccarrone M, Cecconi S, Rossi G, Battista N, Pauselli R, Finazzi-Agrò A. Anandamide activity and degradation are regulated by early postnatal aging and follicle-stimulating hormone in mouse Sertoli cells. Endocrinology 2003;144:20–28.

[45] Grimaldi P, Orlando P, Di Siena S, Lolicato F, Petrosino S, Bisogno T, Geremia R, De Petrocellis L, Di Marzo V. The endocannabinoid system and pivotal role of the CB2 receptor in mouse spermatogenesis. Proc Natl Acad Sci USA 2009;106:11131–11136.

[46] Cacciola G, Chioccarelli T, Fasano S, Pierantoni R, Cobellis G. Estrogens and spermiogenesis: new insights from type1 cannabinoid receptor knockout mice. Int J Endocrinol 2013;2013:501350.

[47] Chianese R, Ciaramella V, Scarpa D, Fasano S, Pierantoni R, Meccariello R. Anandamide regulates the expression of GnRH1, GnRH2, and GnRH-Rs in frog testis. Am J Physiol Endocrinol Metab 2012;303:E475–487.

[48] Chianese R, Ciaramella V, Scarpa D, Fasano S, Pierantoni R, Meccariello R. Endocannabinoids and endovanilloids: a possible balance in the regulation of the testicular GnRH signalling. Int J Endocrinol 2013;2013:904748.

[49] Meccariello R, Chianese R, Chioccarelli T, Ciaramella V, Fasano S, Pierantoni R, Cobellis G. Intra-testicular signals regulate germ cell progression and production of qualitatively mature spermatozoa in vertebrates. Front Endocrinol (Lausanne) 2014;5:69.

[50] Di Giacomo D, De Domenico E, Sette C, Geremia R, Grimaldi P. Type 2 cannabinoid receptor contributes to the physiological regulation of spermatogenesis. FASEB J 2016;30:1453–1463.

[51] Ricci G, Cacciola G, Altucci L, Meccariello R, Pierantoni R, Fasano S, Cobellis G. Endocannabinoid control of sperm motility: the role of epididymus. Gen Comp Endocrinol 2007;153:320–322.

[52] Cobellis G, Ricci G, Cacciola G, Orlando P, Petrosino S, Cascio MG, et al. A gradient of 2-arachidonoylglycerol regulates mouse epididymal sperm cell start-up. Biol Reprod 2010;82:451–458.

[53] Chioccarelli T, Cacciola G, Altucci L, Lewis SE, Simon L, Ricci G, Ledent C, Meccariello R, Fasano S, Pierantoni R, Cobellis G. Cannabinoid receptor 1 influences chromatin remodeling in mouse spermatids by affecting content of transition protein 2 mRNA and histone displacement. Endocrinology 2010;151:5563.

[54] Battista N, Meccariello R, Cobellis G, Fasano S, Di Tommaso M, Pirazzi V, Konje JC, Pierantoni R, Maccarrone M. The role of endocannabinoids in gonadal function and fertility along the evolutionary axis. Mol Cell Endocrinol 2012;355:1–14.

[55] Cacciola G, Chioccarelli T, Altucci L, Ledent C, Mason JI, Fasano S, et al. Low 17beta-estradiol levels in Cnr1knock-out mice affect spermatid chromatin remodeling by interfering with chromatin reorganization. Biol Reprod 2013;88:152.

[56] Sun X, Wang H, Okabe M, Mackie K, Kingsley PJ, Marnett LJ, Cravatt BF, Dey SK. Genetic loss of Faah compromises male fertility in mice. Biol Reprod 2009;80:235–242.

[57] Rossato M. Endocannabinoids, sperm functions and energy metabolism. Mol Cell Endocrinol. 2008;286:S31–35.

[58] Wenger T, Ledent C, Csernus V, Gerendai I. The central cannabinoid receptor inactivation suppresses endocrine reproductive functions. Biochem Biophys Res Commun 2001;284:363–368.

[59] Chianese R, Ciaramella V, Fasano S, Pierantoni R, Meccariello R. Hypothalamus–pituitaryaxis: an obligatory target for endocannabinoids to inhibit steroidogenesis in frog testis. Gen Comp Endocrinol 2014;205:88–93.

[60] Cacciola G, Chioccarelli T, Mackie K, Meccariello R, Ledent C, Fasano S, Pierantoni R, Cobellis G. Expression of type-1 cannabinoid receptor during rat postnatal testicular development: possible involvement in adult leydig cell differentiation. Biol Reprod 2008;79:758–765.

[61] Rossi G, Gasperi V, Paro R, Barsacchi D, Cecconi S, Maccarrone M. Follicle-stimulating hormone activates fatty acid amide hydrolase by protein kinase A and aromatase-dependent pathways in mouse primary Sertoli cells. Endocrinology 2007;148:1431–1439.

[62] Bernabò N, Barboni B, Maccarrone M. The biological networks in studying cell signal transduction complexity: The examples of sperm capacitation and of endocannabinoid system. Comput Struct Biotechnol J 2014;11:11–21.

[63] Lewis SE, Maccarrone M. Endocannabinoids, sperm biology and human fertility. Pharmacol Res 2009;60:126–131.

[64] Schuel H, Burkman LJ. A tale of two cells: endocannabinoid-signaling regulates functions of neurons and sperm. Biol Reprod 2005;73:1078–1086.

Chapter 2

Endocannabinoid Signaling in Neural Circuits of the Olfactory and Limbic System

Thomas Heinbockel, Ze-Jun Wang,
Edward A. Brown and Paul T. Austin

Additional information is available at the end of the chapter

http://dx.doi.org/10.5772/63214

Abstract

The endocannabinoid system with cannabinoid receptors, specifically cannabinoid receptor type 1 (CB1R), and their endogenous activators, the endocannabinoids, has emerged as an important neuromodulator system. Our understanding of the endocannabinoid system has significantly advanced in limbic system areas such as the hippocampus and the amygdala. However, the study of this signaling system in the olfactory pathway is still in its infancy. Here, we review the role of endocannabinoids as signaling molecules in activity-dependent regulation of dynamically changing neural networks in the limbic and olfactory system and the relevance of the endocannabinoid system for synaptic plasticity. We highlight the prospects for cannabinoid-based therapies in the treatment of various brain disorders and the role of endocannabinoids as neuroprotective agents. An increased understanding of cannabinoid signaling has the potential to pave the way for developing cannabis-related substances as medications.

Keywords: amygdala, hippocampus, olfactory bulb, neuroprotection, retrograde signaling, neural plasticity

1. Introduction

Over the past decade, the endocannabinoid system with cannabinoid receptors, specifically cannabinoid receptor type 1 (CB1R), and their endogenous activators, the endocannabinoids, has been implicated as an important modulatory system in function and dysfunction of many brain areas. Endocannabinoids are small lipids that regulate normal behaviors, including pain reception [1] and feeding [2, 3]. Likewise, cannabinoids have therapeutic potential [4]. Endocannabinoids show a neuroprotective role against acute excitotoxicity [5] and facilitate functional recovery after brain injury [6]. They regulate human airway function and provide a means to treat respiratory pathologies [1]. Cannabinoids are widely used as recreational and psychoactive drugs and interact with other drugs of abuse, indicating the need to understand the endocannabinoid system and the neurobiological substrate of its mood-altering capacity [7, 8]. Furthermore, the endocannabinoid system is crucially involved in processes of learning and memory, for example, in the extinction of aversive memories [9]. Endocannabinoids influence synaptic transmission and different forms of short- and long-term plasticity [10–12]. They also influence growth and development such as synapse formation and neurogenesis. Other biological functions and human behaviors modulated by endocannabinoids include eating and anxiety [2, 3, 13].

A hallmark feature of endocannabinoids is their ability to serve as retrograde signaling molecules between activated postsynaptic principal neurons and presynaptic interneurons that express CB1R [10, 12, 14]. While the breadth of endocannabinoid function has become increasingly clear over the past years, we still have much to learn about their detailed signaling mechanisms.

Our understanding of the endocannabinoid system has significantly advanced in limbic system areas such as the hippocampus and the amygdala. However, the study of this signaling system in the olfactory pathway is still in its infancy. Recent work has started to shed light on the role of the endocannabinoid system in the olfactory pathway, specifically in the olfactory bulb as well as for its output to higher order olfactory centers and its centrifugal input [3, 15]. Here, we review the role of endocannabinoids as signaling molecules in activity-dependent regulation of dynamically changing neural networks in the limbic and olfactory system and the relevance of the endocannabinoid system for synaptic plasticity. We highlight the prospects for cannabinoid-based therapies in the treatment of various brain disorders such as epilepsy [16, 17]. An increased understanding of cannabinoid signaling may pave the way for developing cannabis-related substances as antiseizure medications.

2. Endocannabinoids as brain-derived signaling molecules

Endocannabinoids are fatty acid-derived endogenous ligands for $G_{i/o}$-protein-coupled CB1Rs [11]. Endocannabinoids are synthesized from membrane lipids [18]. They can diffuse through cellular membranes and are thus able to activate receptors in the same manner as exogenously applied cannabinoids such as the plant-derived compound Δ^9-tetrahydrocannabinol, THC, the bioactive ingredient of the drugs marijuana and hashish. Marijuana (cannabis) is a commonly abused illicit and recreational drug. The brain produces two endogenous cannabinoids, N-arachidonoylethanolamide (anandamide (AEA)) and 2-arachidonoylglycerol (2-AG). The two endocannabinoids bind to CB1R and have the same functional activity as marijuana. Based on the structural similarity between THC and endocannabinoids, THC is able to activate CB1R and, thereby, hijack this brain communication system. The evolutionary origin of this communication system rests with endogenously produced cannabinoids that bind and activate

CB1R. The discovery of AEA and 2-AG occurred in the 1990s ([19–21], for review see [22]). It took another decade before the function of these two cannabinoids in brain signaling was discovered. It is now well known that endocannabinoids serve as retrograde messengers. Endocannabinoids diminish excitatory and inhibitory transmission. Numerous studies have established their function as retrograde signals in various brain regions: the hippocampus [23–28], cerebellum [29–31], neocortex [32, 33], amygdala [34, 35], and olfactory bulb [15]. Furthermore, in the mediobasal hypothalamus, retrograde endocannabinoid signaling represents a key mechanism under physiological and pathological conditions whereby gonadotropin-releasing hormone (GnRH) neurons control their excitatory GABAergic inputs [36, 37]. Endocannabinoid signaling is terminated by reuptake into neurons and glia. AEA is hydrolyzed enzymatically inside the cell by fatty acid amide hydrolase (FAAH), whereas 2-AG is hydrolyzed by monoacylglycerol lipase (MAGL) [38].

Endocannabinoids serve as important signaling molecules throughout the body including the nervous system [10, 12, 39–44]. Endocannabinoids play important roles in bodily processes during both health and disease [45–48]. Their role in bodily functions has been shown for vertebrates and invertebrates [48]. Pharmacological and physiological experiments in brain slices have described novel aspects of classic brain signaling mechanisms and/or revealed unknown mechanisms of cellular communication involving the endocannabinoid system [41, 49–51]. Endocannabinoids are involved in several forms of cellular signaling [49]. The most distinguishing feature of endocannabinoids is their ability to act as retrograde messengers in neural circuits as first shown in the hippocampus [10, 26, 52].

3. Distribution of cannabinoid receptors in the CNS

Endocannabinoids, together with their G-protein-coupled cannabinoid receptors, form the endocannabinoid system. This system also includes an associated biochemical machinery with endocannabinoid precursors, synthetic and degradative enzymes for these lipidic neurotransmitters, and transporters [10, 12, 14, 40]. Cannabinoid receptors exist in all normal brains and serve many essential brain functions when activated by their natural ligands. Two types of cannabinoid receptors, CB1 (CB1R) and CB2 receptors with 44% amino acid sequence homology, have been described [53, 54]. They are not homogeneously expressed throughout the body; rather, CB1R is the most abundant G-protein-coupled receptor in the brain [55]. In contrast, CB2R is found mainly in immune cells and peripheral tissues [54]. More recent evidence suggests that CB2R is also present in the brainstem, cortex, and cerebellar neurons and microglia [56, 57]. CB1R has a high level of expression in the brain [58, 59], with a particularly strong presence at presynaptic axons terminals [60, 61]. THC, the bioactive ingredient of the drugs marijuana and hashish [62], and other cannabis-derived drugs are potent activators of CB1R. These drugs artificially activate CB1R and act as exogenous cannabinoids. CB1R is found in normal brains and carries out critical brain functions [55, 58, 59] principally through a $G_{i/o}$-protein-coupled mechanism with CB1R.

4. Mechanism of endocannabinoid action: retrograde signaling

Endocannabinoids mediate an unconventional type of neuronal communication, called DSI, **d**epolarization-induced **s**uppression of **i**nhibition (reviewed in [10, 22, 39]). In this communication system, a depolarized postsynaptic principal neuron releases endocannabinoids to regulate neurotransmitter release of presynaptic interneuron. Experimentally, a short rise in intracellular calcium concentration in a principal neuron, for example, a pyramidal cell of the hippocampus, results in a transient decline of incoming inhibitory signals in the form of the neurotransmitter GABA arriving from other neurons. During DSI, endocannabinoids travel from the postsynaptic neuron to the presynaptic GABA-releasing interneuron and turn off neurotransmitter release through activation of potassium channels and blockade of calcium channels. Classical chemical synapses are comprised of a presynaptic, neurotransmitter-releasing neuron and an activated postsynaptic neuron. For example, synaptic GABA release from an inhibitory hippocampal interneuron inhibits glutamatergic pyramidal cells. In contrast, in DSI, the inhibitory input onto an activated pyramidal cell is reduced. In DSI, endocannabinoids are retrograde signaling molecules. They communicate between postsynaptic pyramidal cells and presynaptic inhibitory interneurons resulting in a reduction of GABA release. Chemically, endocannabinoids are lipids. Therefore, their ability to diffuse in the watery extracellular environment of neurons is limited. Subsequently, DSI is a temporary phenomenon to allow individual neurons to pharmacologically break synaptic connections from their neighbors and, thereby, encode information [10]. DSI was mimicked by activating cannabinoid receptors whereas blockade of cannabinoid receptors prevented DSI [24, 26]. A corresponding phenomenon, DSE, **d**epolarization-induced **s**uppression of **e**xcitation, mediated by retrograde action of endocannabinoids, was identified at cerebellar excitatory synapses [28]. DSI and DSE are based on a presynaptic effect as shown by an increase in calcium in the postsynaptic cells and corresponding changes in paired pulse ratio of neurotransmitter release.

5. Endocannabinoids in the olfactory system

The main olfactory bulb offers an ideal platform for investigating how the endocannabinoid system modulates a functional neural network to achieve an integrated outcome. On the one side, the olfactory bulb directly receives sensory input from the nasal epithelium, and on the other side, it receives strong centrifugal cortical input that even outnumbers the cortical projections from the olfactory bulb. This structural organization makes the olfactory bulb preparation significantly different from the hippocampus, amygdala, neocortex, and cerebellum to address functional questions of CB1R modulation in the brain.

As detailed below, new evidence demonstrates that CB1R-mediated retrograde signaling exists among olfactory bulb glomerular neurons such that endocannabinoids released from glomerular neurons function as retrograde messengers to control the excitability of presynaptic neurons and to regulate their transmitter release [15]. Endocannabinoids have a distinct effect on sensory input, that is, they are involved in gain control through regulating presynaptic inhibition. Another new work emphasizes the relevance of cortical feedback to the olfactory bulb as a means to control odor detection and establishes the relationship of food intake and olfactory processing [3]. The endocannabinoid system is a key player in these signaling pathways.

Odorants in the air that we breathe in activate olfactory receptor cells in the nasal epithelium. Each receptor cell sends an axon to the ipsilateral main olfactory bulb which serves as the first relay station in the central nervous system for processing olfactory sensory information. Cannabinoid receptors are expressed at high levels in the olfactory bulb, specifically in the input region, the glomerular layer [58, 63–65]. Furthermore, neurons in the glomerular layer are immunoreactive for enzymes that synthesize endocannabinoids [66–68]. Electrophysiological evidence has now established that the endocannabinoid system plays a functional role in regulating neuronal activity and signaling in olfactory bulb glomeruli [15].

Three types of neurons are housed in the glomerular layer of the main olfactory bulb, that is, these neurons have their cell bodies in the glomerular layer: periglomerular (PG), external tufted (eTC), and short-axon (SA) cells, reviewed in Ref. [49]. PG cells are neurochemically and functionally heterogeneous [69–71]. They are GABAergic, whereas SA cells express both GABA and dopamine and eTC cells are glutamatergic [71–73]. PG cells receive input from the olfactory nerve or dendrodendritic glutamatergic input from eTC or mitral cells, for example, as spontaneous bursts of excitatory postsynaptic currents (EPSCs) [70, 74, 75]. PG cells presynaptically inhibit olfactory receptor neurons through GABAergic transmission [76, 77]. eTC cells receive spontaneous bursts of inhibitory postsynaptic currents (sIPSCs) from PG cells at inhibitory GABAergic synapses as well as spontaneous glutamatergic EPSCs [77, 78]. Endocannabinoids are likely to be released by activated eTC cells in the glomerular layer.

Membrane properties of PG cells are potently regulated by cannabinoid drugs such as the CB1R antagonist AM251 and the potent CB1R agonist WIN 55,212-2 (WIN) [15, 49]. Cannabinoid receptors directly regulate PG cells since the effects of AM251 and WIN persist in the presence of ionotropic glutamate and $GABA_A$ receptor blockers (synaptic blockers: CNQX, APV, gabazine) [15], indicating that CB1R is expressed in PG cells. AM251 increases action potential firing of PG cells and triggers release of GABA. eTC cells are synaptic targets of PG cells such that CB1R-mediated effects on PG cells are affecting chemical synaptic transmission to eTC cells. CB1R is also expressed in eTC cells and may participate in modulating eTC cell activity.

Cannabinoid drugs such as AM251 or WIN have no effect on membrane properties such as firing frequency or membrane potential in eTC cells [15, 49]. In the presence of synaptic blockers, cannabinoid drugs have a modest effect on eTC cells such that AM251 slightly increases the firing rate of eTC cells without membrane depolarization. WIN slightly decreases firing of eTC cells in synaptic blockers without a clear change in membrane potential. The effects of AM251 and WIN in the presence of synaptic blockers, that is, during pharmacological isolation of eTC cells, indicate that CB1R mediates a direct effect on eTC cells. The direct excitatory effect of AM251 is relatively weak and contrasted by strong GABAergic input from PG cells onto eTC cells, namely, the enhanced GABA release from PG cells. The strong inhibitory effect mediated by AM251 acting on PG cells overshadows the direct AM251-evoked excitation of eTC cells.

Experimental evidence indicates direct and indirect effects of cannabinoid drugs on glomerular neurons [15]. In order to determine if endocannabinoids are involved in retrograde signaling in the glomerular neural circuitry, that is, if DSI is present, eTC cells are activated by a 5 s depolarizing voltage step from a holding potential of −60 mV to 0 mV. In eTC cells DSI is visible as a decrease in the amplitude and frequency of sIPSCs. A single depolarizing step evokes a suppression of sIPSC area by ~40% of control which then gradually recovers. Projection or output neurons in the main olfactory bulb can show regular action potential firing or burst firing. eTC cells exhibit a distinct intrinsic bursting pattern [73]. In order to mimic their spontaneous rhythmic bursting, a train of depolarizing steps can be applied to an eTC cell which allows determining a possible functional role of DSI in olfactory glomeruli. A train of depolarizing steps results in a transient 60% reduction in sIPSC area (20 steps, 0.75 Hz). DSI can be completely eliminated in the presence of AM251, indicating that DSI is mediated by CB1R. eTC cells burst at a range from 0.5 to 6.5 Hz with a mean frequency of 2.7 bursts/s [73]. Depolarizing voltage pulses at 2 Hz (20 steps, pulse duration: 250 ms) evoke DSI as a reduction of sIPSCs in eTC cells, similar to the results obtained with voltage steps at 0.75 Hz to 0 mV. In eTC cells, single depolarizing voltage steps as well as a train of voltage steps evoke suppression of inhibition (DSI). The evidence suggests that spontaneous rhythmic bursting of eTC cells triggers the release of endocannabinoids which function as retrograde messengers to reduce GABA release from PG cells [15, 49]. This, in turn, regulates the activity of PG cell synaptic targets such as eTC cells.

The results indicate that endocannabinoids regulate neuronal activity and signaling in olfactory bulb glomeruli and function in DSI through CB1R-mediated retrograde signaling among glomerular neurons [15, 49]. Endocannabinoids are synthesized and released from neuronal cell bodies as a result of cellular excitation [11]. Endocannabinoids in the olfactory bulb are likely to be synthesized and released from neurons that synapse with presynaptic cells, that is, PG cells, and receive feedback synaptic input from them. eTC cells could be a potential endocannabinoid source in the olfactory bulb which is supported by the fact that DSI is found in eTC cells. The extent of DSI in eTC cells is subject to the level of cellular activation, that is, voltage step duration and step number. DSI cannot be evoked with step durations of 1 s or less, while a step duration closer to 5 s evokes transient DSI. Likewise, increasing the number of number steps to more than three evokes strong DSI and inhibits sIPSCs. When eTC cells are activated and show rhythmic burst firing, endocannabinoids are released which in turn affects glomerular activity. Bursting is an intrinsic property of eTC cells [73, 78] and regulates the release of endocannabinoids from principal olfactory bulb neurons such as eTC cells. Bursting-induced endocannabinoid release may also occur also in other brain systems and represent a general phenomenon of endocannabinoid signaling.

Recently, the endocannabinoid system has been placed in a behavioral context by linking an internal metabolic state (hunger) to sensory perception and subsequent behavior, namely, food intake [3]. CB1 receptor-dependent control of excitatory drive from centrifugal feedback projections to the main olfactory bulb determines the efficiency of olfactory processes and food intake in fasted mice. This study focuses on neural processes deeper in the olfactory bulb, primarily involving those olfactory bulb neurons (GABAergic granule cells) that receive heavy

CNS feedback rather than direct sensory input from the nasal epithelium. Given this structural organization of the main olfactory bulb, the authors integrate three separate neural components: sensory (olfactory) input, central processing in the main olfactory bulb, and behavioral output in terms of feeding in the overall framework of the internal state of the animal (hunger). Cortical feedback to the main olfactory bulb is a means to control odor detection. The relationship of food intake and olfactory processing implicates the endocannabinoid system as a key player in this signaling pathway. Thereby, the endocannabinoid system helps to resolve the old question of how the smell of a cookie makes us want to eat it and which brain mechanism allows us to find food more rapidly and reliably when we are hungry. CB1 receptor-dependent control of olfactory processes has a determinant role in coupling the internal state of hunger with the execution of the behavior such as increased food intake. THC has an effect on both olfactory detection thresholds and habituation, while the latter effect had no correlation to food intake. The authors suggest that enhancement of olfactory detection is likely the main mechanism linking (endo)cannabinoid signaling in the main olfactory bulb to increased food intake. Possibly, by reducing overall granule cell-mediated inhibition of mitral cells, the key output neurons of the main olfactory bulb, mitral cells become more sensitive and that would lower the odor detection threshold. The authors suggest that activation of CB1R on terminals of feedback cortical centrifugal glutamatergic neurons in the main olfactory bulb directly reduces the excitatory drive onto granule cells, thereby regulating mitral cell activity to increase odor detection and food intake [3]. However, other cellular mechanisms might come into play as well. These mechanisms could work in the peripheral input region of the main olfactory bulb rather than in the deeper granule cell layer. Also, glutamatergic input to the main olfactory bulb is not the only centrifugal input. Rather, other areas of the brain also provide feedback cortical projections with cholinergic, dopaminergic, serotonergic, or noradrenergic input [69, 79] and might be subject to CB1R modulation.

6. Cannabinoid receptors and hippocampal neural plasticity

Our understanding of the endocannabinoid system has greatly benefited from studies of limbic system areas such as the hippocampus. Work in hippocampal slices first established the role of endocannabinoids as retrograde signaling molecules [26, 80]. One of the main functions of the hippocampus is to convert short-term memory into long-term memory [81]. A hippocampal formation exists in both hemispheres of the brain and is made up of the hippocampus, the dentate gyrus, and the parahippocampal gyrus. The hippocampus is composed of four regions called *cornu ammonis*, or CA1, CA2, CA3, and CA4. The parahippocampal gyrus contains the entorhinal cortex and the subiculum. The entorhinal cortex is connected to parts of the cerebral cortex; and the thalamus, the hypothalamus, and the brain stem send axons into the entorhinal cortex [82]. The organization of the hippocampal formation lends itself to the flow of information. Information flows along the perforant pathway in the hippocampus. Pyramidal cells, originating in the entorhinal cortex, extend axons into the granule cells of the dentate gyrus with secondary outputs into the CA1 and CA3 regions. They extend from the dentate gyrus into the CA3 region through granule cell axons (mossy fiber pathway). CA3 pyramidal cell axons extend into the CA1 region and connect to fibers from the contralateral hippocampus. CA1 pyramidal cells project back into the entorhinal cortex and into the subiculum. The afferent fibers then extend from the subiculum and travel to the entorhinal cortex where other output fibers travel in pathways throughout the cerebrum, completing the pathway and flow of information [82].

Olfactory information is processed into long-term memory though the hippocampus. Sensory olfactory and synaptic information that is processed in the main olfactory bulb is sent to the piriform cortex and close to the orbital prefrontal cortex (PFC). The main olfactory bulb and these cortices project into the entorhinal cortex and the perirhinal area which relays the information through the perforant pathway to the hippocampus. Projections from the parahippocampal region extend to the piriform cortex, enabling a reciprocal and interconnected neural linkage [83].

Neural plasticity changes neuronal connectivity in the hippocampus. Through long-term potentiation and long-term depression (LTP), synaptic connections in the hippocampus are strengthened or weakened, respectively. Intracellular calcium release in postsynaptic neuron determines the level of neural plasticity. Receptors for CB1 are found throughout the hippocampus and are central to calcium-induced inhibition. The presence of the CB1R indicates that the hippocampus can be subject to depolarization-induced suppression of inhibition (DSI) which conversely affects the release of GABA from GABAergic neurons [10]. When endocannabinoids, 2-AG, and AEA are released by postsynaptic hippocampal neurons, GABAergic interneurons are inhibited, thus relieving principal neurons such as hippocampal pyramidal cells from inhibition [26]. This affects the information flow along the perforant pathway. The presence of more GABA increases the level of LTP and less GABA increases the amounts of long-term potentiation [26, 81] which affects memory production and learning. Unlike classical neurotransmitters, endocannabinoids can function as retrograde synaptic messengers. After release from postsynaptic neurons, they travel backward across synapses, activate CB1R on presynaptic axons, and suppress neurotransmitter release in order to modulate their inputs. The transient suppression of GABA-mediated transmission that follows depolarization of hippocampal pyramidal neurons is mediated by retrograde signaling through release of endogenous cannabinoids. Mechanistically, activation of CB1R inhibits presynaptic calcium channels through direct G-protein inhibition [27]. These synapses are unusual among brain synapses in that they use N- but not P/Q-type calcium channels for neurotransmitter release. A combination of patch-clamp electrophysiology in cultured hippocampal slices, calcium measurements, and flash photolysis of caged compounds, such as caged AEA, has allowed determining the temporal kinetics of the hippocampal endocannabinoid signaling cascade [15]. AEA and, by extension, other lipid signaling molecules do not simply serve long-term neuromodulatory functions but they are sufficiently fast to exert moment-to-moment control of synaptic transmission indicating that endocannabinoids are highly selective, rapid modulators of hippocampal inhibition.

7. Cannabinoid receptors as regulators of emotional memory

The amygdala is an almond-shaped nuclear structure located within the temporal lobe. It can be subdivided into three major nuclei: the basolateral nuclear complex, the central nucleus, and the medial nucleus. At the neuronal level, the emotional memory and emotional processes involve a brain network with limbic circuits including the amygdala, the medial PFC, and the anterior insula [84–87]. The amygdala is typically activated in response to emotional events, for example, dangerous situations by triggering and processing anger and fear [88]. Fear-conditioning experiments have delineated an amygdala-hippocampal-cortico-striatal circuit as a key brain circuit responsible for processing and storing fear-related memories and for coordinating fear-related behaviors [89, 90].

The basolateral amygdala is a critical component in the learning of conditioned fear responses [91], emotional processing, and encoding of associative memories with an affective component [92–95]. Animals with lesions to the basolateral amygdala complex produce serious deficits in learning new fear responses in a number of different conditioning tasks [96–99].

High levels of CB1R expression in the amygdala are observed in adult, fetal, and neonatal brains [58, 100–103] including GABAergic axonal terminals of the amygdala [104]. Endocannabinoids are known to retrogradely activate presynaptic CB1 receptors and modulate the release of several neurotransmitters (glutamate and GABA) [7, 15, 105]. Endocannabinoids regulate anxiety- and depressive-like behaviors mostly *via* stimulation of CB1R in emotion-related circuits of the PFC, amygdala, hippocampus, and cerebellum [7, 9, 87, 106–108]. Experiments with CB1R knockout mice revealed anxiogenic- and depressive-like phenotypes [109–111]. CB1 receptors play an important role in social interaction and aggressive behavior [107]. CB1 receptors in the amygdala and other brain areas such as the PFC have been shown to be critically involved in emotional learning and memory [112–117] and in fear learning, consolidation, retrieval, and extinction [118]. Using the fear-potentiated startle (FPS) paradigm, fear memory consolidation and retrieval, as well as extinction, were observed to be regulated differentially by amygdaloid and cortical CB1Rs [118]. Amygdala CB1Rs are involved in the development and maintenance of nicotine abstinence-related social anxiety-like behavior following a behaviorally sensitizing nicotine regimen. This suggests that changes in CB1R expression may contribute to perpetuation of nicotine relapse in vulnerable high responders, that is, in a rat model of novelty-seeking phenotype where animals respond with high locomotor reactivity to novelty [119].

It was found that CB1R expression is sensitive to stressful experiences, as animals submitted to a fear-conditioning paradigm presented CB1R upregulation in the PFC [90, 120]. Exposure to shock or stressful environments leads to an increase in endocannabinoids [121] and increased endocannabinoid release [9, 122] in the amygdala. Therefore, CB1R was considered as being a significant modulator for amygdala responses in social emotional negative situations [87].

The neuronal endocannabinoid system modulates synaptic transmission and plasticity *via* its two principal signaling lipids, AEA and 2-AG. It is commonly thought that both endocannabinoid-mediated short- and long-term plasticities are mediated through synaptic retrograde mechanisms with presynaptic CB1Rs [11, 68, 122–124]. However, polymodal activation of the endocannabinoid system has recently been found in the extended amygdala [125], that is, AEA and 2-AG are responsible for different forms of synaptic plasticity. Release of 2-AG triggered CB1R-mediated, retrograde, short-lasting inhibition of transmitter release, whereas mGluR5-dependent release of AEA activated postsynaptic TRPV1 receptors (transient receptor potential V1) and resulted in LTP [125]. The production of both endocannabinoids and different signaling pathways allows a single BNST (bed nucleus of the stria terminalis) neuron to take on two different forms of synaptic plasticity *via* the release of either 2-AG or AEA such that the endocannabinoid system acts as a polymodal signal integrator to diversify synaptic plasticity at the level of individual neurons [125].

It has been reported that in the amygdala FAAH, the enzyme that degrades AEA aggravates stress, whereas AEA protects and helps with recovery from stress [126]. Exposure to stress rapidly mobilizes FAAH to deplete the available pool of AEA and increases neuronal excitability in the basolateral amygdala, an anxiety-mediating region [126]. When FAAH is genetically deleted and pharmacologically inhibited, stress-induced reductions in AEA are prevented. Along the same line, long-term fear extinction is facilitated when FAAH is inhibited suggesting that the restoration of AEA levels in the basolateral amygdala by blocking FAAH with drugs might be clinically relevant to treat traumatic stress disorders.

The endocannabinoid system has become a major focus in the search for pharmacological interventions for fear extinction (for review see [91, 127, 128]). CB1R agonists and antagonists generate diverse cognitive effects and change extinction learning. CB1R is implicated in the sensory processing and learning. CB1R is expressed at high levels in the medial PFC, hippocampus, and basolateral amygdala. CB1R affects synaptic transmission and plasticity such as LTP in these brain areas.

Impairment of CB1R signaling affects the neuronal excitatory/inhibitory balance with effects on emotional function and anxiety- or depressive-like behaviors [129–132]. Drug use often starts during adolescence. During this time, the structure and function of the developing brain are particularly receptive to external stimuli such as cannabis. Adolescence is critical in the emergence of mental illness prior to its manifestation in adults but how does adolescent cannabis use affect brain development and function? Indeed, synaptic CB1R expression in adult mouse brain amygdala regions is downregulated by adolescent THC exposure, that is, it affects brain structure and function [133]. A recent study shows broad CB1R/b-arrestin2 co-expression in the medial PFC, amygdala, and hippocampus. This is paralleled by impairment of extracellular signal-regulated kinase signaling and elevation of vesicular glutamate transporter (VGluT1) at CB1R-expressing excitatory terminals in the medial PFC or vesicular GABA transporter (VGAT) at CB1R-expressing inhibitory terminals in the amygdala and hippocampus [132]. These alterations play a key role in the etiology of anxiety-like behaviors when occurring in the PFC, amygdala, and hippocampal circuits [129, 131].

Emotional dysfunction has been considered a hallmark of schizophrenia dating back to early days of research. Emotional disturbances in brain circuits, especially the amygdala, play a key part in symptoms of schizophrenia [134]. Adolescent cannabis use is an environmental risk to exacerbate cognitive and emotional behavioral abnormalities in individuals with genetic vulnerabilities [133].

Deficiency of CB1R signaling is associated with anxiety and persistence of negative memories [135]. Endocannabinoid-CB1R signaling is reduced with pharmacologic antagonists or genetic deletion [136–138]. Blockade of endocannabinoid-CB1R signaling with CB1R antagonists results in increased anxiety-like behaviors [135, 139] and also results in delayed and ineffective extinction of fearful memories in an animal model [9]. Administration of CB1R antagonist to healthy humans increases anxiety [140]. Indeed, anxiety is a main adverse effect in humans treated with a CB1R antagonist for metabolic disorder and obesity [141]. Patients, particularly those with prior depressive symptoms, exhibit increased depressive symptoms, including suicidality after treatment with CB1R antagonists [142].

Endocannabinoids are strongly linked to stress, fear, and anxiety, which has led to a growing interest in developing novel medication for anxiety and other psychological disorders targeting the endocannabinoid system [126]. Robusting endocannabinoid-CB1R signaling is vital for appropriate stress responses and for the maintenance of emotional homeostasis, particularly in the face of chronic stress. Understanding the underlying mechanisms of endocannabinoids in controlling stress, fear, and anxiety has grown considerably in recent years, with some targets already having been advanced to preliminary clinical trials in patients [126].

8. Endocannabinoids as neuroprotective agents

Studies highlighting the effects of endocannabinoids point to their neuroprotective role in the brain. Endocannabinoid-like compounds such as arachidonoyl serine (AraS), which has a similar structure to the endocannabinoid 2-AG, have been found to reduce lesion size following the induction of traumatic brain injury in mice [143]. Brain diseases have been shown to cause alterations to endocannabinoid synthesis. In Alzheimer's disease, FAAH, the enzyme which terminates endocannabinoid signaling, is epigenetically regulated. Patients with late-onset Alzheimer's disease, LOAD patients, display an increase in FAAH, whereas other components of the endocannabinoid system remain unchanged [144]. Another example of alteration of FAAH resulting in an increase in endocannabinoid system activation has been shown through application of an FAAH inhibitor. Use of the FAAH inhibitor, PF3845, in a mouse model helped to relieve traumatic brain injury-induced impairments including impairments of fine motor movement, hippocampus-dependent working memory, and anxiety-like behaviors. An FAAH inhibitor can result in the promotion of neuronal survival, attenuation of inflammation, and improvement of functional recovery following traumatic brain injury [145]. Traumatic brain injury is the leading cause of death in young people in the USA. Therefore, studies on FAAH potentially have great benefit to society in terms of treating traumatic brain injury.

The endocannabinoid system has also been shown to be neuroprotective during neurological diseases such as Alzheimer's disease, amyotrophic lateral sclerosis, and drug addiction. A role of endocannabinoids has been shown in Alzheimer's disease when WIN 55,212-2, a CB1R agonist, was tested on the effect of the toxic peptide Aβ1–42 in cultured astrocytes. Peptide Aβ1–42 accumulates during Alzheimer's disease causing cellular damage. Treatment with WIN 55,212-2 resulted in an increase in cellular viability of astrocytes and a decrease in inflammation [146]. An area of current investigation is the role of endocannabinoids as neuroprotectants in motor degeneration diseases. In one study, endocannabinoids played a neuroprotective role in amyotrophic lateral sclerosis [147]. In addition to endogenous cannabinoids assisting in ameliorating the effects of disease such as traumatic brain injury and neuropathic pain, research has also shown that endocannabinoids help to reduce the effects of drugs of abuse on the brain, in particular amphetamine abuse. THC, an exogenous form of cannabinoid, has been shown to reduce the neurotoxicity of methamphetamine by reducing the methamphetamine-induced overexpression of neuronal nitric oxide synthase in the caudate putamen [148].

Endocannabinoids have been shown to play a neuroprotective role in the limbic system. CB1R in both the hippocampus and amygdala is sufficient for synaptic and behavioral functions. In a study using conditional CB1R knockout mice, genetic restoration of wild-type CB1R function, specifically in dorsal telencephalic glutamatergic neurons, fully restored hippocampus-dependent neuroprotection from chemically induced epileptic-like seizures [149]. Dopamine receptor (D3 receptor) null mice have been shown to exhibit changes in levels of endocannabinoid and TRPV1 (transient receptor potential cation channel subfamily V member 1, also known as the capsaicin receptor and the vanilloid receptor 1), but not in CB1R in the hippocampus, nucleus accumbens, amygdala, and striatum. This change is related to less anxious-like behavior when mice underwent the elevated maze plus test. Hence, the endocannabinoid and endovanilloid systems may interact with dopamine receptors in order to produce normal responses to excitotoxic or anxiogenic stimuli [150]. Following exposure to foot shocks and situational reminders which mimic post-traumatic brain disorder in mice, treating mice with WIN 55,212-2, leads to normalization of CB1R upregulation in the PFC and CA1 of the hippocampus. Consequently, cannabinoids aid in emotional processing by preventing the distraction of foot shock followed by situation reminders [90].

The endocannabinoid AEA has been shown to protect HT22 cells exposed to hydrogen peroxide. This occurs *via* inhibition of NADPH oxidase 2 (Nox2). Activation of neuronal Nox2 enhances oxidative damage of the brain, and inhibition of Nox2 can attenuate cerebral oxidative stress [151]. Using a mouse model of oxidative stress by exposing hippocampal HT22 cells (mouse hippocampal neuron cell line HT22) to hydrogen peroxide, researchers tested whether AEA can attenuate the effects of oxidative stress on the brain. Cells exposed to hydrogen peroxide and treated with AEA were shown to experience fewer symptoms of oxidative stress such as morphological changes, decreased lactate dehydrogenase (LDH) release, reduced metabolic activity, increased levels of intracellular reactive oxygen species (ROS) and oxidized glutathione (GSSG), reduced levels of superoxide dismutase (SOD) and neuronal glutathione (GSH), and increased expression of neuronal Nox2, a contributor to oxidative damage to the brain. AEA was shown to prevent the oxidative stress effects unless the CB1R antagonist AM251 is simultaneously administered [151].

http://dx.doi.org/10.5772/63214

Endocannabinoid action is needed for normal activation of focal adhesion kinase (FAK) and extracellular signal-regulated kinase (ERK ½, ERK1/ERK2 subtypes) induced synaptic integrity in the hippocampus. This has been determined by treating hippocampal cells with endocannabinoid antagonist AM281, resulting in FAK and ERK ½ activation being blocked. The blocking of FAK and ERK ½ results in a decrease in synaptic markers. These results support the notion that the endocannabinoid system is the key for the integrity and maintenance of synapses in the hippocampus [152]. Endocannabinoid signaling can be modulated not only through direct activation of CB1 receptors but also through inhibition of endocannabinoid transport and FAAH, two mechanisms of endocannabinoid inactivation. Dual modulation of endocannabinoid transport and the enzyme FAAH results in protection against excitotoxicity. When hippocampal slices are exposed to excitotoxic insult and then treated with endocannabinoid transport blocker AM404 and FAAH blocker AM374, neuroprotection occurs against cytoskeleton damage and a decrease of synaptic decline. Likewise, the blockers protect against behavioral impairment and memory impairment characteristic of excitotoxic insult [153]. In the hippocampus THC has been shown to protect neurons from excitotoxicity. Both WIN 55122, a full CB1R agonist, and THC, a partial CB1R agonist, elicit a neuroprotective effect on rat hippocampal cells when the cells are excitotoxically stimulated to mimic disease-generated excitotoxic neuronal death [154]. CB1R also plays a role in neural progenitor proliferation and neurogenesis induced by excitotoxicity. During excitotoxicity the brain will attempt to repair damage by stimulating neural progenitor cells. When CB1R is inhibited in the hippocampus, both basic fibroblast growth factor (bFGF) and epidermal growth factor (EGF), key factors in neural progenitor stimulation, are blocked [155]. Excitotoxicity results in an increase in CB1R-positive and bFGF-positive cells, which proceeds neural progenitor cell proliferation. These results point to the importance of the endocannabinoid system in cellular regeneration from excitotoxic cellular damage in the hippocampus [155]. The endocannabinoid N-arachidonoyldopamine (NADA) has been shown to exert a neuroprotective effect in response to excitotoxic neuronal damage [156]. The neuronal damage occurs *via* CB1R. Excitotoxic lesioning of hippocampal slices by applying N-methyl-D-aspartate (NMDA), and subsequent treatment with NADA, determines whether endocannabinoids can be neuroprotective. NADA treatment protects dentate gyrus cells in organotypic hippocampal slice cultures. At the same time, the number of phagocytic microglia, which are attracted to sites of brain injury, decreases slightly [156].

Additionally, endocannabinoids have been shown to be neuroprotective in other disorders and anatomical systems such as obesity, endocannabinoid deficiency syndrome, and anti-inflammation. The endocannabinoid system has a direct relation with obesity because rimonabant (SR141716, trade names Acomplia, Zimulti), an anorectic anti-obesity drug, is an inverse agonist for CB1R. Rimonabant is a selective CB1 receptor blocker that was originally approved for use but has been withdrawn from the market because of potentially negative side effects. Since rimonabant has been shown to be an anti-obesity drug by inactivating the endocannabinoid system, it can be argued that the endocannabinoid system when activated can assist with weight gain, an issue faced by people experiencing weight-compromising diseases including cancer and people facing food absorption diseases including Crohn's disease [157]. The endocannabinoid system can potentially be used in clinical interventions. A growing area of research documents the "endocannabinoid deficiency syndrome" which is linked to migraine, fibromyalgia, irritable bowel syndrome, and psychological disorders [158]. Activation of nuclear receptor protein peroxisome proliferator-activated receptor-gamma has been shown to play a key role in the neuroprotective anti-inflammatory role of 2-AG in the brain [159].

Endocannabinoids and their receptors are expressed through the central nervous system and immune system suggesting a critical functional role for endocannabinoids in the operation of these systems. Activation of the endocannabinoid system is directly related to bodily recovery from a disease state such that endocannabinoids play a neuroprotective role in the nervous and immune system. This neuroprotective effect can be seen specifically in response to neurological disorders and injury such as Alzheimer's disease and traumatic brain injury. Likewise, endocannabinoids show neuroprotective effects following spinal cord injury. These data suggest that the endocannabinoid system as a neuroprotective agent has the potential for new therapeutic interventions during diseases of the nervous system and immune system.

Acknowledgements

This work was supported in part by grants from NIH (MD007597) and NSF (IOS-1355034) to TH. PTA was supported through The Advanced Research Training Corps: A Novel Initiative for URM Students, NIH-NIGMS [GM101997].

Author details

Thomas Heinbockel*, Ze-Jun Wang, Edward A. Brown and Paul T. Austin

*Address all correspondence to: theinbockel@howard.edu

Department of Anatomy, Howard University College of Medicine, Washington, DC, USA

References

[1] Calignano A, Katona I, Desarnaud F, Giuffrida A, La Rana G, Mackie K, Freund TF, Piomelli D. Bidirectional control of airway responsiveness by endogenous cannabinoids. Nature 2000; 408:96–101.

[2] Cota D, Marsicano G, Lutz B, Vicennati V, Stalla GK, Pasquali R, Pagotto. Endogenous cannabinoid system as a modulator of food intake. Int J Obesity 2003; 27:289–301.

[3] Soria-Gómez E, Bellocchio L, Reguero L, Lepousez G, Martin C, Bendahmane M, Ruehle S, Remmers F, Desprez T, Matias I, Wiesner T, Cannich A, Nissant A, Wadleigh

A, Pape HC, Chiarlone AP, Quarta C, Verrier D, Vincent P, Massa F, Lutz B, Guzmán M, Gurden H, Ferreira G, Lledo PM, Grandes P, Marsicano G. The endocannabinoid system controls food intake *via* olfactory processes. Nat Neurosci 2014; 17:407–415. doi: 10.1038/nn.3647.

[4] Iversen L, Chapman V. Cannabinoids: a real prospect for pain relief. Curr Opin Pharmacol 2002; 2:50–55.

[5] Marsicano G, Goodenough S, Monory K, Hermann H, Eder M, Cannich A, Azad SC, Cascio MG, Gutierrez SO, van der Stelt M, Lopez-Rodriguez ML, Casanova E, Schutz G, Zieglgansberger W, Di Marzo V, Behl C, Lutz B. CB1 cannabinoid receptors and on-demand defense against excitotoxicity. Science 2003; 302:84–88.

[6] Panikashvili D, Simeonidou C, Ben-Shabat S, Hanus L, Breuer A, Mechoulam R, Shohami E. An endogenous cannabinoid (2-AG) is neuroprotective after brain injury. Nature 2001; 413:527–531.

[7] Katona I, Rancz EA, Acsady L, Ledent C, Mackie K, Hajos N, Freund TF. Distribution of CB1 cannabinoid receptors in the amygdala and their role in the control of GABAergic transmission. J Neurosci 2001; 21:9506–9518.

[8] Valjent E, Mitchell JM, Besson MJ, Caboche J, Maldonado R. Behavioural and biochemical evidence for interactions between Delta9-tetrahydrocannabinol and nicotine. Br J Pharmacol 2002; 135:564–578.

[9] Marsicano G, Wotjak CT, Azad SC, Bisogno T, Rammes G, Cascio MG, Hermann H, Tang J, Hofmann C, Zieglgansberger W, Di Marzo V, Lutz B. The endogenous cannabinoid system controls extinction of aversive memories. Nature 2002; 418:530–534.

[10] Alger BE. Retrograde signaling in the regulation of synaptic transmission: focus on endocannabinoids. Prog Neurobiol 2002; 68:247–286.

[11] Kano M, Ohno-Shosaku T, Hashimotodani Y, Uchigashima M, Watanabe M. Endocannabinoid-mediated control of synaptic transmission. Physiol Rev 2009; 89:309–380.

[12] Freund TF, Katona I, Piomelli D. Role of endogenous cannabinoids in synaptic signaling. Physiol Rev 2003; 83:1017–1066.

[13] Soria-Gomez E, Bellocchio L, Marsicano G. New insights on food intake control by olfactory processes: the emerging role of the endocannabinoid system. Mol Cell Endocrinol 2014; 397(1–2):59–66. doi: 10.1016/j.mce.2014.09.023.

[14] Howlett AC, Breivogel CS, Childers SR, Deadwyler SA, Hampson RE, Porrino LJ. Cannabinoid physiology and pharmacology: 30 years of progress. Neuropharmacology 2004; 47:345–358.

[15] Wang Z-J, Sun L, Heinbockel T. Cannabinoid receptor-mediated regulation of neuronal activity and signaling in glomeruli of the main olfactory bulb. J Neurosci 2012; 32:8475–8479. doi: 10.1523/JNEUROSCI.5333-11.2012.

[16] Alger BE. Seizing an opportunity for the endocannabinoid system. Epilepsy Curr 2014; 14(5):272–276. doi: 10.5698/1535-7597-14.5.272.

[17] Soltesz I, Alger BE, Kano M, Lee SH, Lovinger DM, Ohno-Shosaku T, Watanabe M. Weeding out bad waves: towards selective cannabinoid circuit control in epilepsy. Nat Rev Neurosci 2015; 16(5):264–277. doi: 10.1038/nrn3937. Erratum in: Nat Rev Neurosci. 2015 Jun; 16(6):372.

[18] Di Marzo V, Melck D, Bisogno T, De Petrocellis L. Endocannabinoids: endogenous cannabinoid receptor ligands with neuromodulatory action. Trends Neurosci 1998; 21:521–528.

[19] Devane WA, Hanus L, Breuer A, Pertwee RG, Stevenson LA, Griffin G, et al. Isolation and structure of a brain constituent that binds to the cannabinoid receptor. Science 1992; 258:1946–1949.

[20] Mechoulam R, Ben-Shabat S, Hanus L, Ligumsky M, Kaminski NE, Schatz AR, Gopher A, Almog S, Martin BR, Compton DR, Pertwee RG, Griffin G, Bayewitch M, Barg J, Vogel Z. Identification of an endogenous 2-monoglyceride, present in canine gut, that binds to cannabinoid receptors. Biochem Pharmacol 1995; 50:83–90.

[21] Sugiura T, Kondo S, Sukagawa A, Nakane S, Shinoda A, Itoh K, Yamashita A, Waku K. 2-Arachidonoylgylcerol—a possible endogenous cannabinoid receptor–ligand in brain. Biochem Biophys Res Commun 1995; 215:89–97.

[22] Nicoll R, Alger BE. The brain's own marijuana. Sci Am 2004; 291:68–75

[23] Maejima T, Ohno-Shosaku T, Kano M. Endogenous cannabinoid as a retrograde messenger from depolarized postsynaptic neurons to presynaptic terminals. Neurosci Res 2001; 40:205–210.

[24] Ohno-Shosaku T, Maejima T, Kano M. Endogenous cannabinoids mediate retrograde signals from depolarized postsynaptic neurons to presynaptic terminals. Neuron 2001; 29:729–738.

[25] Varma N, Carlson GC, Ledent C, Alger BE. Metabotropic glutamate receptors drive the endocannabinoid system in hippocampus. J Neurosci 2001; 21:RC188.

[26] Wilson RI, Nicoll RA. Endogenous cannabinoids mediate retrograde signalling at hippocampal synapses. Nature 2001; 410:588–592.

[27] Wilson RI, Kunos G, Nicoll RA. Presynaptic specificity of endocannabinoid signaling in the hippocampus. Neuron 2001; 31:1–20.

[28] Makara JK, Mor M, Fegley D, Szabó SI, Kathuria S, Astarita G, Duranti A, Tontini A, Tarzia G, Rivara S, Freund TF, Piomelli D. Selective inhibition of 2-AG hydrolysis enhances endocannabinoid signaling in hippocampus. Nat Neurosci 2005; 8:1139–1141.

[29] Kreitzer AC, Regehr WG. Cerebellar depolarization-induced suppression of inhibition is mediated by endogenous cannabinoids. J Neurosci 2001; 21:RC174.

[30] Maejima T, Hashimoto K, Yoshida T, Aiba A, Kano M. Presynaptic inhibition caused by retrograde signal from metabotropic glutamate to cannabinoid receptors. Neuron 2001; 31:463–475.

[31] Yoshida T, Hashimoto K, Zimmer A, Maejima T, Araishi K, Kano M. The cannabinoid CB1 receptor mediates retrograde signals for depolarization-induced suppression of inhibition in cerebellar Purkinje cells. J Neurosci 2002; 22:1690–1697.

[32] Trettel J, Levine ES. Endocannabinoids mediate rapid retrograde signaling at interneuron pyramidal neuron synapses of the neocortex. J Neurophys 2003; 89:2334–2338.

[33] Trettel J, Fortin DA, Levine ES. Endocannabinoid signalling selectively targets perisomatic inhibitory inputs to pyramidal neurones in juvenile mouse neocortex. J Physiol (Lond) 2004; 556:95–107.

[34] Zhu PY, Lovinger DM. Retrograde endocannabinoid signaling in a postsynaptic neuron/synaptic bouton preparation from basolateral amygdala. J Neurosci 2005; 25:6199–6207.

[35] Kodirov SA, Jasiewicz J, Amirmahani P, Psyrakis D, Bonni K, Wehrmeister M, Lutz B. Endogenous cannabinoids trigger the depolarization-induced suppression of excitation in the lateral amygdala. Learn Mem 2009; 17:43–49.

[36] Farkas I, Kalló I, Deli L, Vida B, Hrabovszky E, Fekete C, Moenter SM, Watanabe M, Liposits Z. Retrograde endocannabinoid signaling reduces GABAergic synaptic transmission to gonadotropin-releasing hormone neurons. Endocrinology 2010; 151:5818–5829.

[37] Meccariello R, Battista N, Bradshaw HB, Wang H. Updates in reproduction coming from the endocannabinoid system. Int J Endocrinol 2014; 2014: 412354.

[38] Muccioli GG. Endocannabinoid biosynthesis and inactivation, from simple to complex. Drug Discov Today 2010; 15:474–483

[39] Alger BE. Endocannabinoids at the synapse a decade after the dies mirabilis (29 March 2001): what we still do not know. J Physiol 2012; 590(10):2203–2212.

[40] Alger BE, Kim J. Supply and demand for endocannabinoids. Trends Neurosci 2011; 34:304–315.

[41] Fonseca BM, Costa MA, Almada M, Correia-da-Silva G, Teixeira NA. Endogenous cannabinoids revisited: a biochemistry perspective. Prostaglandins Lipid Mediat 2013; 102–103:13–30.

[42] Howlett AC, Breivogel CS, Childers SR, Deadwyler SA, Hampson RE, Porrino LJ. Cannabinoid physiology and pharmacology: 30 years of progress. Neuropharmacology 2004; 47:345–358.

[43] Heinbockel, T. Electrophysiological recording and imaging of neuronal signals in brain slices. In: Heinbockel T, ed., Neuroscience, vol. 2. Intech Open Access Publisher: Rijeka, Croatia. 2012; pp. 19–48.

[44] Piomelli, D. More surprises lying ahead. The endocannabinoids keep us guessing. Neuropharmacology 2014; 76:228–234.

[45] Hill AJ, Williams CM, Whalley BJ, Stephen GJ. Phytocannabinoids as novel therapeutic agents in CNS disorders. Pharmacol Ther 2012; 133:79–97.

[46] Hofmann ME, Frazier CJ. Marijuana, endocannabinoids, and epilepsy: potential and challenges for improved therapeutic intervention. Exp Neurol 2013; 244:43–50.

[47] Pertwee RG. Targeting the endocannabinoid system with cannabinoid receptor agonists: pharmacological strategies and therapeutic possibilities. Philos Trans R Soc B 2012; 367:3353–3363.

[48] Elphick, M.R. The evolution and comparative neurobiology of endocannabinoid signaling. Philos Trans R Soc B 2012; 367:3201–3215.

[49] Heinbockel T. Neurochemical communication: the case of endocannabinoids. In: Heinbockel T, ed., Neuroscience. Intech Open Access Publisher: Rijeka, Croatia. 2014; pp. 179–198 (ch. 6, ISBN: 978-953-51-1237-2).

[50] Kano M. Control of synaptic function by endocannabinoid-mediated retrograde signaling. Proc Jpn Acad Ser B 2014; 90:235–250.

[51] Castillo PE, Younts TJ, Chavez AE, Hashimotodani Y. Endocannabinoid signaling and synaptic function. Neuron 2012; 76:70–81.

[52] Heinbockel T, Brager DH, Reich C, Zhao J, Muralidharan S, Alger BE, Kao JPY. Endocannabinoid signaling dynamics probed with optical tools. J Neurosci 2005; 25:9449–9459.

[53] Matsuda LA, Lolait SJ, Brownstein MJ, Young AC, Bonner TI. Structure of a cannabinoid receptor and functional expression of the cloned cDNA. Nature 1990; 346:561–564.

[54] Munro S, Thomas KL, Abu-Shaar M. Molecular characterization of a peripheral receptor for cannabinoids. Nature 1993; 365:61–65.

[55] Herkenham M, Lynn AB, Little MD, Johnson MR, Melvin LS, de Costa BR, Rice KC. Cannabinoid receptor localization in brain. Proc Natl Acad Sci U S A 1990; 87:1932–1936.

[56] Van Sickle MD, Duncan M, Kingsley PJ, Mouihate A, Urbani P, Mackie K, et al. Identification and functional characterization of brainstem cannabinoid CB2 receptors. Science 2005; 310:329–332.

[57] Núñez E, Benito C, Pazos MR, Barbachano A, Fajardo O, González S, et al. Cannabinoid CB2 receptors are expressed by perivascular microglial cells in the human brain: an immunohistochemical study. Synapse 2004; 53:208–213.

[58] Herkenham M, Lynn AB, Johnson MR, Melvin LS, de Costa BR, Rice KC. Characterization and localization of cannabinoid receptors in rat brain: a quantitative in vitro autoradiographic study. J Neurosci 1991; 11:563–583.

[59] Matsuda LA, Bonner TI, Lolait SJ. Localization of cannabinoid receptor mRNA in rat brain. J Comp Neurol 1993; 327:535–550.

[60] Katona I, Sperlagh B, Sik A, Kafalvi A, Vizi ES, Mackie K, Freund TF. Presynaptically located CB1 cannabinoid receptors regulate GABA release from axon terminals of specific hippocampal interneurons. J Neurosci 1999; 19:4544–4558.

[61] Tsou K, Mackie K, Sanudo-Pena MC, Walker JM. Cannabinoid CB1 receptors are localized primarily on cholecystokinin-containing GABAergic interneurons in the rat hippocampal formation. Neurosci 1999; 93:969–975.

[62] Ameri A. The effects of cannabinoids on the brain. Prog Neurobiol 1999; 58:315–348.

[63] Pettit DA, Harrison MP, Olson JM, Spencer RF, Cabral GA. Immunohistochemical localization of the neural cannabinoid receptor in rat brain. J Neurosci Res 1998; 51:391–402.

[64] Tsou K, Brown S, Sanudo-Pena MC, Mackie K, Walker JM. Immunohistochemical distribution of cannabinoid CB1 receptors in the rat central nervous system. Neurosci 1998; 83:393–411.

[65] Moldrich G, Wenger T. Localization of the CB1 cannabinoid receptor in the rat brain. An immunohistochemical study. Peptides 2000; 21:1735–1742.

[66] Allen Institute for Brain Science. Allen Mouse Brain Atlas [Online]. Allen Institute: Seattle, WA. 2009; http://mouse.brain-map.org.

[67] Okamoto Y, Wang J, Morishita J, Ueda N. Biosynthetic pathways of the endocannabinoid anandamide. Chem Biodivers 2007; 4:1842–1857.

[68] Piomelli D. The molecular logic of endocannabinoid signaling. Nat Rev Neurosci 2003; 4:873–884.

[69] Ennis M, Hayar A, Hamilton KA. Neurochemistry of the main olfactory system. In: Lajtha A, ed., Handbook of Neurochemistry and Molecular Neurobiology, Johnson DA ed., Sensory Neurochemistry. Springer: Heidelberg. 2007; pp. 137–204.

[70] Shao Z, Puche AC, Kiyokage E, Szabo G, Shipley MT. Two GABAergic intraglomerular circuits differentially regulate tonic and phasic presynaptic inhibition of olfactory nerve terminals. J Neurophysiol 2009; 101:1988–2001.

[71] Kiyokage E, Pan YZ, Shao Z, Kobayashi K, Szabo G, Yanagawa Y, Obata K, Okano H, Toida K, Puche AC, Shipley MT. Molecular identity of periglomerular and short axon cells. J Neurosci 2010; 30:1185–1196.

[72] Hayar A, Karnup S, Ennis M, Shipley MT. External tufted cells: a major excitatory element that coordinates glomerular activity. J Neurosci 2004; 24:6676–6685.

[73] Hayar A, Karnup S, Shipley MT, Ennis M. Olfactory bulb glomeruli: external tufted cells intrinsically burst at theta frequency and are entrained by patterned olfactory input. J Neurosci 2004; 24:1190–1199.

[74] Hayar A, Shipley MT, Ennis M. Olfactory bulb external tufted cells are synchronized by multiple intraglomerular mechanisms. J Neurosci 2005; 25:8197–8208.

[75] Aroniadou-Anderjaska V, Zhou F-M, Priest CA, Ennis M, Shipley MT. GABA-B receptor-mediated presynaptic inhibition of sensory input to the olfactory bulb. J Neurophysiol 2000; 84:1194–1203.

[76] Murphy GJ, Darcy DP, Isaacson JS. Intraglomerular inhibition: signaling mechanisms of an olfactory microcircuit. Nat Neurosci 2005; 8:354–364.

[77] Hayar A, Ennis M. Endogenous GABA and glutamate finely tune the bursting of olfactory bulb external tufted cells. J Neurophysiol 2007; 98:1052–1056.

[78] Liu S, Shipley MT. Multiple conductances cooperatively regulate spontaneous bursting in mouse olfactory bulb external tufted cells. J Neurosci 2008; 28:1625–1639.

[79] Shipley MT, Ennis M. Functional organization of olfactory system. J Neurobiol 1996; 30:123–176.

[80] Wilson RI, Nicoll RA. Endocannabinoid signaling in the brain. Science 2002; 296:678–682.

[81] Strange BA, Witter MP, Lein ES, Moser EI. Functional organization of the hippocampal longitudinal axis. Neuroscience 2014; 15:655–669.

[82] Kenney J, Gould T. Modulation of hippocampus-dependent learning and synaptic plasticity by nicotine. Mol Neurobiol 2008; 38:101–121.

[83] Eichenbaum H, Schoenbaum G, Young B, Bunsey M. Functional organization of the hippocampal memory system. Proc Natl Acad Sci U S A 1996; 93(24):13500–13507.

[84] Adolphs, R. Is the human amygdala specialized for processing social information? Ann N Y Acad Sci 2003; 985:326–340.

[85] Adolphs R, Tranel D. Amygdala damage impairs emotion recognition from scenes only when they contain facial expressions. Neuropsychologia 2003; 41:1281–1289.

[86] Grosbras MH, Paus T. Brain networks involved in viewing angry hands or faces. Cereb Cortex 2006; 16:1087–1096.

[87] Ewald A, Becker S, Heinrich A, Banaschewski T, Poustka L, Bokde A, Büchel C, Bromberg U, Cattrell A, Conrod P, Desrivières S, Frouin V, Papadopoulos-Orfanos D, Gallinat J, Garavan H, Heinz A, Walter H, Ittermann B, Gowland P, Paus T, Martinot JL, Paillère Martinot ML, Smolka MN, Vetter N, Whelan R, Schumann G, Flor H, Nees F, IMAGEN consortium. The role of the cannabinoid receptor in adolescents' processing of facial expressions. Eur J Neurosci 2016; 43:98–105. doi: 10.1111/ejn.13118.

[88] Tahmasebi AM, Artiges E, Banaschewski T, Barker GJ, Bruehl R, Buechel C, Conrod PJ, Flor H, Garavan H, Gallinat J, Heinz A, Ittermann B, Loth E, Mareckova K, Martinot JL, Poline JB, Rietschel M, Smolka MN, Stroehle A, Schumann G, Paus T, IMAGEN Consortium. Creating probabilistic maps of the face network in the adolescent brain: a multicentre functional MRI study. Hum Brain Mapp 2012; 33:938–957.

[89] Neumeister A, Seidel J, Ragen BJ, Pietrzak RH. Translational evidence for a role of endocannabinoids in the etiology and treatment of posttraumatic stress disorder. Psychoneuroendocrinology 2015; 51:577–584. doi: 10.1016/j.psyneuen.2014.10.012.

[90] Korem N, Akirav I. Cannabinoids prevent the effects of a footshock followed by situational reminders on emotional processing. Neuropsychopharmacology 2014; 39:2709–2722. doi: 10.1038/npp.2014.132.

[91] Chhatwal JP, Ressler KJ. Modulation of fear and anxiety by the endogenous cannabinoid system. CNS Spectr 2007; 12:211–220.

[92] Rosenkranz JA, Grace AA. Regulation of conditioned responses of basolateral amygdala neurons. Physiol Behav 2002; 77(4–5):489–493

[93] Rosenkranz JA, Grace AA. Affective conditioning in the basolateral amygdala of anesthetized rats is modulated by dopamine and prefrontal cortical inputs. Ann N Y Acad Sci 2003; 985:488–491

[94] Laviolette SR, Lipski WJ, Grace AA. A subpopulation of neurons in the medial prefrontal cortex encodes emotional learning with burst and frequency codes through a dopamine D4 receptor-dependent basolateral amygdala input. J Neurosci 2005; 25(26):6066–6075.

[95] McLaughlin RJ, Gobbi G. Cannabinoids and emotionality: a neuroanatomical perspective. Neuroscience 2012; 204:134–144. doi: 10.1016/j.neuroscience.2011.07.052.

[96] LeDoux JE. Emotion circuits in the brain. Annu Rev Neurosci 2000; 23:155–184.

[97] Davis M. The role of the amygdala in fear and anxiety. Annu Rev Neurosci 1992; 15:353–375.

[98] Maren S. The amygdala, synaptic plasticity, and fear memory. Ann N Y Acad Sci 2003; 985:106–113.

[99] Quirk GJ, Gehlert DR. Inhibition of the amygdala: key to pathological states? Ann N Acad Sci 2003; 985:263–272.

[100] Glass M, Dragunow M, Faull RL. Cannabinoid receptors in the human brain: a detailed anatomical and quantitative autoradiographic study in the fetal, neonatal and adult human brain. Neuroscience 1977; 77:299–318.

[101] Mackie K. Distribution of cannabinoid receptors in the central and peripheral nervous system. Handb Exp Pharmacol 2005; 168:299–325.

[102] Trezza V, Damsteegt R, Manduca A, Petrosino S, Van Kerkhof LW, Pasterkamp RJ, Zhou Y, Campolongo P, Cuomo V, Di Marzo V, Vanderschuren LJ. Endocannabinoids in amygdala and nucleus accumbens mediate social play reward in adolescent rats. J Neurosci 2012; 32:14899–14908.

[103] Grewen K, Salzwedel AP, Gao W. Functional connectivity disruption in neonates with prenatal marijuana exposure. Front Hum Neurosci 2015; 9:601. doi: 10.3389/fnhum.2015.00601

[104] Azad SC, Kurz J, Marsicano G, Lutz B, Zieglgänsberger W, Rammes G. Activation of CB1 specifically located on GABAergic interneurons inhibits LTD in the lateral amygdala. Learn Mem 2008; 15:143–152.

[105] Jung KM, Mangieri R, Stapleton C, Kim J, Fegley D, Wallace M, Mackie K, Piomelli D. Stimulation of endocannabinoid formation in brain slice cultures through activation of group I metabotropic glutamate receptors. Mol Pharmacol 2005; 68:1196–1202.

[106] Crowe MS, Nass SR, Gabella KM, Kinsey SG. The endocannabinoid system modulates stress, emotionality, and inflammation. Brain Behav Immun 2014; 42:1–5. doi: 10.1016/j.bbi.2014.06.007.

[107] Rodriguez-Arias M, Navarrete F, Daza-Losada M, Navarro D, Aguilar MA, Berbel P, Miñarro J, Manzanares J. CB1 cannabinoid receptor-mediated aggressive behavior. Neuropharmacology 2013; 75:172–180. doi: 10.1016/j.neuropharm.2013.07.013.

[108] Valverde O, Torrens M. CB1 receptor-deficient mice as a model for depression. Neuroscience 2012; 204:193–206. doi: 10.1016/j.neuroscience.2011.09.031.

[109] Haller J, Bakos N, Szirmay M, Ledent C, Freund TF. The effects of genetic and pharmacological blockade of the CB1 cannabinoid receptor on anxiety. Eur J Neurosci 2002; 16:1395–1398.

[110] Maccarrone M, Valverde O, Barbaccia ML, Castañé A, Maldonado R, Ledent C, Parmentier M, Finazzi-Agrò A. Age-related changes of anandamide metabolism in CB1 cannabinoid receptor knockout mice: correlation with behaviour. Eur J Neurosci 2002; 15:1178–1186.

[111] Urigüen L, Pérez-Rial S, Ledent C, Palomo T, Manzanares J. Impaired action of anxiolytic drugs in mice deficient in cannabinoid CB1 receptors. Neuropharmacology 2004; 46:966–973.

[112] Laviolette SR, Grace AA. Cannabinoids potentiate emotional learning plasticity in neurons of the medial prefrontal cortex through basolateral amygdala inputs. J Neurosci 2006; 26:6458–6468.

[113] Laviolette SR, Grace AA. The roles of cannabinoid and dopamine receptor systems in neural emotional learning circuits: implications for schizophrenia and addiction. Cell Mol Life Sci 2006; 63(14):1597–1613.

[114] Azad SC, Monory K, Marsicano G, et al. Circuitry for associative plasticity in the amygdala involves endocannabinoid signaling. J Neurosci 2004; 24:9953–9961.

[115] Roche M, O'Connor E, Diskin C, Finn DP. The effect of CB(1) receptor antagonism in the right basolateral amygdala on conditioned fear and associated analgesia in rats. Eur J Neurosci 2007; 26:2643–2653.

[116] Kim MJ, Loucks RA, Palmer AL, Brown AC, Solomon KM, Marchante AN, et al. The structural and functional connectivity of the amygdala: from normal emotion to pathological anxiety. Behav Brain Res 2011; 223:403–410.

[117] Tan H, Lauzon NM, Bishop SF, et al. Integrated cannabinoid CB1 receptor transmission within the amygdala-prefrontal cortical pathway modulates neuronal plasticity and emotional memory encoding. Cerebral Cortex 2010; 20:1486–1496.

[118] Kuhnert S, Meyer C, Koch M. Involvement of cannabinoid receptors in the amygdala and prefrontal cortex of rats in fear learning, consolidation, retrieval and extinction. Behav Brain Res 2013; 250:274–284. doi: 10.1016/j.bbr.2013.05.002.

[119] Aydin C, Oztan O, Isgor C. Long-term effects of juvenile nicotine exposure on abstinence-related social anxiety-like behavior and amygdalar cannabinoid receptor 1 (CB1R) mRNA expression in the novelty-seeking phenotype. Behav Brain Res 2012; 228:236–239. doi: 10.1016/j.bbr.2011.11.015.

[120] Lisboa SF, Reis DG, da Silva AL, Corre^a F, Guimaraes FS, Resstel L. Cannabinoid CB1 receptors in the medial prefrontal cortex modulate the expression of contextual fear conditioning. Int J Neuropsychopharmacol 2010; 13:1163–1173.

[121] Hill MN, Ho W-SV, Meier SE, Gorzalka BB, Hillard CJ. Chronic corticosterone treatment increases the endocannabinoid 2-arachidonoylglycerol in the rat amygdala. Eur J Pharmacol 2005; 528:99–102.

[122] Morena M, Hauer D, Ratano P, Scaccianoce S, Trezza V, Pecci C, et al. The endocannabinoid system and the regulation of memory consolidation for emotionally arousing experiences. FENS Abstract 2012; 6:0.45.14.

[123] Heifets BD, Castillo PE. Endocannabinoid signaling and long-term synaptic plasticity. Annu Rev Physiol 2009; 71:283–306.

[124] Katona I, Freund TF. Endocannabinoid signaling as a synaptic circuit breaker in neurological disease. Nat Med 2008; 14:923–930.

[125] Puente N, Cui Y, Lassalle O, Lafourcade M, Georges F, Venance L, Grandes P, Manzoni OJ. Polymodal activation of the endocannabinoid system in the extended amygdala. Nat Neurosci 2011; 14(12):1542–1547. doi: 10.1038/nn.2974.

[126] Gunduz-Cinar O, Hill MN, McEwen BS, Holmes A. Amygdala FAAH and anandamide: mediating protection and recovery from stress. Trends Pharmacol Sci 2013; 34: 637–644. doi: 10.1016/j.tips.2013.08.008.

[127] Kaplan GB, Moore KA. The use of cognitive enhancers in animal models of fear extinction. Pharmacol Biochem Behav 2011; 99:217–228. doi: 10.1016/j.pbb.2011.01.009.

[128] Varvel SA, Wise LE, Lichtman AH. Are CB(1) receptor antagonists nootropic or cognitive impairing agents? Drug Dev Res 2009; 70(8):555–565.

[129] Chiba S, Numakawa T, Ninomiya M., Richards MC, Wakabayashi C, Kunugi H. Chronic restraint stress causes anxiety and depression-like behaviors, down regulates glucocorticoid receptor expression, and attenuates glutamate release induced by brain-derived neurotrophic factor in the prefrontal cortex. Prog Neuropsychopharmacol Biol Psychiatry 2012; 39:112–119.

[130] den Boon FS, Werkman TR, Schaafsma-Zhao Q, Houthuijs K, Vitalis T, Kruse CG, Wadman WJ, Chameau P. Activation of type-1 cannabinoid receptor shifts the balance between excitation and inhibition towards excitation in layer II/III pyramidal neurons of the rat prelimbic cortex. Pflugers Arch 2014; 20:2–8.

[131] Prager EM, Pidoplichko VI, Aroniadou-Anderjaska V, Apland JP, Braga MF. Pathophysiological mechanisms underlying increased anxiety after soman exposure: reduced GABAergic inhibition in the basolateral amygdala. Neurotoxicology 2014; 44:335–343.

[132] Imperatore R, Morello G, Luongo L, Taschler U, Romano R, De Gregorio D, Belardo C, Maione S, Di Marzo V, Cristino L. Genetic deletion of monoacylglycerol lipase leads to impaired cannabinoid receptor CB1R signaling and anxiety-like behavior. J Neurochem 2015; 135:799–813. doi: 10.1111/jnc.13267.

[133] Ballinger MD, Saito A, Abazyan B, Taniguchi Y, Huang CH, Ito K, Zhu X, Segal H, Jaaro-Peled H, Sawa A, Mackie K, Pletnikov MV, Kamiya A. Adolescent cannabis exposure interacts with mutant DISC1 to produce impaired adult emotional memory. Neurobiol Dis 2015; 82:176–184. doi: 10.1016/j.nbd.2015.06.006.

[134] Aleman A, Kahn RS. Strange feelings: do amygdala abnormalities dysregulate the emotional brain in schizophrenia? Prog Neurobiol 2005; 77:283–298.

[135] Hillard CJ. Stress regulates endocannabinoid-CB1 receptor signaling. Semin Immunol 2014; 26:380–388. doi: 10.1016/j.smim.2014.04.001.

[136] Hill MN, McLaughlin RJ, Morrish AC, Viau V, Floresco SB, Hillard CJ, et al. Suppression of amygdalar endocannabinoid signaling by stress contributes to activation of the hypothalamic-pituitary-adrenal axis. Neuropsychopharmacology 2009; 34:2733–2745.

[137] Hill MN, McLaughlin RJ, Pan B, Fitzgerald ML, Roberts CJ, Lee TT, et al. Recruitment of prefrontal cortical endocannabinoid signaling by glucocorticoids contributes to termination of the stress response. J Neurosci 2011; 31:10506–10515.

[138] Patel S, Roelke CT, Rademacher DJ, Cullinan WE, Hillard CJ. Endocannabinoid signaling negatively modulates stress-induced activation of the hypothalamic-pituitary-adrenal axis. Endocrinology 2004; 145:5431–5438.

[139] Patel S, Hillard CJ. Pharmacological evaluation of cannabinoid receptor ligands in a mouse model of anxiety: further evidence for an anxiolytic role for endogenous cannabinoid signaling. J Pharmacol Exp Ther 2006; 318:304–311.

[140] Bergamaschi MM, Queiroz RH, Chagas MH, Linares IM, Arrais KC, de Oliveira DC, et al. Rimonabant effects on anxiety induced by simulated public speaking in healthy humans: a preliminary report. Hum Psychopharmacol 2014; 29:94–99.

[141] Moreira FA, Grieb M, Lutz B. Central side-effects of therapies based on CB1 cannabinoid receptor agonists and antagonists: focus on anxiety and depression. Best Pract Res Clin Endocrinol Metab 2009; 23:133–144.

[142] Christensen R, Kristensen PK, Bartels EM, Bliddal H, Astrup A. Efficacy and safety of the weight-loss drug rimonabant: a meta-analysis of randomised trials. Lancet 2007; 370:1706–1713.

[143] Mann A, Cohen-Yeshurun A, Trembovler V, Mechoulam R, Shohami E. Are the endocannabinoid-like compounds N-acyl aminoacids neuroprotective after traumatic brain injury? J Basic Clin Physiol Pharmacol 2015. doi: 10.1515/jbcpp-2015-0092.

[144] D'Addario C, Di Francesco A, Arosio B, Gussago C, Dell'Osso B, Bari M, Galimberti D, Scarpini E, Altamura AC, Mari D, Maccarrone M. Epigenetic regulation of fatty acid amide hydrolase in Alzheimer disease. PLoS One 2012; 7:e39186. doi: 10.1371/journal.pone.0039186.

[145] Tchantchou F, Tucker LB, Fu AH, Bluett RJ, McCabe JT, Patel S, Zhang Y. The fatty acid amide hydrolase inhibitor PF-3845 promotes neuronal survival, attenuates inflammation and improves functional recovery in mice with traumatic brain injury. Neuropharmacology 2014; 85:427–439. doi: 10.1016/j.neuropharm.2014.06.006.

[146] Aguirre-Rueda D, Guerra-Ojeda S, Aldasoro M, Iradi A, Obrador E, Mauricio MD, Vila JM, Marchio P, Valles SL. WIN 55,212-2, agonist of cannabinoid receptors, prevents amyloid β1–42 effects on astrocytes in primary culture. PLoS One 2015; 10:e0122843. doi: 10.1371/journal.pone.0122843.

[147] de Lago E, Moreno-Martet M, Espejo-Porras F, Fernández-Ruiz J. Endocannabinoids and amyotrophic lateral sclerosis. In: Fattore L, ed., Cannabinoids in Neurologic and Mental Disease. Elsevier Inc.. 2015; pp. 99–123.

[148] Castelli MP, Madeddu C, Casti A, Casu A, Casti P, Scherma M, Fattore L, Fadda P, Ennas MG. Δ9-tetrahydrocannabinol prevents methamphetamine-induced neurotoxicity. PLoS One 2014; 9:e98079. doi: 10.1371/journal.pone.0098079.

[149] Ruehle S, Remmers F, Romo-Parra H, Massa F, Wickert M, Wörtge S, Häring M, Kaiser N, Marsicano G, Pape HC, Lutz B.Cannabinoid CB1 receptor in dorsal telencephalic glutamatergic neurons: distinctive sufficiency for hippocampus-dependent and amygdala-dependent synaptic and behavioral functions. J Neurosci 2013; 33: 10264–10277.

[150] Micale V, Cristino L, Tamburella A, Petrosino S, Leggio GM, Drago F, Di Marzo V. Altered responses of dopamine D3 receptor null mice to excitotoxic or anxiogenic stimuli: possible involvement of the endocannabinoid and endovanilloid systems. Neurobiol Dis 2009; 36:70–80. doi: 10.1016/j.nbd.2009.06.015.

[151] Jia J, Ma L, Wu M, Zhang L, Zhang X, Zhai Q, Jiang T, Wang Q, Xiong L. Anandamide protects HT22 cells exposed to hydrogen peroxide by inhibiting CB1 receptor-mediated type 2 NADPH oxidase. Oxid Med Cell Longev 2014; 2014:893516. doi: 10.1155/2014/893516.

[152] Karanian DA, Brown QB, Makriyannis A, Bahr BA. Blocking cannabinoid activation of FAK and ERK1/2 compromises synaptic integrity in hippocampus. Eur J Pharmacol 2005; 508:47–56.

[153] Karanian DA, Brown QB, Makriyannis A, Kosten TA, Bahr BA. Dual modulation of endocannabinoid transport and fatty acid amide hydrolase protects against excitotoxicity. J Neurosci 2005; 25:7813–7820.

[154] Gilbert GL, Kim HJ, Waataja JJ, Thayer SA. Delta9-tetrahydrocannabinol protects hippocampal neurons from excitotoxicity. Brain Res 2007; 1128:61–69.

[155] Aguado T, Romero E, Monory K, Palazuelos J, Sendtner M, Marsicano G, Lutz B, Guzmán M, Galve-Roperh I. The CB1 cannabinoid receptor mediates excitotoxicity-induced neural progenitor proliferation and neurogenesis. J Biol Chem 2007; 282:23892–23898.

[156] Grabiec U, Koch M, Kallendrusch S, Kraft R, Hill K, Merkwitz C, Ghadban C, Lutz B, Straiker A, Dehghani F. The endocannabinoid N-arachidonoyldopamine (NADA) exerts neuroprotective effects after excitotoxic neuronal damage *via* cannabinoid receptor 1 (CB(1)). Neuropharmacology 2012; 62:1797–1807. doi: 10.1016/j.neuropharm.2011.11.023.

[157] McPartland JM. Obesity, the endocannabinoid system, and bias arising from pharmaceutical sponsorship. PLoS One 2009; 4:e5092. doi: 10.1371/journal.pone.0005092

[158] McPartland JM, Guy GW, Di Marzo V. Care and feeding of the endocannabinoid system: a systematic review of potential clinical interventions that upregulate the endocannabinoid system. PLoS One 2014; 9:e89566. doi: 10.1371/journal.pone.0089566.

[159] Xu JY, Chen C. Endocannabinoids in synaptic plasticity and neuroprotection. Neuroscientist 2015; 21:152–168. doi: 10.1177/1073858414524632.

[160] Skaper, S.D.; Di Marzo, V. Endocannabinoids in nervous system health and disease: the big picture in a nutshell. Philos Trans R Soc B 2012; 367:3193–3200.

Chapter 3

The Potential Therapeutic Role of the Cannabinoid System in Neurological Disorders of the Basal Ganglia: An Overview

Gabriela Aguilera and Abel Santamaría

Additional information is available at the end of the chapter

http://dx.doi.org/10.5772/63375

Abstract

Cannabinoid pharmacology has been explored as a therapeutic option for handling pathologies and conditions of varying nature. In regard to neurological disorders, cannabinoid chemistry has been explored for the regulation of hyperkinetic symptoms, anti-inflammation, neuroprotection, and neurodegeneration, a collective goal of many preclinical studies. The enhancement and improvement of the endogenous cannabinergic responses of the human body in both physiological and pathological conditions, together with the overall consequential effects of the modulation of its elements, are currently under strict scrutiny and undeniably possess incalculable value that might support the hypothesis aiming to improve the endocannabinoid tone with therapeutic purposes. Therefore, this chapter reviews the mechanisms known to be present in the course of several disorders of the basal ganglia, as well as the available treatments exploring this novel approach.

Keywords: Alzheimer's disease, Parkinson's disease, Huntington's disease, multiple sclerosis, amyotrophic lateral sclerosis, organic acidemias, endocannabinoid system

Article Note

Doctoral student from the Experimental Biology Ph.D. Program, Metropolitan Autonomous University—Iztapalapa, supported with fellowship CVU 486539 from CONACYT.

1. Introduction

Cannabinoid signaling has been reported to play an active role in a number of neurological diseases. Its functions begin with the constitutive expression of receptors within the central nervous system (CNS), as well as inducible expression of such upon inflammatory processes; in addition, endogenous ligands and the enzymes in charge of the synthesis and degradation of endocannabinoids complete the arrangement. Therefore, the study of the cannabinoid circuitry is currently directed towards the description of the events that typically take place as part of the onset and development of disease, as well as the exploitation of the experimental evidence that supports and enables novel and promising therapies. Given the poor effectiveness of existing treatments in matter of neurological diseases, the interest of the vast majority of such approaches involves strategies that aim to describe and explain common alterations that occur at early stages of a number of disorders. Basal ganglia, comprising complex nuclei such as caudate, putamen, globus pallidus, or the substantia nigra, are intimately associated with the endocannabinoid system (ECS) through the expression of its receptors, inducement of synthesis of such compounds and, therefore, exert a prominent modulatory motor function and some rewarding processes [1–4].

Such findings have greatly encouraged the study of the implications of cannabinoid-derived compounds in neurological diseases from the basal ganglia. From motor-related striatal disorders such as catalepsy or dystonias, to neurodegenerative diseases such as Alzheimer's disease (AD), Parkinson's disease (PD), Huntington's disease (HD), or even low-incidence disorders such as glutaric or propionic acidemias, the efficacy of cannabinoids has and is still being demonstrated in a number of pathological schemes, particularly through the reduction of oxidative stress, neuroinflammation, and excitotoxicity, therefore enhancing intrinsic restoration mechanisms [2, 5–7].

Nowadays, the progress towards effective therapeutic approaches involves mainly the manipulation of the cannabinoid pathway through pharmacological means, with particular emphasis in models capable of evoking neuronal cell death and impaired cell communication; on the other hand, the exploration of cannabinoid compounds able to trigger endogenous responses has gained popularity given several hypotheses claiming promissory neuroprotective qualities of endocannabinoids, despite the heterogeneous data that has been retrieved so far. Nevertheless, the therapeutic use of cannabinoid compounds has raised and will most surely continue to raise questions regarding its capacity in long-term outlines, as well as the potential risks acquired when dealing with the design of therapies, all of which need to be addressed accurately. The challenge remains, and contemporary therapeutic advances must respond to these questions; therefore, this chapter will provide with punctual evidence of the known mechanisms that underlie the onset and development of the aforementioned diseases of the basal ganglia and the available treatment regimes, and together with a current overview of the mechanisms of action of endocannabinoids under physiological and pathological conditions, will contribute to paint a realistic picture of the area of competence of cannabinoids in basal ganglia disease, and its perspectives in short and long term.

http://dx.doi.org/10.5772/63375

2. Neurological diseases and the potential cannabinoid therapies

2.1. Alzheimer's disease

Since the first description of AD over a 100 years ago, our knowledge of the mechanisms underlying this condition has evolved and enriched ever since. Consistent pathological traits of AD include the presence of extracellular deposits of β-amyloid peptide which, through several mechanisms, are thought to play a relevant role in the origins of the disease by inducing cell death and consequent memory, behavioral and cognitive detriment. A second feature encompasses the formation of intracellular neurofibrillary tangles of tau protein, which eventually impairs neuronal communication [6, 8, 9]. In addition, such hallmarks are accompanied by influential conditions that have attracted increasing interest by acquiring value as causal agents of the disease. First, oxidative stress; as expected, an imbalance between pro-oxidant and antioxidant systems leads to the accumulation of reactive oxygen species (ROS) produced by the mitochondria, and, therefore, to unequivocal damage to lipids, proteins, and nucleic acids. Second, a number of excitotoxicity events take place, especially when considering that AD patients exhibit a considerable reduction in glutamate transporter activity, hence easing neurodegeneration. In fact, several stressing stimuli (dysregulation of intracellular Ca^{2+} homeostasis, mitochondrial dysfunction, exposure to aberrant Aβ/tau proteins, oxidative stress, and inflammation itself) are thought to run simultaneously and lead to AD progression. While the vast majority of AD cases are idiopathic and with unknown etiology, a minority have a genetic basis; the aforementioned conditions are involved thoroughly with its genesis and evolution, and the disease is currently recognized as multifactorial.

From a different perspective, recent reports indicate that AD constitutes nowadays a noteworthy threat to the elder as it is a highly frequent condition among people over the age of 65 years (affecting up to 5–8% of individuals over 65 years, as high as 15–20% of individuals over 75 years, or an alarming 25–50% of individuals over 85 years) [10]; also, it accounts as the most prevalent disease among the dementias [11], accounting for 50–75% of the total number of dementias [10]. As a consequence of the late onset of the disease, it occurs with other major age-related pathologies, and therefore, an early and accurate diagnosis represents a great challenge added to the consolidation of an effective therapy. As a result of such complexity, substantial amount of efforts have been set towards the comprehension and treatment of this condition.

Existing pharmacological therapies include cholinesterase inhibitors such as donepezil, galantamine or rivastigmine [8], statins, and memantine. Unfortunately, all of those fail to modify the course of the disease or reverse its progression. Moreover, current approved drugs can only ameliorate symptoms in a limited number of patients facing initial features of the disease; consequently, to improve the strategy, symptomatic therapies must be accurately managed with patient's comorbidities. Activated microglia at the periphery of senile plaques is known to contribute greatly with the antioxidant defense in brains of patients suffering from the disease, and for that reason, anti-inflammation and antioxidant strategies are likely to cast a feasible alternative for early stages of the disease. Also, research efforts have begun to explore drug delivery vehicles and bioimaging at nanoscale, which despite comprising revolutionary nanotech-based developments, still face impediments linked to its biological toxicity, bioavailability, stability, and efficacy to name a few. Undoubtedly, the challenge into the proposal and consolidation of an effective therapy still remains, and great emphasis has been put into the study of therapeutic targets of AD and other neurodegenerative diseases.

2.2. Parkinson's disease

PD is a neurodegenerative disorder characterized by several motor and non-motor signs resulting from a progressive loss of dopaminergic neurons from the *substantia nigra pars compacta* (SNpc) [12] and a selective degeneration of the nigrostriatal pathway [13]. Neuronal death occurs in other brain regions, such as locus coeruleus, the dorsal nucleus of the vagus nerve, and the nucleus basalis of Meynert and might be even more acute than the neuronal death from the SNpc [14]. However, the pathological processes of this disease involve far more events than cell loss, primarily in routes in which non-dopaminergic neurotransmitters are affected (and include noradrenalin, serotonin, glutamate, or acetylcholine in the basal ganglia and cortex) [2]. PD accounts for the second most common neurodegenerative disorder among the elder people worldwide, and hence, science has focused great amount of effort into its comprehension. Along with the knowledge of the causes that lead to this illness, several pathogenic mechanisms have been suggested; these include oxidative stress, mitochondrial deficiency, proteolytic stress, and neuroinflammation [12, 15]. Also, it is now considered the dopaminergic metabolism itself as another crucial factor in the cell death, taking into account that it is the intracellular key source of ROS and that dopamine oxidation can generate endogenous neurotoxins. To control the dopaminergic homeostasis, several enzymes such as tyrosine hydroxylase (TH) or dopamine decarboxylase (DDC) play a very important role in preventing the excessive oxidative stress; however, nigrostriatal levels of glutathione and superoxide dismutase activity in PD' patients are diminished, and therefore, cells are more vulnerable to damage by oxidative stress. Together with ROS overload, some effects such as lipid oxidation or electron transport chain decoupling take place, which are later translated into cell death [2]. Taking into consideration that dopamine does not cross the blood–brain barrier (BBB), drug therapy in this matter is palliative [16] and is mainly oriented to increase dopamine levels through oral dopamine-replacement therapies. Such treatments include L-dopa, dopamine agonist receptors, monoaminooxidase B inhibitors, and catechol-o-methyl-transferase (COMT) inhibitors. From the previous examples, L-dopa remains in our day as the most prescribed treatment, as well as the most functional therapy to lessen motor symptoms. Unfortunately, the neurodegenerative nature of this disease implies the progression of symptoms with time, and frequently motor fluctuations and dyskinesias go on and accentuate; this ends up by promoting alternate periods with decreased motion and abnormal involuntary movements [12]. In addition, L-dopa loses effectiveness and causes dyskinesias and conduct abnormalities in many patients [17]; on the other hand, some patients do not tolerate adequately dopaminergic agonists and need to substantially reduce dosage [2], and even patients receiving other dopaminergic therapies develop abnormal conducts such as impulse-controlled disorders or dopamine deregulation syndrome; furthermore, some non-motor symptoms such as hallucinations may even accentuate with dopaminergic treatment [12]. The motor and non-motor abnormalities presented by the effect of these limitations reduce drastically the quality of life of the patients suffering from this disease and intensify the need of an efficient treatment.

2.3. Huntington's disease

HD is a neurodegenerative disorder which follows an autosomal dominant inheritance and exhibits choreic movements and adverse psychiatric and cognitive signs. The disease holds grounds on a gene coding for the protein huntingtin, in which an abnormality exhibits from 40 up to 125 trinucleotide repeats (from a 38-trinucleotide repetitions in normal conditions); hence leading to a toxic protein. Significant cognitive and psychiatric detriment and abnormal involuntary movements occur as part of the distinctive features of the condition; the aforementioned symptoms are explained by the degeneration and cell death at the level of globus pallidus, cortex, or striatum, all of which are accented with the progress over time [18]. The neurodegenerative quality of this pathology is attributed partially to the toxicity of the mutant Htt, condition characterized by abnormal folding, abnormal proteolysis, aggregation/ protein deposition, to name a few. Nonetheless, despite the progress achieved in the definition of the pathogenic mechanism that encloses this disease, the clinical expression, the evolution, or even its genesis cannot be merely explained through the mutation of the Htt protein [19], since oxidative events, excitotoxicity, glial activation, and local inflammatory events converge with the onset and progression of the disease [3].

HD is a rare, chronic, and neurodegenerative disorder in which clinical symptoms start typically once past 40 years; nevertheless, slight symptoms may be present even for decades before diagnosis is met [1]. Recent epidemiologic data on the matter reveals that HD has an incidence of 1–100 cases per million in Europe and North America only, while Japan, Hong Kong or Taiwan has only up to 7 cases per million. In accordance with the stated figures, high-incidence regions or "hot spots" have been identified, and correspond to each of the following: British Columbia and Canada, the city of Maracaibo in Venezuela, and South Wales region in the United Kingdom [20]. Despite this scenario, current therapeutics lack of an effective option to stop the progression of the disease; as a consequence, available treatments consist mainly of antipsychotics, antidepressants, and sedatives, as well as psychological treatment and rehabilitation [20–27]. For these reasons, notorious efforts to elucidate the pathophysiological mechanisms that underlie this condition were executed intensely during the last decade.

2.4. Multiple sclerosis

Multiple sclerosis (MS) is a demyelinating disorder of the CNS that is characterized by a number of progressive and disabling symptoms of inflammatory and degenerative nature; affecting up to 2.5 million people worldwide, MS accounts as one of the most common cause of neurological disability in young adults (from 20 to 40 years). MS has accompanied human beings for about 150 years, time in which the disorder has been target of enormous endeavors that have aimed to describe and understand the underlying mechanisms. In regard to the causes that lead to this illness, strong evidence indicates that a particular genotype plus environmental or somewhat random stimulus may led individuals more prone to develop the disorder [5, 28, 29]. MS patients experience immune attack to the CNS, exerting acute damage to the glial cells that form myelin, the oligodendrocytes. In addition, the autoimmune acute inflammation can be spotted along brain matter and meninges. In this form, loss of neurons is eventually reached as the demyelination process turns chronic and is convoyed by severe degeneration of axons; as expected, neuronal loss is linked with the disability manifested throughout the disease, a condition that lessens dramatically the quality of life of patients. MS can portray neuronal dysfunction, and states of accumulated or irreversible disability, and even some cases exhibit both [30].

Central manifestations of the disease involve "relapses," or exacerbation periods, which are often followed by "remissions," which are partial or complete recovery periods. Primary-progressive MS, PPMS, is considered the only phase of this condition and estimated to affect around 10% of the people with MS. A high percentage of MS patients are likely to be initially diagnosed with a relapsing–remitting disease course, or RRMS, a stage that will most surely shift to the so-called secondary-progressive MS, or SPMS. Unfortunately, the neurodegenerative nature of the disease implies that after a period of relapses and remissions, MS' steady progression will be reached either with or without relapses. Consequently, the distressing outcome that characterizes MS has drawn the attention of the medical fields in order to improve the quality of life of patients who endure it through valid therapeutic options; unfortunately, the etiology remains unknown, and to this date, there is no definite treatment. Moreover, despite a myriad of efforts and even after a century of awareness and constant research, MS therapeutics still face major challenges as a proper diagnose is hard to meet given the lack of a leading and straightforward test that prevents from missed and incorrect diagnoses.

Thus, while we face the lack of a cure or effective treatment, research has offered several disease-modifying drugs (DMDs), which help reducing MS activity and improve the overall course of the disease. Approved treatments for MS are diverse and include glatiramer acetate, immunomodulatory compound approved by the FDA for the reduction of the frequency of relapses of MS and, however, does not reduce progression of disability; on the other hand, mitoxantrone is an antineoplastic agent that has shown effectiveness in slowing the progression of secondary-progressive MS, a stage of the disease that follows the relapsing–remitting disease course; although this therapy provides some benefit, the use of agents of this nature carries several adverse reaction of varying severity, which limits usage in MS patients; lastly fingolimod, a selective immunosuppressive drug currently approved in the United States as a first-line treatment, or otherwise approved in countries of the European Union as a second-line treatment given safety clauses [30]. The previously stated therapies are effective to some extent and mainly regulate the immune system activity but have no competence to repair immune-mediated damage to the myelin sheaths, turning them worthless for neurodegenerative scenarios. Alternatively, with remyelination therapies, neuronal function can be restored, and some future neuronal loss can be prevented. A therapy of this class is substantiated with the proposal that a treatment that enhances remyelination might be even more effective in reducing long-term disability due to the increase in neuronal survival. For these purposes, monoclonal antibodies such as alemtuzumab and BIIB033 are few examples of novel attempts on the mater, and so far, the promotion of remyelination has proven to reduce overall clinical severity in animal models of the disease [31]. Despite moving towards clinical studies, several factors have been found to contribute to failure of the approach, as sporadically oligodendrocytes do not remyelinate axons effectively; moreover, oligodendrocyte precursor cells (OPC) are not always recruited into the lesions at functional levels [28, 31].

2.5. Amyotrophic lateral sclerosis

Amyotrophic lateral sclerosis (ALS) is a motor neuron disorder with a fatal outcome, and accounts as one of the most devastating disorders in adults, as approximately 70% of patients die within 3 years from the beginning of symptoms. Often referred to as "Lou Gehrig's disease," ALS brain exhibits severe damage on motor neurons in brain, brainstem, and spinal cord; the disease is clinically characterized by a high-degree of cognitive impairment, as well as progressive motor manifestations such as muscular atrophy and consequential respiratory complications and paralysis, all of which constitute possible and unfortunate death causes for those who suffer from it. With an indefinite pathogenesis, ALS is known to comprise environmental and genetic factors. In this form, the highest percentage of ALS cases are sporadic, while only 10% are familial with dominant inheritance. Aberrant folding of Cu/Zn superoxide dismutase (*SOD1*) is a pathological change known to be present in the familial form of ALS (fALS) caused by several mutations in the *SOD1* gene; such alterations are still under scrutiny and current hypotheses state that such result in protein misfolding and fibrillary aggregation observed as part of the hallmarks of ALS. As expected, the assessment of the environmental factors that may be associated to the disease is imperative; however, many more studies from different sources are needed to judge appropriately such relationship and determine accurately the risk factors that come along with it. Early diagnosis of ALS is based mainly on the neurologist judgment of clinical signs and symptoms and constitutes a crucial element to ensure quality of life; nevertheless, diagnosis is often met a year, or up to 3 years, before the first symptoms, creating an obstacle to adequate medical care. Besides, very few therapeutic alternatives are currently licensed as treatment for the ALS; a great example is riluzole, a potent inhibitor of glutamate release used recurrently to delay the onset of particular symptoms, but which does not result in substantial benefit in terms of therapeutic effects. Still, emerging evidence indicates that numerous factors may contribute strongly with the degenerative process of the disorder; primarily, the influence of enhanced oxidative stress and neuroinflammation events, which is also hypothesized as causative agents for other high-incidence diseases such as AD or PD; additionally, glutamate toxicity, mitochondrial dysfunction, or excessive apoptosis contribute actively to the progression of the disease and entail the basis of proposed therapies to delay neural loss and prolong cell survival [32–36].

Likewise, numerous evidence is implicating the receptor for advanced glycation end-products, or RAGE, as part of the genesis of several disorders. RAGE is known to be part of cell surface immunoglobulins, and its role as a factor of oxidative stress, inflammation, and cellular detriment in neurodegenerative diseases is gaining attention over the years. The precise mechanisms underlying the involvement of RAGE in neurodegeneration and its detrimental effects remain unknown, and yet some studies have provided valuable suggestions of RAGE as a crucial contributor of the pathogenesis of ALS; of special interest are those works that demonstrate the upregulation of AGE receptors and its ligands, revealing an interesting trace to further look into on experimental approaches [33]. In this form, many more hypotheses and experiments are needed to reach definite understanding of the etiopathogenesis of ALS.

2.6. Organic acidemias

Organic acid disorders are autosomal-recessive inherited metabolic disorders that appear as a result of an aberrant step in the catabolic route of branched-chain amino acids, usually the consequence of deficient enzyme activity. In this form, organic acids tend to accumulate in fluids and tissues, followed by various pathological effects such as overdosage of toxic chemical compounds, as well as shortage of essential compounds omitted with the interruption of inner pathways. Examples of disorders under the latter classification include propionic acidemia, methylmalonic acidemia (MMA), homocystinuria, 3-hydroxy-3-methylglutaryl-CoA (HMG-CoA) lyase deficiency, and type I glutaric acidemia (GA I). A recurrent clinical manifestation of such disorders comprises encephalopathy, which consist of neurologic symptoms as seizures, lethargy, and malnutrition, all of which progress over time and lead to coma. Therefore, the term "organic acidemia" (OAs) has been applied to a group of disorders characterized by the excretion of nonamino organic acids in urine and accounts as the most frequent metabolic disorders among severely ill children. In this way, those who endure it often present acute symptoms early in life; prompt diagnosis is thus a crucial element to avoid irreversible brain damage, as lack, tardy, or incorrect treatment would lead to low quality of life and permanent neurological consequences. Likewise, several organizations working towards the awareness and understanding of metabolic diseases have emphasized the importance of prenatal diagnosis for cases with elevated risk factors through the analysis of amniotic fluid, enzyme activity, or DNA testing. Such efforts have thrown some sampling and tests that have been useful for this purpose, such as very long chain fatty acids or lysosomal enzymes; however, the elevated costs along with the lack of consciousness of the implied consequences have slowed the progress in the matter.

The hereditary element of the disease signalizes the increased number of risk factors of offspring presenting an OAs; in this form, as OAs are considered rare, adequate assessment of the prevalence of the disease would need to rely on rigorous and periodic reports; however, the reportage of its presence among the population is irregular. Thereby, high prevalence has been theorized in Porto Alegre, Brazil, and South Indian regions, as well as some Western countries; in addition, several cases have been followed closely at health institutions from Damascus, Syria. Luckily, the elevated presence of these disorders over the past 20 years increased noticeably the efforts towards its study. So that the diagnostic elements and clinical features of these disorders of metabolic nature are increasingly being documented. Considering the poor prognosis faced by patients, lots of efforts have been placed into the treatment of the manifestations of these disorders. Options imply the restoration of the biochemical homeostasis in regard to the specific aberrant element, usually through complete treatment schedules of dietary restriction of the precursor amino acids, administration of adjunctive compounds to dispose the toxic metabolites, or enhancement of the deficient enzymes. Additionally, patients often require liver transplantation given the high demand on this organ;

however, only a minority has access to such alternatives, and even less patients find success with this alternative [37–40].

In spite of its concrete aberrations, search of new clinical options has reached this neurometabolic disorders. Along with the accumulation of several metabolites, including glutaric, methylmalonic, and propionic acid, a severe neurodegenerative process takes place in OAs brain of children; the latter, as known, is associated with many other damage mechanisms from oxidative stress to excitotoxicity. In this form, the benefits and multiple advantages or proposed neuroprotective therapies could provide invaluable input for such disorders.

3. The role of the cannabinoid system in neurodegenerative diseases

The ECS has been formally recognized as such for around 20 years, and its study has yielded information that reveals the close relationship of this system in the brain. As known, type 1 cannabinoid receptors (CB1r) are widely expressed within the CNS, in particular in the motor cortex, thalamus, hypothalamus, and hippocampus to name a few. On the other hand, type 2 cannabinoid receptors (CB2r) are found in the CNS as well as peripheral tissue. Cannabinoid circuitry is associated with a number of physiological processes, as endogenous cannabinoids such as 2-arachidonoyl glycerol (2-AG) or anandamide (AEA) interact with the G-protein-coupled receptors, CB1r and CB2r, and are known to regulate the neurotransmitter-release inhibition through the adenylate cyclase inhibition [41].

Given the foregoing in regard to the current status of AD and its therapeutics, the high density of CB1r in the basal ganglia tipped the balance towards a scenario in which particularly this receptor could provide evidence that highlight the therapeutic potential of the ECS in the AD. Moreover, subpopulations of the CB1r located at the hippocampus are well-known to contribute to the effect in memory and learning, processes that face great detriment during the progression of AD and are also features of the AD brain [42]. It is strongly suggested that cannabinoids hold anti-inflammatory and antioxidant properties that result in an overall neuroprotective effect; this is hypothesized to occur through the promotion of several intrinsic repair mechanisms able to reduce oxidative stress or apoptotic events. A number of studies have supported the fact that neuronal survival is intimately related with cannabinoid circuitry, hence diminishing the deleterious effect of harmful molecules such as Aβ in AD. Neuronal damage is known to trigger the endogenous production of cannabinoids such as AEA [43]. Also, Aβ is known to evoke hippocampal degeneration and cognitive impairment, but would also be responsible of inducing an increase in the production of 2-AG; as a consequence, ECS would exert its neuroprotective actions from Aβ-induced dent [44]. On the other hand, the overactivation of the N-methyl-D-aspartate receptor (NMDAr) and dysregulation of intracellular Ca^{2+} homeostasis portray the unique hallmarks of the disease and ultimately hold great potential for novel therapeutic strategies. Such an outline implies the manipulation of the ECS to promote a response which ideally involve the upregulation in the endocannabinoid synthesis, or the reduction of the Ca^{2+} influx and the consequent suppression in the excitotoxic events to confer neuroprotection. Conveying those coveted effects, evidence suggests that the activation of the CB1r is capable of exerting protective actions in cells in the hippocampal region, action that would be completed through the inhibition of Ca^{2+} entry and reduction of the glutamatergic activity [45]; in this matter, several experiments with inhibitors of the NMDAr have shown to protect cell cultures from excitotoxic damage; in addition, it is now known that the synthesis of the two main cannabinoids of endogenous nature, AEA and 2-AG, is dependent of Ca^{2+} influx, and thus, levels of compounds of cannabinoid basis would be determined in response to the intracellular Ca^{2+} load. On the other hand, CB2r is also of interest, and so far, its anti-inflammatory properties and neurogenesis stimulation have been proven as well. In conclusion, the promissory potential of the ECS satisfies the demands of a neurodegenerative condition with no cure or adequate treatment to this date. The abovementioned strategies represent interesting actions of the cannabinoids; until now, the manipulation of the ECS has yielded promising results and might be more efficient than the present choices. Cannabinoids have shown to reduce oxidative stress and neuroinflammation markers, typically Aβ-related, while fundamental restoration mechanisms are increased [8]. In this way, the AD therapeutics strongly call for further research to demonstrate conclusively such properties, in order to respond accordingly to the needs of those who endure it.

On the other hand, current pharmacological therapy in PD relies on formulations unable to attain suitable efficiency; in response to this condition, the potential of cannabinoid compounds has attracted attention to the field, as well as the possible applications with countless clinic value. As known, cannabinoid receptors are currently being associated to a number of neuropathogenic processes as various reports affirm that such molecules may act as ideal means for pathologies with inflammatory components. In regard to these events, the development of dyskinesias constitutes a disabling complication shown by most PD′ patients; for that reason, CB1r antagonists are proposed as an accurate treatment for parkinsonian symptoms (bradykinesia, rigidity, tremor, and so on) as well as levodopa-induced dyskinesias through the inhibition of such abnormal movements [46]. Furthermore, increasing evidence has disclosed that ECS goes through a number of alterations during brain disorders and PD is not an exception. To this point, it is known that dopamine depletion imposes great impact into the ECS and causes an upregulation of the CB1r and endocannabinoids in basal ganglia, which of course fundaments the multiple hypothesis regarding cannabinoid applications. In fact, published data states that an early pre-symptomatic phase in PD would display desensitization or downregulation of CB1r, and which ultimately lead to excitotoxicity, oxidative stress, and inflammatory events; on the other hand, advanced phases of the disease would exhibit upregulation of CB1r consistently with the hyperkinesia manifested by patients [18]; in this form, the opportunity area in the different stages is evident. In regard to the experimental revisions, several studies report that the use of rimonabant, another antagonist of the CB1r, could trigger positive effects on parkinsonian motor inhibition; the results, however, seem to be related to low-dose schemes [47]. Then again, the prompt administration of inhibitors of the degradation of endogenous cannabinoids may be able to reduce typical motor symptoms of the disease, as it has been found that cerebrospinal fluid contains high levels of endogenous cannabinoids such as AEA [48] in patients' treatment-naïve; this constitutes a remarkable finding, and such an approach represents a feasible challenge for clinicians. In this way, research on the matter has disclosed so far that both agonists and antagonists of cannabinoid receptors are likely to improve some but not all motor symptoms, and further clinical trials might provide additional information needed to appropriately identify such compounds and migrate from research to clinic. However, some studies have not found noteworthy effects of cannabinoids in PD; a remarkable example is the orally administered *cannabis*, as it did not produce either qualitative or quantitative improvement in dyskinesias or parkinsonism [48]. Over the same goal, innovative experimental designs determined that the administration of Δ^9-tetrahydrocannabinol (Δ^9-THC) or cannabidiol, both full agonists of CB1r, lead to significant protection of dopaminergic neurons of the nigrostriatal pathway after great toxic insult with 6-hydroxydopamine (6-OHDA). Likewise, Δ^9-THC and cannabidiol weakened the dopaminergic depletion resulting from a toxic insult with 6-OHDA toxin and lessened the tyrosine hydroxylase deficits [21]. Then again, the dramatic loss of neurons in substantia nigra and striatum that distinguishes PD from the rest entails consequences besides the alterations in the dopaminergic transmission. Glutamatergic excitation is known to be mediated strongly by NMDAr with located at such brain regions, and as known, overactivation of NMDAr leads to excitotoxicity events and great cellular damage. In this form, antagonists of NMDAr of cannabinoid nature such as rimonabant hold viable qualities for the treatment applications by reducing its elevated activity and reducing drastically inflammatory events. Although exciting and promising, these new approaches revealed somewhat conflicting results as a positive outcome was not always reached; therefore, the proposal of clinical strategies to accurately treat PD must be followed by supplementary research that provides grounds for its migration towards the clinic.

Research has expanded to low-incidence diseases such as HD, and so far, it is known that initial phases display a downregulation of CB1r, a stage mostly pre-symptomatic and usually prediagnose [24]. As part of the degenerative process, advanced states of the disease exhibit an important loss of the CB1r in the striatum, GP, and SNpc in particular, but which might spread further [27, 49].

It is well known that cannabinoid signalling pathways face great alterations as part of the ruling elements of the disease; to start with, CB1r show evidence of deregulation and hypofunction in basal ganglia. Such findings differed with the traditional paradigm in which the receptor loss was attributed as a secondary effect of the progressive loss of GABAergic neurons; however, recent evidence has revealed that such loss is present also in models without striatal lesion. Hence, it has been established that decrease and functional loss of CB1r may perhaps be related with the pathogenesis of HD and not a mere consequence in the line of events; moreover, alterations and overall detriment in CB1r may actually contribute with the onset and progression by rendering neurons more vulnerable to oxidative stress and excitotoxicity [3].

A strong exploration of plentiful strategies under this understanding started a few years ago, and so far, the power of cannabinoids as toxicity modulators has been challenged. It was recently reported that tetrahydrocannabivarin (Δ^9-THCV) delays disease progression and reduces motor inhibition through changes in glutamatergic transmission [50]. Preclinical models of the disease have been used as platforms to explore the scope and limitations of cannabinoid derivatives in therapy. Administration of cannabigerol (CBG) was capable of reducing reactive microgliosis and counteracted the overregulation of inflammatory markers in preclinical models with neurotoxin administration, and all of which were explained through a cannabinoid receptor-dependent mechanism [51]; likewise, R6/1 transgenic mice expressing ≥115 CAG repetitions displayed lower toxicity markers after the administration of synthetic cannabinoids such as WIN 55,212-2 or HU210 through a CB1r coupling mechanism [52].

While a number of alternatives continue to justify its benefits and disadvantages in the run for the establishment as competent therapies, new hypotheses have raised in regard to the involvement of the ECS in neurodegenerative diseases, and MS is not an exception. Unlike cannabinoid applications on AD or HD in which data suggests a definite trend of positive outcomes, MS deals with rather differing data in terms of the etiopathogenesis of the disease. The immune attack that takes place in MS is reported to come along with the decrease in endocannabinoid levels due to the alteration of receptors in purinergic signalling induced by some cytokines, hence declining the endocannabinoid tone [10]; in this form, such alterations may contribute with both the onset and progression of the disease by reducing endocannabinoid protection. On the other hand, several reports state that immune attack comes along with endocannabinoid increase in several models of the disease (encephalomyelitis, or EAE), arrangement in which cannabinoids would serve, once again, as neuroprotectors [5]. Despite conflicting, strategies involving the ECS encompass a wide range of approaches; up to this date, several studies currently evaluate the role of synthetic cannabinoids on the improvement of symptoms. For example, spasticity was proven to be dependent on the complete action of CB1r, but not CB2r in preclinic studies with CB1-knockout mice [53]. In fact, the motor disability nature of MS is conferred partly by spasticity, reason why this symptom has been target of novel hypothesis; while a great number of such still stand preclinical evaluations, some have reached further stages. Several clinical trials have confirmed the results obtained previously, given that beneficial effects on spasticity symptoms were reached when patients received experimental therapies with dronabinol [54]. Sativex®, a mixture of Δ^9-THC and cannabidiol in 50% ethanol solution, is currently approved in countries such as Canada, Germany, and the United Kingdom to alleviate spasticity in patients with MS that was somewhat unresponsive to standard therapies [55, 56]. As far as this, the applications born from the exploitation of cannabis derivatives and the overall study of the ECS are vast and have yielded valuable insights that help clarify the events that take place in the MS brain, as well as the future outlook in terms of treatment and care. However, supplementary data are needed to ascertain innovative cannabinoid therapies, as well as to ensure efficacy and safety of those already under study.

Accordingly, several preclinical studies involving animal models of ALS have evaluated the efficacy of CB2r activation in terms of motor symptom reduction and overall cell survival. for example, regular administration of the selective antagonist of CB2r AM-1241 was found to significantly decrease degeneration of motor neurons in a transgenic mouse model of ALS; more importantly, motor function was preserved under schemes of early administration after the onset of symptoms [57]. Experimental approaches using a mouse model of ALS, the *SOD1**G93A, disclosed congruent results with the above statements, given that noteworthy delay on progression of the disease was reached under treatment with WIN 55,212-2. This potent CB1r agonist is going under strict scrutiny as many analgesic and anti-neurotoxic effects have been attributed to its chemical structure; thus, the exploitation of the vast properties of this molecule is currently at its height and further research will surely follow. A genetic model of the disease comprising the ablation of the FAAH was also tested, and revealed valuable information in regard to the same animal model approach; as such, the consequential increase of endogenous levels of AEA led to weakening of ALS symptoms and disease progression on the *SOD1* aged-animal model, results that, however, did not spread to the overall life-span [36]. The previous are only few examples that emphasize the necessity of supplementary studies that challenge the actual properties of cannabinoids and ECS management for therapeutic means. Expressly, the definite process of neuroprotection in animal models of the disease is controversial, given that some reports suggest non-CB receptor-dependent mechanisms. In this form, pharmacological usage of cannabinoids would provide the needed pieces to elucidate the pathogenesis of ALS, as well as thoroughly justify its applications.

In contrast, though metabolic disorders such as OAs could get enormous benefit from a renewed clinical outlook, data in regard to the link between the pathophysiology of the disease and the potential uses of elements of the ECS are still incipient, and studies comprising both variables are scarce. Oxidative stress and excitotoxicity are known to be implicated among several processes stimulated during the development of OAs. Under this understanding, an experimental approach determined the effects of WIN 55,212-2, a synthetic agonist of cannabinoid receptors known for eliciting analgesic properties on several animal models. This preclinical study reported that an experimental design administrating WIN 55,212-2 as pretreatment was sufficient to induce protective effects on early markers of endogenous metabolites that tend to be produced and accumulated in OAs; in addition, decrease in levels of ROS was also noted [58]. Despite limited, such emerging data can substantiate further research under the same paradigm, with the aims of assembling an alternative capable of preventing the formation of ROS, as well as lipid peroxidation, systematic events found to be exerted by toxic metabolites of OAs.

4. Concluding remarks

Neurological illnesses, such as the ones mentioned in this chapter, pose exceptional challenges for therapy and technology while conversely carry great predicaments for human quality of life and morbidity (See **Figure 1**). Oxidative stress, inflammation, excitotoxicity, and degeneration itself conform the basis of many diseases addressed in this revision; moreover, such factors constitute harbingers of mortality. Thus, diverse treatment paths need to be followed to advance towards fruitful options. In this form, the understanding of the physiological and functional consequences of the molecular changes comprised during health and disease is crucial. In this journey, the involvement of the ECS and its many angles has arisen, and the therapeutic approximations resulting from its employment have found a counterpart in many diseases that bear scenarios of great defies for both patients and clinicians, and unfortunately, many roadblocks lie ahead. Ideally such obstacles would be overcome through the establishment of compatible tests and measures for accurate and timely diagnosis, the addressing of the actual mechanisms of its pathogenesis, the proposal, and assessment of future protective therapies, and the development of prevention strategies for individuals at risk if applicable. Novel developments have driven scientific excitement to a new high; in this form, the pace of experimental research shows that neuroscience is headed towards the integration of the current clinical needs, with novel discoveries and technology. For these reasons, numerous researches cast a spotlight into the ECS, given the intimate relationship of these and pathological processes; in addition, its lipophilic qualities along with the remarkable low toxicity of its derivatives enable exogenous and synthetic cannabinoids as suitable strategies, hence avoiding common inconveniences and side effects commonly presented with traditional therapies. Besides, the challenges facing a future implementation to thwart neurodegenerative diseases are vast, and needless to say, misleading information in regard to safety and efficacy of cannabinoid-based therapies overwhelms general public, and appropriate studies must allow the substantiation of the viability of the endocannabinoid modulation as a strategy against neurodegeneration, and more importantly, would determine if the overall benefits outweigh all realistic disadvantages.

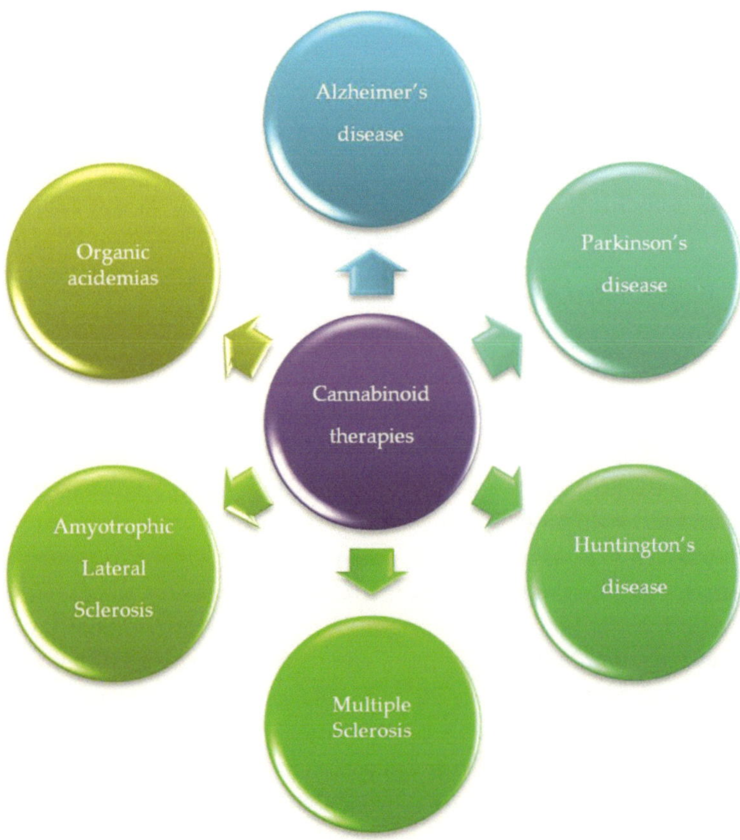

Figure 1. Schematic representation of the neurological diseases acquiring therapeutic options based on cannabinoid chemistry.

Author details

Gabriela Aguilera and Abel Santamaría*

*Address all correspondence to: absada@yahoo.com

Laboratory of Excitatory Amino Acids, National Institute of Neurology and Neurosurgery, S. S. A., Mexico City, Mexico

References

[1] Di lorio G, Lupi M, Sarchione F, Matarazzo I, Santacroce R, Petruccelli F, Martinotti G, Di Giannantonio M. The endocannabinoid system: a putative role in neurodegenerative diseases. Int J High Risk Behav Addict. 2013;2(3):100–6. doi:10.5812/ijhrba.9222.

[2] Dray A. Neuropathic pain: emerging treatments. Br J Anaesth. 2008;101(1):48–58. doi: 10.1093/bja/aen107.

[3] Marsciano G, Goodenough S, Monory K, Hermann H, Eder M, Cannich A, Azad SC, Cascio MG, Gutiérrez SO, van der Stelt M, López-Rodríguez ML, Casanova E, Schutz G, Zieglgansberg W, Di Marzo V, Behl C, Lutz B. CB1 cannabinoid receptors and on-demand defense against excitotoxicity. Science. 2003;302(5642):84–8.

[4] Sanchez-Mut JV, Graff J. Epigenetic alterations in Alzheimer's disease. Front Behav Neurosci. 2015;9:347. doi:10.3389/fnbeh.2015.00347.

[5] Aso E, Ferrer I. Cannabinoids for treatment of Alzheimer's disease: moving toward the clinic. Front Pharmacol. 2014;5:37. doi:10.3389/fphar.2014.00037.

[6] Grotenhermen F, Muller-Vahl K. The therapeutic potential of cannabis and cannabinoids. Dtsch Arztebl Int. 2012;109(29–30):495–501. doi:10.3238/arztebl.2012.0495

[7] Leung L. Cannabis and its derivatives: review of medical use. J Am Board Fam Med. 2011;24(4):452–62. doi:10.3122/jabfm.2011.04.100280.

[8] Cabranes A, Venderova K, de Lago E, Fezza F, Sánchez A, Mestre L, Valenti M, García-Merino A, Ramos JA, Di Marzo V, Fernández-Ruiz J. Decreased endocannabinoid levels in the brain and beneficial effects of agents activating cannabinoid and/or vanilloid receptors in a rat model of multiple sclerosis. Neurobiol Dis. 2005;20(2):207–17. doi: 10.1016/j.nbd.2005.03.002.

[9] Pazos MR, Sagredo O, Fernández-Ruiz J. The endocannabinoid system in Huntington's disease. Curr Pharm Des. 2008;14(23):2317–25. doi:10.2174/138161208785740108.

[10] Riedel G, Davies SN. Cannabinoid function in learning, memory and plasticity. Handb Exp Pharmacol. 2005;(168):445–77. doi:10.1007/3-540-26573-2_15.

[11] Shoemaker JL, Seely KA, Reed RL, Crow JP, Prather PL. The CB2 cannabinoid agonist AM-1241 prolongs survival in a transgenic mouse model of amyotrophic lateral sclerosis when initiated at symptom onset. J Neurochem. 2007;101(1):87–98. doi: 10.1111/j.1471-4159.2006.04346.x.

[12] Lastres-Becker I, Molina-Holgado F, Ramos JA, Mechoulam R, Fernández-Ruiz J. Cannabinoids provide neuroprotection against 6-hydroxydopamine toxicity in vivo and in vitro: relevance to Parkinson's disease. Neurobiol Dis. 2005;19(1):96–107. doi: 10.1016/j.nbd.2004.11.009

[13] Malek N, Kucharczyk M, Starowicz K. Alterations in the anandamide metabolism in the development of neuropathic pain. Biomed Res Int. 2014;2014:686908. doi: 10.1155/2014/686908.

[14] Salama M, Arias-Carrión O. Natural toxins implicated in the development of Parkinson's disease. Ther Adv Neurol Disord. 2011;4(6):361–73. doi: 10.1177/1756285611413004.

[15] Bates GP, Dorsey R, Gusella JF, Hayden MR, Kay C, Leavitt BR, Nance M, Ross CA, Scahill RI, Wetzel R, Wild EJ, Tabrizi SJ. Huntington's disease. Nat Rev Dis Primers. 2015;1:15052. doi:10.1038/nrdp.2015.52.

[16] Di Marzo V, De Petrocellis L. Why do cannabinoid receptors have more than one endogenous ligand? Philos Trans R Soc Lond B Biol Sci. 2012;367(1607):3216–28. doi: 10.1098/rstb.2011.0382.

[17] Malek N, Kucharczyk M, Starowicz K. Alterations in the anandamide metabolism in the development of neuropathic pain. Biomed Res Int. 2014;2014:686908. doi: 10.1155/2014/686908

[18] Takahashi KA, Castillo PE. The CB1 cannabinoid receptor mediates glutamatergic synaptic supression in the hippocampus. Neuroscience. 2006;139(3):795–802. doi: 10.1155/2014/686908.

[19] Karanian DA, Brown QB, Makriyannis A, Kosten TA, Bahr BA. Dual modulation of endocannabinoid transport and fatty acid amide hydrolase protects against excitotoxicity. J Neurosci. 2005;25(34):7813–20. doi:10.1523/JNEUROSCI.2347-05.2005.

[20] Bari M, Battista N, Valenza M, Mastrangelo N, Malaponti M, Catanzaro G, Centonze D, Finazzi-Agro A, Cattaneo E, Maccarrone M. In vitro and in vivo models of Huntington's disease show alterations in the endocannabinoid system. FEBS J. 2013;280(14):3376–88. doi:10.1111/febs.12329.

[21] González S, Scorticati C, García-Arencibia M, de Miguel R, Ramos JA, Fernández-Ruiz J. Effects of rimonabant, a selective cannabinoid CB1 receptor antagonist, in a rat model of Parkinson's disease. Brain Res. 2006;1073–1074:209–19. doi:10.1016/j.brainres.2005.12.014.

[22] Mayer IM, Orth M. Neurophysiology in Huntington's disease: an update. Neurodegener Dis Manag. 2014;4(2):155–64. doi:10.2217/nmt.14.1.

[23] Narayanan MP, Kannan V, Vinayan KP, Vasudevan DM. DIagnosis of major organic acidurias in children: two years experience at a tertiary care centre. Indian J Clin Biochem. 2011;26(4):347–53. doi:10.1007/s12291-011-0111-9.

[24] Domaradzki J. The impact of Huntington disease on family carers: a literature overview. Psychiatr Pol. 2015;49(5):931–944. doi:10.12740/PP/34496.

[25] Costantino G. Inhibitors of quinolinic acid synthesis: new weapons in the study of neuroinflammatory diseases. Future Med Chem. 2014;6(8):841–3. doi:10.4155/fmc.14.35.

[26] Colín-González AL, Paz-Loyola AL, Serratos IN, Seminotti B, Ribeiro CA, Leipnitz G, Souza DO, Wajner M, Santamaría A. The effect of WIN 55,212-2 suggests a cannabinoid-sensitive component in the early toxicity induced by organic acids accumulating in glutaric acidemia type I and in related disorders of propionate metabolism in rat brain synaptosomes. Neuroscience. 2015;310:578–88. doi:10.1016/j.neuroscience.2015.09.043.

[27] Baker D, Jackson SJ, Pryce G. Cannabinoid control of neuroinflammation related to multiple sclerosis. Br J Pharmacol. 2007;152(5):649–54. doi:10.1038/sj.bjp.0707458.

[28] García C, Palomo-Garo C, García-Arencibia M, Ramos JA, Pertwee RG, Fernández-Ruiz J. Symptom-relieving and neuroprotective effects of the phytocannabinoid Δ9-THCV in animal models of Parkinson's disease. Br J Pharmacol. 2011;163(7):1495–1506. doi:10.1111/j.1476-5381.2011.01278.x.

[29] Leung L. Cannabis and its derivatives: review of medical use. J Am Board Fam Med. 2011;24(4):452–62. doi:10.3122/jabfm.2011.04.100280.

[30] Fernández-Ruiz F. The endocannabinoid system as a target for the treatment of motor dysfunction. Br J Pharmacol. 2009;156(7):1029–1040. doi:10.1111/j.1476-5381.2008.00088.x.

[31] Brotchie JM. CB1 cannabinoid receptor signalling in Parkinson's disease. Curr Opin Pharmacol. 2003;3(1):54–61. doi:10.1016/S1471-4892(02)00011-5.

[32] Obeso JA, Rodíguez-Oroz MC, Goetz CG, Marin C, Kordower JH, Rodriguez M, Hirsch EC, Farrer M, Schapira AH, Halliday G. Missing pieces in the Parkinson's disease puzzle. Nat Med. 2010;16(6):653–61. doi:10.1038/nm.2165.

[33] Giacoppo S, Mandolino G, Galuppo M, Bramanti P, Mazzon E. Cannabinoids: new promising agents in the treatment of neurological diseases. Molecules. 2014;19(11): 18781–816. doi:10.3390/molecules191118781.

[34] Feng LR, Maguire-Zeiss KA. Gene therapy in Parkinson's disease: rationale and current status. CNS Drugs. 2010;24(3):177–92. doi:10.2165/11533740-000000000-00000.

[35] Fernández-Ruiz J, Sagredo O, Pazos MR, García C, Pertwee R, Mechoulam R, Martínez-Orgado J. Cannabidiol for neurodegenerative disorders: important new clinical applications for this phytocannabinoid? Br J Clin Pharmacol. 2013;75(2):323–33. doi: 10.1111/j.1365-2125.2012.04341.x.

[36] Blázquez C, Chiarlone A, Sagredo O, Aguado T, Pazos MR, Resel E, Palazuelos J, Julien B, Salazar M, Borner C, Benito C, Carrasco C, Diez-Zaera M, Paoletti P, Díaz-Hernández M, Ruiz C, Sendtner M, Licas JJ, de Yébenes JG, Marsciano G, Monory K, Lutz B, Romero J, Alberch J, Ginés S, Kraus J, Fernández-Ruiz J, Galve-Roperh I, Guzmán M. Loss of striatal type 1 cannabinoid receptors is a key pathogenic factor in Huntington's disease. Brain. 2011;134:119–136. doi:10.1093/brain/awq278.

[37] Piomelli D, Tarzia G, Duranti A, Tontini A, Mor M, Compton TR, Dasse O, Monaghan EP, Parrot JA, Putman D. Pharmacological profile of the selective FAAH inhibitor KDS-4103 (URB597). CNS Drug Rev. 2006;12(1):21–38. doi:10.1111/j.1527-3458.2006.00021.x.

[38] Lewerenz J, Maher P. Chronic glutamate toxicity in neurodegenerative diseases- What is the evidence? Front Neurosci. 2015;9:469. doi:10.3389/fnins.2015.00469.

[39] Pryce G, Baker D. Control of spasticity in a multiple sclerosis model is mediated by CB1, not CB2, cannabinoid receptors. Br J Pharmacol. 2007;150(4):519–525. doi:10.1038/sj.bjp.0707003.

[40] Vaidyanathan K, Narayanan MP, Vasudevan DM. Organic acidurias: an updated review. Indian J Clin Biochem. 2011;26(4):319–325. doi:10.1007/s12291-011-0134-2.

[41] Sanchez-Mut JV, Graff J. Epigenetic alterations in Alzheimer's disease. Front Behav Neurosci. 2015;9:347. doi:10.3389/fnbeh.2015.00347.

[42] Panlilio LV, Justinova Z, Goldberg SR. Animal models of cannabinoid reward. Br J Pharmacol. 2010;160(3):499–510. doi:10.1111/j.1476-5381.2010.00775.x.

[43] Juranek JK, Daffu GK, Wojtkiewicz J, Lacomis D, Kofler J, Schmidt AM. Receptor for advanced glycation end products and its inflammatory ligands are upregulated in amyotrophic lateral sclerosis. Front Cell Neurosci. 2015;9:485. doi:10.3389/fncel.2015.00485.

[44] Scotter EL, Goodfellow CE, Graham ES, Dragunow M, Glass M. Neuroprotective potential of CB1 receptor agonists in an in vitro model of Huntington's disease. Br J Pharmacol. 2010;160(3):747–61. doi:10.1111/j.1476-5381.2010.00773.x.

[45] Renton AE, Chio A, Traynor BJ. State of play in amyotrophic lateral sclerosis genetics. Nat Neurosci. 2014;17(1):17–23. doi:10.1038/nn.3584

[46] Belbasis L, Bellou V, Evangelou E. Environmental risk factors and amyotrophic lateral sclerosis: an umbrella review and critical assessment of current evidence from systematic reviews and meta-analyses of observational studies. Neuroepidemiology. 2016;46(2):96–105. doi:10.1159/000443146.

[47] Galvin M, Madden C, Maguire S, Heverin M, Vajda A, Staines A, Hardiman O. Patient journey to a specialist amyotrophic lateral sclerosis multidisciplinary clinic: an exploratory study. BMC Health Serv Res. 2015;15:571. doi:10.1186/s12913-015-1229-x

[48] Meissner WG, Frasier M, Gasser T, Goetz CG, Lozano A, Piccini P, Obeso JA, Rascol O, Schapira A, Voon V, Weiner DM, Tison F, Bezard E. Priorities in Parkinson's disease research. Nat Rev Drug Discov. 2011;10(5):377–93. doi:10.1038/nrd3430.

[49] Gajofatto A, Turatti M, Monaco S, Benedetti MD. Clinical efficacy, safety, and tolerability of fingolimod for the treatment of relapsing-remitting multiple sclerosis. Drug Healthc Patient Saf. 2015;7:157–167. doi:10.2147/DHPS.S69640.

[50] Fox SH. Non-dopaminergic treatments for motor control in Parkinson's disease. Drugs. 2013;73(13):1405–15. doi:10.1007/s40265-013-0105-4.

[51] Seashore MR. The organic acidemias: an overview. In: Pagon RA, Bird TD, Dolan CR, Stephens K, Adam MP, editors. GeneReviews. New Haven, CT: University of Washington, Seattle; 2009.

[52] Pisani A, Fezza F, Galati S, Battista N, Napolitano S, Finazzi-Agro A, Bernardi G, Brusa L, Pierantozzi M, Stanzione P, Maccarrone M. High endogenous cannabinoid levels in the cerebrospinal fluid of untreated Parkinson's disease patients. Ann Neurol. 2005;57(5):777–9. doi:10.1002/ana.20462.

[53] Morandi E, Tarlinton RE, Gran B. Multiple Sclerosis between genetics and infections: human endogenous retroviruses in monocytes and macrophages. Front Immunol. 2015;6:647. doi:10.3389/fimmu.2015.00647.

[54] Duthey B. Alzheimer's disease and other Dementias: update on 2004 Background paper written by Saloni Tanna. Priority Medicines for Europe and the World "A Public Health Approach to Innovation". 2013

[55] Shennar HK, Al-Asmar D, Kaddoura A, Al-Fahoum S. Diagnosis and clinical features of organic acidemias: a hospital-based study in a single center in Damascus, Syria. Qatar Med J. 2015;2015(1):9. doi:10.5339/qmj.2015.9.

[56] Furukawa Y, Anzai I, Akiyama S Imai M, Consul-Cruz FJ, Saio T, Nagasawa K, Nomura T, Ishimori K. Conformational disorder of the most immature Cu,Zn-Superoxide Dismutase leading to Amyotrophic Lateral Sclerosis. J Biol Chem. 2016;291(8):4144–55. doi:10.1074/jbc.M115.683763.

[57] Ramaswamy S, McBride JL, Kordower JH. Animal models of Huntington's disease. ILAR J. 2007;48(4):356–73. doi:10.1093/ilar.48.4.356.

[58] Carroll CB, Bain PG, Teare L, Liu X, Joint C, Wroath C, Parkin SG, Fox P, Wright D, Hobart J, Zajicek JP. Cannabis for dyskinesia in Parkinson disease: a randomized double-blind crossover study. Neurology. 2004;63(7):1245–50. doi:10.1212/01.WNL.0000140288.48796.8E.

Chapter 4

Cannabinoids and Motor Control of the Basal Ganglia: Therapeutic Potential in Movement Disorders

Teresa Morera-Herreras, Cristina Miguelez,
Asier Aristieta, María Torrecilla,
José Ángel Ruiz-Ortega and Luisa Ugedo

Additional information is available at the end of the chapter

http://dx.doi.org/10.5772/62431

Abstract

Cannabinoid receptors in the brain appear to be intimately involved in the motor control. Cannabinoid CB1 receptors are densely located in the basal ganglia (BG), a forebrain system that integrates cortical information to coordinate motor activity regulating signals. In fact, the administration of plant-derived, synthetic or endogenous cannabinoids produces several effects on motor function. These effects are paralleled to changes in the levels of different neurotransmitters in the BG, including GABA, dopamine and glutamate, all of which are important players in movement control.

Cannabinoid receptors also participate in the etiopathology of movement disorders such as Parkinson's disease (PD) or Huntington's disease (HD). In fact, both CB receptors and endocannabinoid levels are altered in the BG of patients with PD and HD and animal models of these diseases. The benefit of cannabinoids in PD or HD is not limited to the symptomatic amelioration, since several publications have revealed interesting neuroprotective and anti-inflammatory effects of these drugs. It has been suggested that cannabinoid modulation may constitute an important component in new therapeutic approaches to the treatment of motor disturbances.

Keywords: Basal Ganglia, endocannabinoids, Parkinson's disease, Huntington's disease, CB1 receptor, CB2 receptor, TRPV1

Abbreviation List

Δ^9-THC: Δ^9-Tetrahydrocannabinol

Δ^9-THCV: Δ^9-Tetrahydrocannabivarin

2-AG: 2-Arachidonoylglycerol

3-NP: 3-nitropropionic acid

6-OHDA: 6-hydroxidopamine

AEA: Anandamide

BDNF: Brain-derived neurotrophic factor

BG: Basal Ganglia

CAG: Cytosine-adenine-guanine

CBD: Cannabidiol

CNS: Central nervous system

ECS: Endocannabinoid system

FAAH: Fatty acid amide hydrolase

HD: Huntington's disease

HTT: huntingtin protein

Internal/external globus pallidus: GPi/GPe

LPS: Lipopolysaccharide

MAGL: Monoacylglycerol lipase

MPTP: 1-methyl-4-phenyl-1,2,3,6-tetrahydropyridine

PD: Parkinson's disease

PEA: Palmitoylethanolamide

SNc: Substantia nigra pars compacta

SNr: Substantia nigra pars reticulata

SPN: Spiny projection neurons

STN: Subthalamic nucleus

TRPV1: Transient receptor potential vanilloid 1

VGLUT1: vesicular glutamate transporter 1

VGLUT2: vesicular glutamate transporter 2

http://dx.doi.org/10.5772/62431

1. Introduction

The identification of more than 60 oxygen-containing aromatic hydrocarbon compounds, known as cannabinoids in the plant *Cannabis sativa*, led to the discovery of the endocannabinoid system (ECS) [1]. This system consists of two well-characterized seven transmembrane G-protein coupled receptors, CB1 [2] and CB2 [3], the transient receptor potential vanilloid 1 (TRPV1) channel, a number of endogenous ligands and associated enzymes for biosynthesis and degradation (for review see [4,5]). The endocannabinoids are lipids localized in the central nervous system (CNS) and peripheral tissue, being anandamide (AEA) and 2-arachidonoylglycerol (2-AG) the best characterized ones [4]. These endocannabinoids are synthesized, on demand, after neuronal depolarization, released into the extracellular space and after CB receptors activation they are uptaken by a specific transport protein located on both neurons and glial cells to be subsequently degraded by intracellular enzymes [6].

The CB1 receptor is one of the most abundant cannabinoid receptor in the neurons from the CNS whereas the CB2 receptor is more predominant in glial cells and peripheral tissues [7]. CB receptors are coupled to Gi/o proteins, negatively to adenylyl cyclase and positively to mitogen-activated protein kinase and ion channels. Thereby activation of these receptors exerts diverse responses as inhibition of neurotransmitter release including GABA, glutamate, noradrenalin and dopamine [6,8,9], gene transcription and cell proliferation, differentiation and survival [10]. Commonly, the ECS is described as a neuromodulatory system which interacts with other neurotransmitter systems and may be implicated in (patho)physiological functions among others, those related to motor activity, neuron proliferation and inflammatory process. Consequently the ECS appears as a promising target for drug development. *Cannabis sativa* derivatives have been used medically for thousands of years, however the psychoactive effects together with tolerance and its potential abuse have limited the clinical application. Nowadays numerous efforts are being made to develop non-psychotropic cannabinoids that could be used in several CNS disorders.

This review will focus on recent studies clarifying the role of the ECS as a target to develop new therapeutic tools to treat movement disorders.

2. Neuroanatomical distribution of the endocannabinoid system in the BG

The ECS is highly expressed in the Basal Ganglia (BG), which is a highly organized network of subcortical nuclei composed of the striatum (caudate and putamen), *subthalamic nucleus* (STN), internal and external *globus pallidus* (or entopeduncular nucleus in rodents, GPi/EP and GPe) and *substantia nigra* (*pars compacta*, SNc, and *pars reticulata*, SNr). The BG connects the cortex with the thalamus, creating the cortico–basal ganglia–thalamo–cortical loop, and plays a crucial role on controlling movement activity.

High levels of CB1 receptors are found in the striatum and motor cortex where they are mainly present in projecting terminals (reviewed in [11]). Thus, CB1 receptors have been observed in glutamatergic corticostriatal afferences [12,13], striatal projections to the GPi/GPe and to the SNr [14,15] and also in subthalamonigral and subthalamopallidal terminals [15,16]. Moderate to dense CB2 immunoreactivity is also present in the cortex, striatum and SN [17] and is increased in several pathological conditions [18,19]. TRPV1 receptors have also been located in nigrostriatal terminals and on tyrosine hydroxylase-positive cells in the SNc [20,21].

The two most important endocannabinoid-synthesizing enzymes (N-acyl phosphatidylethanolamine phospholipase D and diacylglycerol lipase-alpha) as well as the endocannabinoid degradative enzymes (fatty acid amide hydrolase (FAAH) and monoacylglycerol lipase (MAGL)) are found in the BG, particularly in the striatum [22–24]. Finally, both AEA and 2-AG are expressed within the BG and modulate the activity of the cortico–basal ganglia–thalamo–cortical loop leading to motor activity modulation (for review see [25]).

3. Motor effects of cannabinoids

Over the last three decades a wide range of experimental and clinical studies have demonstrated that the ECS plays a key role controlling motor function. Specifically, three lines of evidence support this idea. First, administration of plant-derived compounds, synthetic cannabinoids and endocannabinoids produces a variety of effects on motor activity in humans and laboratory animals. Second, endocannabinoids and their receptors are abundant in the BG and the cerebellum, two brain areas that exert direct control of motor function. Third, biochemical and functional alterations of the ECS have been related to the etiology of several movement disorders, since overactivity of the ECS signaling is associated with the progression of the nigral degeneration in patients with Parkinson's disease (PD) [26–28] and down-regulation of CB1 receptors has been reported in brain samples collected from patients with Huntington's disease (HD) [29–31].

Marijuana consumption affects psychomotor skills clearly reflected in poor performance of highly demanding tasks and potent impairment of motor coordination [32–34], interfering with driving skills and increasing the risk of injuries [35]. In experimental animal models, the motor effects of the endogenous ligand AEA are similar to those induced by the plant-derived cannabinoid agonist Δ^9-tetrahydrocannabinol (Δ^9-THC), but less pronounced and of shorter duration. The main motor outcomes of cannabinoid agonists are hypoactivity and catalepsy, however biphasic effects have been described depending on the drug and dose used. While relatively low doses of Δ^9-THC and AEA have been associated with a transient increase in motor activity, high doses produce motor inhibition and catalepsy [36–45]. Additionally, both drugs AEA and Δ^9-THC potentiate the catalepsy induced by a local administration of muscimol into the GP [46] and reduce stereotyped behaviors [40–42]. Δ^9-THC reduces the amphetamine-induced hyperlocomotion [47] and impairs fine motor control in rats [48].

Interestingly, cannabidiol (CBD), other plant-derived cannabinoid, has been proposed as a modulator of the effects induced by Δ^9-THC (reviewed in [49]). Several studies conclude that CBD attenuates some Δ^9-THC motor side effects such as catalepsy [50–52], while others show that high doses of CBD fail to prevent or exacerbate the pharmacological effects of Δ^9-THC, including hypoactivity [45,53]. Nevertheless, the influence of CBD on spontaneous locomotion seems to be limited [45,53–55] and it may be unrelated to the CB receptors interaction [49].

Preclinical studies using synthetic cannabinoid agents have highlighted the role of the ECS on the control of motor function. Thus, systemic administration of the agonists WIN 55,212-2, CP55,940 and HU210 usually causes inhibition of motor activity [45,56–61] and produces basal catalepsy [52,62–64]. Activation of CB1 receptors by the agonist CP55,940 enhances the catalepsy induced by dopaminergic antagonists [65] and genetic inactivation of either dopamine D2 receptors or adenosine A2A receptors reduces the motor depression produced by CP55,940 [63]. In fact, the inhibitory motor effects caused by an intrastriatal injection of the CB1 agonist WIN 55,212-2 are mediated by a functional interaction between the adenosine A2A and the CB1 receptors [66], which are present as heteromers in the rat corticostriatal terminals [67]. In line with this, the specific adenosine A2A receptor antagonist MSX-3 blocks the inhibitory effect of the CB1 receptor agonist CP 55,940 on the hyperactivity induced by the dopamine D2 receptor agonist quinpirole [58]. Although, a strong functional interaction between striatal A2A and CB1 receptors is accepted, the mechanisms of this interaction are still not clear since it has been proposed a stimulatory role as well as an inhibitory role of A2A receptors on CB1 receptor-dependent effects [68].

Pharmacological agents that indirectly elevate endocannabinoid levels by inhibiting either their uptake or the intracellular degradation have been proposed as promising therapeutic agents for the treatment of diverse diseases including movement disorders (for review see [69]). These pharmacological agents are also referred as indirect agonists and they also elicit some cannabimimetic motor effects, including hypoactivity. On one hand, the selective and potent inhibition of the endocannabinoids transport by the arachidonic acid derivative, UCM707 potentiates the hypokinetic effects caused by a non-efficacious dose of AEA [70]. Similarly, the selective blockade of the AEA transport by AM404 elevates circulating levels of the endocannabinoid and causes hypoactivity [71,72], likely by activating TRPV1 [73]. On the other hand, selective inhibition of the endocannabinoids metabolizing enzymes has brought interesting results suggesting the differential role of the endogenous agents, AEA and 2-AG, in the unwanted motor effects induced by cannabinoid compounds. Specifically, inhibition of MAGL, but not FAAH, causes CB1 receptor-mediated hypoactivity. However, neither FAAH nor MAGL produce cataleptic effects usually elicited by direct agonists [74,75]. Thus, the FAAH inhibitor URB597 does not significantly alter motor function at doses that induces analgesia [74] and a single or repeated administration of PF-04457845, a specific and irreversible FAAH inhibitor, is well tolerated in healthy humans [76]. Conversely, the MAGL inhibitor JZL184 reduces locomotor activity [77,78], and dual inhibitors JZL195 and AS-57 induce also catalepsy [75,79].

From a general point of view, the motor effects of direct and indirect agonists are usually mediated by stimulation of CB1 receptor since its pharmacological blockade prevents the above mentioned effects [64,72,75,80,81]. In addition, a high dose of the CB1 receptor antagonist SR141716A causes hyperlocomotion by itself [82,83] while a lower dose does not affect motor activity [84]. Also the CB1 receptor antagonist AM251 administrated alone fails to alter basal locomotion but diminishes the psychomotor effects induced by the co-administration of amphetamine [85]. In agreement with these observations, mice lacking CB1 receptors exhibit several motor anomalies [86,87] and show less sensitivity to the psychomotor stimulants and sensitizing effects of the psychostimulants [88,89].

Although these findings provide evidence for the involvement of CB1 receptor-related mechanisms in motor control, other reports demonstrate that also the TRPV1 receptors can mediate effects of certain cannabinoids such as AEA [90]. The potential beneficial effects of cannabinoid agents in movement disorders are further reviewed here.

4. Alterations of the endocannabinoid system in movement disorders

4.1. Endocannabinoid system in Parkinson's disease

PD is the second most common neurodegenerative disorder, after Alzheimer's disease. It is a chronic and progressive neurodegenerative illness and its etiology is interpreted as a combination of genetic, environmental, and aging-related processes, although the exact cause of this degeneration is unknown. Clinical manifestation of the disease includes tremor at rest, worsening of voluntary movements, bradykinesia, muscle rigidity and postural instability [91,92]. All of these symptoms appear as a result of pathological processes, including neuroinflammation, mitochondrial dysfunction, oxidative stress, kinase pathways and calcium dysregulation, protein aggregation and prion-like processes, which result in a degeneration of dopamine neurons in the SNc and a subsequent dopaminergic depletion in the striatum, the main input nucleus of the BG neural circuit. [93].

Several components of the ECS are altered in movement disorders which have led to consider it as a possible target for developing new treatments for these disorders. The effects of cannabinoid compounds and their potential utility in PD has been tested, but inconsistent data have been produced, as there are many complex responses elicited by dopamine and its interaction with different cannabinoid mechanisms [94].

4.1.1. Endocannabinoid levels

The ECS in the BG becomes overactivated in PD. For instance, the cerebrospinal fluid of untreated patients with PD has at least two-fold higher levels of AEA, compared to controls, being this increase independent of either disease stage or progression [27]. Overall, results from preclinical studies support the clinical findings.

In 1-methyl-4-phenyl-1,2,3,6-tetrahydropyridine (MPTP)-lesioned monkeys, the levels of both AEA and 2-AG were determined throughout the BG after induction of parkinsonism and L-DOPA treatment. Both AEA and 2-AG levels were elevated in the striatum of untreated parkinsonian monkeys and returned to those found in the striatum of normal monkeys after treatment with L-DOPA [95]. These results are similar to those reported in rodent models of PD, where AEA levels were estimated to be higher in the BG output regions, as compared to the striatum or GPe, while 2-AG levels were similar throughout the BG regions analyzed [96]. Similarly, in a rat model of PD induced by unilateral nigral lesion with 6-hydroxidopamine

http://dx.doi.org/10.5772/62431

(6-OHDA), striatal levels of AEA, but not 2-AG levels, were increased. Moreover, decreased activity of the AEA membrane transporter and FAAH was observed, whereas the binding of AEA to CB receptors was unaffected [97]. In studies with reserpine-treated rats an increase of 2-AG levels in output BG regions, such as GP and SNr has been reported compared to other brain regions like the cortex, cerebellum, hippocampus, and striatum [98]. In mutant models of the disease, as the homozygous *Pink1* knockout mice, the levels of 2-AG and AEA were not altered in striatum, and no change was observed as for the activity of FAAH and MAGL, responsible for endocannabinoids hydrolysis. Although the levels of 2-AG remains unchanged in PD, this endocannabinoid has revealed its neuroprotective role in the MPTP mouse model [99] as well as palmitoylethanolamide (PEA) [100].

4.1.2. Cannabinoid receptors

CB1 availability is unevenly modified in patients with PD, which is decreased in the SN but relatively increased in nigrostriatal, mesolimbic, and mesocortical dopaminergic projection areas [101]. In *post-mortem* samples from patients with PD increased CB1 receptor binding in the caudate-putamen was found and a higher stimulation by CB1 receptor agonists of [35S]GTPγS binding was measured in the same brain areas [26]. Other studies performed in PD human brain have shown that the expression of CB1 receptor mRNA was decreased in the caudate nucleus, anterior dorsal putamen and GPe, but remained unchanged in the other brain areas examined [102]. When the relationship between CB1 receptors and dopamine D2/D3 receptor densities was analyzed by receptor autoradiography, unchanged CB1 receptor density in the putamen and caudate of patients with PD (treated with L-DOPA) was found together with a parallel decreased in the density levels of dopamine D2/D3 receptors in the same nuclei [103].

Studies in animal models also show disparity of results concerning CB1 receptors. In MPTP-lesioned marmosets, increase in CB1 receptor binding was also confirmed in the caudate-putamen [26]. In contrast, in the reserpine-treated rat model of PD a topographically organized reduction in CB1 receptor mRNA expression in the striatum was found [98]. However, in other studies with 6-OHDA-lesioned rats, no significant change in CB1 receptor expression or binding was detected, although an increase in CB1 receptor mRNA levels in the striatum was found [104,105]. In *Pink1* knockout mice, however, a significant reduction of binding ability of CB1 receptor agonists was found [106].

Regarding CB2 receptors, in neurotoxin rat models of PD, when 6-OHDA or lipopolysaccharide (LPS) is injected into the striatum, increased expression of the CB2 receptor and proportionally increased microglial activation was found [107]. Other CB receptors may have a role in PD treatment, thus the pharmacological blockade of TRPV1 receptors, which have been implicated in the modulation of dopamine transmission in the BG, attenuates the 6-OHDA induced hypokinesia [108]. TRPV1 receptors, where AEA binds, may play opposite roles to CB1 receptors in order to treat L-DOPA-induced dyskinesia [94,109]. Although it seem that the ECS suffers dramatic modifications in PD, so far clinical and preclinical studies show no conclusive results.

4.2. Endocannabinoid system in Huntington's disease

HD is a rare autosomal-dominant progressive neurodegenerative disease that affects 4–10 per 100,000 people in Western countries [110]. It is caused by the mutation in the IT15 gene (*HTT)* that encodes the huntingtin protein(HTT) and consists in an expanded cytosine-adenine-guanine (CAG) repeat that yields an abnormally long polyglutamine sequence in HTT [111]. Healthy subjects have less than 35 CAG repeats, while genes with more than 39–40 CAG repeats (or more) encode pathogenic HTT. Although physiological HTT is widely found in the brain, the mutation leads to the expression of the aberrant protein harmful only to specific neuron populations. Indeed, the prominent degeneration of GABAergic spiny projecting neurons (SPN) in the striatum [112] and to a lesser extent, of glutamatergic cortical pyramidal neurons [113,114] are the hallmarks of the disease. In late stages of the disease other brain areas and neurons may also be affected, producing a complex disease. The clinical manifestation can appear early, at the ages of 30–50 years, and progressively worsen over the following years. On the course of the disease, the patient can suffer from movement disorders, cognitive disability and psychiatric symptoms such as personality changes, depression or memory loss, among others [115]. The early stages of the disease are characterized by choreic involuntary movements and cognitive impairment, which are related to mutant HTT aggregation and aberrant neurotransmission in the striatopallidal SPN and corticostriatal neurons, respectively (reviewed in [116]). In more advanced phases of the disease, when the direct pathway in the BG is also affected, the patients display parkinsonian-like symptoms, as bradykinesia and rigidity [117].

4.2.1. Endocannabinoid levels

As mentioned for PD, in HD The ECS also suffers notorious modifications on the course of the disease in the BG [30,31,118]. In *post-mortem* tissue, higher expression of FAAH was observed in the caudate-putamen from HD brains [119] while the opposite effect was found in the cortex [120].

The activity of the ECS has also been investigated in animal models of HD without consistent results, probably due to the different models and ages selected for the studies. In the R6/1 transgenic model of HD, significant decrease in AEA levels were detected in the hippocampus in contrast to increased 2-AG concentrations only found in the cortex at 12 weeks of age, prior to the motor disturbances [121]. Another study in R6/2 transgenic mice, which differ in CAG repeats number from R6/1 mice and show severe motor and cognitive defects at earlier ages, also reported decreased in cortical 2-AG during motor presymptomatic stages [122]. In symptomatic R6/2 mice, AEA, 2-AG and PEA were markedly decreased in the striatum and in a lesser extent in the hippocampus or cortex [122]. Other study performed also in R6/2 mice found increased 2-AG but unchanged AEA levels in the striatum [123]. As for the enzymes' activity, Bari et al. found increased FAAH and decreased MAGL activity in the cortex together with reduced activity of AEA and 2-AG metabolic-enzymes at different ages in the striatum, which disagrees with the higher expression of FAAH reported by others [119]. The use of other animal models, such us the 3-nitropropionic acid (3-NP)-lesion rat, showed decreased AEA and 2-AG in the striatum but suggested increased AEA levels in the SN [124].

So far studies regarding enzyme activity and endocannabinoid levels in HD are limited and offer inconsistent results although overall endocannabinoid levels seem to be reduced in different brain areas. More homogeneous preclinical studies together with clinical investigations will be needed for clarifying these founds.

4.2.2. Cannabinoid receptors

Autoradiographical and immunohistochemical studies in human *post-mortem* tissue demonstrated that early stages of the disease are characterized by a loss of CB1, dopamine D2 and adenosine A2A receptors in the caudate nucleus, putamen and GPe, which corresponds to the deterioration of striatopallidal SPNs [30,118,125]. Later in the disease, when the striatonigral pathway also degenerates, even greater down-regulation of striatal and nigral CB1 receptors is observed [30]. *In vivo* imaging of CB1 in patients confirmed the down-expression of these receptors in cortical and subcortical structures, starting early in the development of the disease [126]. Despite the variety of animal models available for studying the disease, most preclinical studies back up the observations from human tissue. In transgenic mice, such as the HD94 or R6/2 transgenic models, loss of mRNA levels, binding, receptor expression and activation of GTP-binding proteins for cannabinoid CB1 receptors have been reported primarily in SPNs belonging to the indirect pathway in the early phases of the disease accompanied or not by cortical and hippocampal alterations [121,123,125,127–129]. In models induced by the administration of 3-NP, where striatal neuronal loss is produced, additional loss of CB1 receptors is also observed [124,130,131]. Small animal PET studies performed in transgenic HD rat and mouse models, have also confirmed reduced CB1 receptor binding in the striatum and GPe in all stages, as well as alterations in the cortex, hippocampus, thalamic nuclei or cerebellum in more advanced phases of the disease [132,133]. Results from human brain and most animal models coincide in reporting down-regulation of striatal CB1 receptors in HD, which has been proposed to be induced by mutant HTT that controls gene promoter activity via repressor element 1 silencing transcription factor [119]. In this respect, genetic CB1 receptor deletion has been proven to worsen motor symptomatology and to exacerbate striatal degeneration by increasing excitotoxic damage and decreasing brain-derived neurotrophic factors [119,134,135]. Although rescuing CB1 receptors prevents the striatal morphological modifications observed in mice models of HD, it failed to improve motor deterioration [136].

Regarding CB2 receptors in the HD brain, studies performed in *post-mortem* human tissue suggest up-regulation of CB2 receptors on CD68-positive microglial cells [137] or slight increase on brain blood vessels [138] but not on astrocytic cells. These results agree in part with preclinical studies where up-regulation of CB2 receptors has been observed in the striatal microglial of R6/2 mice and striatal microglia and astrocytes in a rat model of HD induced by intrastriatal injection of malonate (mitochondrial complex II inhibitor) [137,139]. This compensatory increase of CB2 receptors may have a neuroprotective effect on the disease [137]. In this line, CB2 agonists have been proposed to decrease striatal neurodegeneration in malonate-lesioned rats [139]. In addition, CB2 depletion has been documented to accelerate the onset of the disease and aggravate the motor disabilities in a mouse model of HD [137,140].

Less attention has been paid to the TRPV1 channels, which also play an important role in the ECS. So far, only one publication has studied these receptors reporting no modification in TRPV1 binding in R6/2 mice at any age [123].

In general, preclinical and clinical studies have well characterized a down-regulation of CB1 receptors at different stages of HD, which may cause a role in the progression of the disease. Less is known about CB2 or TRPV1 receptors and further investigations are required to clarify their role in the neuropathology of the disease.

5. Potential therapeutic role of cannabinoids in movement disorders

5.1. Parkinson's disease

Currently, pharmacological treatment for PD is focused on dopaminergic replacement, which controls the symptoms in both early and advanced stages [141]. However, its chronic use is limited due to the development of severe and disabling side effects, such as motor fluctuations or L-DOPA-induced dyskinesia. Besides, none of the available treatments are capable of slowing or stopping the disease progression. Cannabinoid-based therapies have been proposed as a promising approach for PD treatment, not only for their antiparkinsonian properties, but also for the neuroprotective and anti-inflammatory effects of these compounds.

5.1.1. Cannabinoids for the treatment of motor symptoms

Studies in animal models and patients with PD have indicated that both CB1 agonists and antagonists used alone or as coadjuvants, could be useful to treat different symptoms of this movement disorder. Thus, CB1 agonists have been shown to improve motor impairment in animal models of PD [142–145] and to reduce tremor associated with the hyperactivity of the STN [145,146]. However, because of the hypokinetic profile of the cannabinoid agonists, it is unlikely that these drugs would be useful for alleviating bradykinesia in PD patients. In fact, the administration of agonists to humans or MTPT-lesioned primates enhanced motor disability (for review [34]).

On the other hand, behavioral changes in parkinsonian rodents also improved with the administration of CB1 antagonists [147–149]. It has been suggested that blocking CB1 receptors could be useful in particular conditions, as when the patients do not respond to dopaminergic therapy or in advanced phases of the disease [147,148,150]. It is also important to consider the therapeutic benefits of TRPV1 receptor antagonists, given their role in regulating dopamine release from nigral neurons [151].

Cannabinoids also may be beneficial in treating L-DOPA-induced dyskinesia. Indeed, administration of CB1 agonists to parkinsonian rats chronically treated with L-DOPA reduced the occurrence of dyskinesia [109,152,153] without reducing the efficacy of L-DOPA to improve motor performance. In MPTP-lesioned monkeys and patients with PD the results are mixed. Indeed, both CB1 agonist and antagonists showed antidyskinetic effect [95,154–157] while plant-derived cannabinoids failed to improve motor disability [158,159].

http://dx.doi.org/10.5772/62431

5.1.2. *Cannabinoids as neuroprotective agents*

In vivo as well as *in vitro* preclinical studies in animal models of PD have revealed that cannabinoid receptor modulation can be potentially useful for protecting dopaminergic neurons from progressive neurodegeneration. Although CB1 receptor-mediated effects cannot be excluded, some authors argue that CB1 receptors may have a minimal implication in neuroprotection [10,160–162]. It seems plausible that neuroprotection is principally mediated by the antioxidant properties of the cannabinoids [160,163,164], given that oxidative stress is a major hallmark in the pathogenesis of PD. The effect of numerous phytocannabinoids, as Δ^9-THC, CBD and Δ^9-Tetrahydrocannabivarin (Δ^9-THCV), has been investigated in experimental models of PD (6-OHDA-lesioned rodents, MPTP or LPS-lesioned mice) [160,163,165]. These studies have showed that cannabinoids could be useful for developing novel neuroprotective therapies in PD due to their CB receptors-independent antioxidant actions. Double-blind trial carried out in patients with PD tried to evaluate the neuroprotective effect of CBD administration but definitive conclusions were not established [166].

Neuroprotection has also been provided by synthetic cannabinoids such as the endocannabinoid transporter inhibitor/vanilloid agonist AM404, or the CB1/CB2 receptors agonist CP55,940, which also produce antioxidant effects via cannabinoid receptor-independent mechanisms [163,167]. By contrast, selective CB1 or CB2 agonists failed to protect these neurons [163].

5.1.3. *Cannabinoids as anti-inflammatory agents*

Substantial evidence supports that inflammation plays a pivotal role in the death of neurons in the BG in PD. Activated microglia has been found in *post-mortem* brains from patients with PD [168] and elevated levels of inflammatory cytokines have been measured in the cerebrospinal fluid of patients [169–171]. Cannabinoid compounds have demonstrated anti-inflammatory properties. Concretely, CB2 receptor agonists are the most promising cannabinoids to treat the inflammatory processes related to neurodegenerative disorders, although other cannabinoid agonists have also showed anti-inflammatory activity [172]. In fact, the selective CB1 receptor agonist arachidonoyl-2-chloroethylamide and other non-selective cannabinoid agonists have revealed strong anti-inflammatory properties [173].

CB2 receptor is expressed on microglia and it is strongly up-regulated when these cells are activated [174]. *In vitro* activation of microglial CB2 receptors leads to suppression of the release of pro-inflammatory cytokines reducing neurotoxicity [175]. The beneficial effect of CB2 receptor stimulation has also been proved in animal models of PD [161,165]. Moreover, an increase of sensitivity to the neurotoxin LPS in CB2 receptor knockout mice has been described [165] and the overexpression of this receptor subtype reduced the recruitment of glial cells to the lesion and decreased the level of various oxidative parameters [176].

Apart from the CB2 receptor, several studies have corroborated the anti-inflammatory potential of targeting CB1 receptor in PD. WIN 55,212-2 or HU 210 administration decreases the number of activated microglia and reduces the mRNA levels of the proinflammatory cytokine IL-6 in MPTP mice and LPS-treated rats [162,177,178]. In another study, 2 week pretreatment with Δ^9-THC and CBD, followed by 6-OHDA injection, decreased the loss of dopaminergic neurons in hemiparkinsonian rats [160].

All these studies suggest that the CB1 and CB2 receptors could be potential targets for anti-inflammatory intervention in PD.

5.2. Huntington's disease

To date, the treatment of HD is merely symptomatic and focuses on the restoration of the neurotransmitter imbalance that occurs in the disease. For this reason, GABA agonists, dopamine depleting agents, neuroleptics, anti-glutamatergic agents, antidepressants or acetylcholinesterase inhibitors are often used for ameliorating the symptoms (for review see [179]), despite not being able to cure or stop the progression of the disease. In this situation cannabinoid compounds may play a promising therapeutic role as it has been proven in other neurodegenerative diseases [180,181]. Indeed, activation of cannabinoid receptors facilitates the activation of intracellular mechanisms related to cell homeostasis, repair and survival. Moreover, several pre-clinical and clinical studies have showed that cannabinoids can be useful in HD. The effects of cannabinoid compounds on HD can be divided in three different actions: improvement of motor symptoms, neuroprotection and anti-inflammatory activity.

5.2.1. Cannabinoids for the treatment of motor symptoms

As mentioned above, the most characteristic feature of HD is the motor impairment which varies along the progression of the disease. In this context, cannabinoid compounds have been tested for treating these motor symptoms in animal models of HD, some of them showing anti-hyperkinetic activity. The administration of the endocannabinoid re-uptake inhibitor, AM404, reduced hyperkinetic movements and restored the neurochemical alterations (dopamine and GABA reduction) in the HD rat model with bilateral striatal injection of 3-NP [130]. However, the anti-hyperkinetic effect showed by AM404 seems to be mainly consequence of TRPV1 receptor activation, and not CB1-dependent [130]. In the same rat model of HD, the administration of UCM707, another endocannabinoid uptake inhibitor, also showed anti-hyperkinetic activity that may be due to the recovery of GABAergic and glutamatergic function in the GP and SN, respectively [182]. In addition, Arvanil, a hybrid endocannabinoid and vanilloid compound, has also demonstrated anti-hyperkinetic activity, although it could not restore the neurochemical alterations in the 3-NP rat model of HD [183]. Similarly, the CB1 receptor agonist CP55,940 has showed anti-hyperkinetic activity, without changing dopamine and GABA levels [184]. Other compounds, VDM11 (endocannabinoid re-uptake inhibitor) and AM374 (endocannabinoid hydrolysis inhibitor), have not demonstrated any significant effect on hyperkinetic movements in the same HD model [184]. The chronic, but not the acute administration of the CB1 receptor agonist WIN 55,212-2 prevented the appearance of motor impairment in the R6/1 transgenic mice model of HD, without improving the social and cognitive deficits [185]. So far, the clinical use of plant-derived cannabinoids and synthetic analogues has shown disappointing results in the treatment of the motor symptoms. A case report and a pilot study of nabilone in patients with HD showed that the effect of this drug on

http://dx.doi.org/10.5772/62431

HD motor symptoms is limited [186,187]. Other studies have demonstrated that the administration of nabilone or CBD did not improve the hyperkinetic alterations associated with HD [188,189]. The lack of therapeutic efficacy may lie on the mechanism of action of the cannabinoid agonists used. These cannabinoid drugs were unable to activate TRPV1 receptors, which have been proven to mediate anti-hyperkinetic in 3-NP-lesioned rats. Thus, the most appropriate compounds for future clinical trials, at least in the early stages of the disease, may be those able to activate both CB1 and TRPV1 receptors [190].

5.2.2. Cannabinoids as neuroprotective agents

The neuroprotective properties of the cannabinoids make them very interesting tools to stop the progression of HD. In fact, cannabinoid compounds may reduce cytotoxic processes that occur in neurons and glial cells in neurodegenerative diseases [181]. The protective effects are consequence of the intracellular signaling pathways activated by cannabinoid compounds [116], and are mediated by the activation of CB1, CB2 or TRPV1 receptors, but also due to CB receptor independent processes [172].

Cannabinoid CB1 receptors are located in neuronal glutamatergic terminals at presynaptic and postsynaptic levels. The activation of these receptors by cannabinoid agonists decreases glutamate release and limits the glutamatergic excitotoxicity in neurodegenerative processes [172]. Furthermore, CB1 receptor stimulation activates the phosphatidylinositol 3-kinase/Akt/mammalian target of rapamycin complex 1 pathway, protecting cells from excitotoxic damage, and facilitating brain-derived neurotrophic factor (BDNF) release [191]. The activation of CB1 receptors also diminishes the activity of voltage-sensitive calcium channels [192], reducing calcium dependent damaging pathways. Moreover, cannabinoid compounds activating CB1 receptors are also involved in some other mechanisms related to cell protection and survival, such as GABAergic signaling [193,194] or blood supply to lesioned brain areas [195]. On the other hand, CB2 receptors are mainly located in glial cells and their activation also supports cannabinoids-mediated neuroprotection. In fact, CB2 receptor activation reduces cytotoxic factors release and generation of reactive oxygen and nitric oxide-derived substances [10]. However, cannabinoids also induce CB receptor independent neuroprotective mechanisms. Some cannabinoid compounds can act on NMDA glutamatergic receptors, reducing high glutamate levels at postsynaptic levels and excitotoxicity. Moreover, cannabinoids restore the balance between oxidative and antioxidant mechanisms, mainly, by blocking reactive oxygen substances [196] but also facilitating endogenous antioxidant activity [163,197].

Several pre-clinical studies have been performed to clarify the role of cannabinoids in CB1 receptors mediated neuroprotection in HD. In PC12 cells expressing HTT, CB1 receptor stimulation showed different effects. Activation of CB1 receptors, coupled to Gi/o, induced cell protection by inhibiting cAMP and ERK phosphorylation. However, CB1 receptors could also couple to Gs, which stimulated cAMP and favored cell death in this HD model [198]. Similar results were also obtained in the *in vitro* model of striatal SPNs expressing wild-type ($STHdh^{Q7/Q7}$) or mutant HTT ($STHdh^{Q111/Q111}$) [199]. Studies in rodent models of HD have showed that cannabinoid compounds acting on CB1 receptors can reduce or delay the neurodegeneration associated with this disease [116]. The striatal injection of quinolinic acid in rats increases the glutamatergic transmission, and therefore, the excitotoxicity, mimicking some of the characteristic features of HD [200]. In this rat model of HD, the administration of the CB1 receptor agonist WIN 55,212-2 diminished the increment of glutamate levels induced by the quinolinic acid. In addition, WIN 55,212-2 also reduced the effect of quinolinic acid on corticostriatal local field potential recordings *in vitro*. The effects of WIN 55,212-2 were blocked by the CB1 receptor antagonist AM 251, demonstrating that the effects observed were CB1-dependent [200]. Thus, WIN 55,212-2 protected the striatum from the damage induced by quinolinic acid, although, this CB1 receptor agonist could not modify the motor abnormalities induced by quinolinic acid [200]. In R6/2 mice, the administration of the Δ^9-THC improved the symptoms, the neuropathology and the molecular pathology related to this HD model, and induced BDNF expression in the striatum [119]. Moreover, the depletion of CB1 receptors in these transgenic mice impaired all the pathological features expressed by this HD model, and reduced BDNF expression [119]. Additionally, in R6/2 mice, the striatal injection of a recombinant adeno-associated viral vector encoding CB1 receptor induced the expression of CB1 receptors and BDNF and normalized the molecular pathological signs observed in this well established transgenic mice model of HD [191]. Interestingly, genetic rescue of CB1 receptors in the SPNs prevented the loss of vesicular glutamate transporter 1 and 2 (VGLUT1 and VGLUT2) and synaptophysin in the striatum, although it did not improve the motor phenotype expressed by R6/2 mice [136]. Moreover, enriched environment delayed the onset of motor alterations and the loss of CB1 receptors in R6/1 mice, slowing the progression of the disease [201,202]. All these studies support the role of CB1 receptors and CB1 agonists as useful therapeutic tools to reduce or delay the progression of HD. However, not all the studies have showed that CB1 receptor agonists induce protective effects. Indeed, chronic administration of HU210, Δ^9-THC or URB597 did not modify the progressive impairment of motor activity in the transgenic R6/1 mice model of HD [203]. Additionally, in the malonate-lesioned rat model of HD, the administration of UCM707 did not delay the degeneration observed in this model [182]. Thus, further studies are needed to investigate and clarify the implication of CB1 receptors in HD and the potential therapeutic effects of CB1 receptor agonists.

Cannabinoid compounds that activate CB2 receptors have showed neuroprotective effects in HD [139]. The administration of the CB2 receptor agonist HU-308 in the quinolinic acid-lesioned mice attenuated glial activation and reduced the neuronal damage in the striatum [137]. Likewise, in the malonate-lesioned rat model of HD, the administration of the selective CB2 receptor agonist HU-308 protected striatal neurons from the apoptotic mechanisms activated by malonate [139]. This neuroprotection was blocked by the administration of the selective CB2 receptor antagonist SR144528, ratifying that the effect observed was CB2-dependent [139]. The neuroprotective effects of CB2 receptor agonists are associated with the reduction of the toxicity caused by reactive microglial cells [116,137]. The activation of CB2 receptors can also induce the expression of pro-survival substances [10,204]. In contrast, CB2 receptor-deficient R6/2 mice showed accelerated progression of the HD phenotype expressed by this model [137]. In fact, the ablation of CB2 receptors in these mice increased the glial activation and the sensitivity to striatal neurodegeneration induced by excitotoxic processes [137]. Thus, both in genetic and in toxin-lesioned rodent models of HD cannabinoids displayed CB2 receptor mediated protective effects [137,139].

http://dx.doi.org/10.5772/62431

Finally, cannabinoid compounds may also exert neuroprotective effects independent of CB1 or CB2 receptor activation in animal models of HD. This CB receptor independent protection displayed by some cannabinoids (i.e. Δ^9-THC or CBC) is related to the blockage of reactive oxygen molecules [172]. The capacity to block reactive oxygen molecules may be due to the phenolic structures of these cannabinoid compounds. Indeed, in 3-NP-lesioned rat model of HD, the administration of CBC reduced the striatal atrophy produced by this toxin [197]. Thus, cannabinoid compounds may be useful to protect cells from the cytotoxicity associated with oxidative processes.

As mentioned above, clinical studies have been developed to examine the effect of cannabinoids on HD. However, most of these studies were designed to analyze the effect of specific cannabinoid compounds on specific symptoms, and not to study the neuroprotective effect of cannabinoids [116]. Moreover, results obtained from animal models of HD have showed that combination of cannabinoids can be more useful to protect neurons than single cannabinoids [116]. In fact, Sativex®, a combination of Δ^9-THC and CBC, has showed protective effect on striatal neurons in some rodent models of HD [205,206]. A clinical trial in patients with HD concluded that Sativex® was safe and well tolerated, but it was not able to stop or slow the progression of the neurodegeneration (see https://clinicaltrials.gov/ct2/show/NCT01502046).

5.2.3. Cannabinoids as anti-inflammatory agents

As mentioned before, CB2 receptors are mainly located in glial cells, and are poorly expressed in the striatum in healthy condition. However, the striatal expression of these receptors is increased in patients with and animal models of HD. In HD, the reactive microglia may release inflammatory cytokines, reactive oxygen substances or nitric oxide [10,207,208]. Cannabinoid compounds activating CB2 receptors in glial cells can reduce the release of these factors, and promote the release of some anti-inflammatory cytokines (i.e. IL-10, IL-1ra) [209,210]. Moreover, it has been demonstrated that CB2 receptor agonists improve striatal inflammation in different rodent models of HD [137,139]. Interestingly, CB2 receptors are not involved in the psychotrophic effects induced by cannabinoid compounds. This property makes CB2 receptor agonists valuable compounds for future therapeutic approaches in HD.

6. Concluding remarks

To date, vast number of preclinical evidence have demonstrated that the ECS controls the motor activity in both physiological and pathological states. Cannabinoid compounds have been proven to ameliorate motor symptoms and drug-induced side effects. In addition, the anti-inflammatory and neuroprotective properties of these agents make them promising drugs to delay the progression of neurodegenerative diseases. For these reasons, further basic and clinical cannabis-based research could bring a new light into the treatment of movement disorders, such as PD and HD.

Author details

Teresa Morera-Herreras[1*], Cristina Miguelez[1], Asier Aristieta[1], María Torrecilla[1], José Ángel Ruiz-Ortega[1,2] and Luisa Ugedo[1]

*Address all correspondence to: teresa.morera@ehu.eus

1 Department of Pharmacology, Faculty of Medicine and Nursing, University of the Basque Country (UPV/EHU), Spain

2 Department of Pharmacology, Faculty of Pharmacy, University of the Basque Country (UPV/EHU), Spain

References

[1] Mechoulam R, Shani A, Edery H, GrunfeldY. Chemical basis of hashish activity. Science. 1970;169(3945):611-2. doi: 10.1126/science.169.3945.611.

[2] Matsuda LA, Lolait SJ, Brownstein MJ, Young AC, Bonner TI. Structure of a cannabinoid receptor and functional expression of the cloned cDNA. Nature. 1990;346(6284): 561-4. doi: 10.1038/346561a0.

[3] Munro S, Thomas KL, Abu-Shaar M. Molecular characterization of a peripheral receptor for cannabinoids. Nature. 1993;365(6441):61-5. doi: 10.1038/365061a0.

[4] Lu HC, Mackie K. An introduction to the endogenous cannabinoid system. Biol Psychiatry. 2015. doi: 10.1016/j.biopsych.2015.07.028.

[5] Cacciola G, Chianese R, Chioccarelli T, Ciaramella V, Fasano S, Pierantoni R, et al. Cannabinoids and reproduction: a lasting and intriguing history. Pharmaceuticals. 2010;3(10):3275. doi: 10.3390/ph3103275.

[6] Wilson RI, Nicoll RA. Endocannabinoid signaling in the brain. Science. 2002;296(5568): 678-82. doi: 10.1126/science.1063545.

[7] Svizenska I, Dubovy P, Sulcova A. Cannabinoid receptors 1 and 2 (CB1 and CB2), their distribution, ligands and functional involvement in nervous system structures–a short review. Pharmacol Biochem Behav. 2008;90(4):501-11. doi: 10.1016/j.pbb.2008.05.010.

[8] Schlicker E, Timm J, Zentner J, Gothert M. Cannabinoid CB1 receptor-mediated inhibition of noradrenaline release in the human and guinea-pig hippocampus. Naunyn Schmiedebergs Arch Pharmacol. 1997;356(5):583-9. doi: 10.1007/PL00005155

[9] Kuepper R, Ceccarini J, Lataster J, van Os J, van Kroonenburgh M, van Gerven JM, et al. Delta-9-tetrahydrocannabinol-induced dopamine release as a function of psycho-

sis risk: 18F-fallypride positron emission tomography study. PLoS One. 2013;8(7):e70378. doi: 10.1371/journal.pone.0070378.

[10] Fernandez-Ruiz J, Romero J, Velasco G, Tolon RM, Ramos JA, Guzman M. Cannabinoid CB2 receptor: a new target for controlling neural cell survival? Trends Pharmacol Sci. 2007;28(1):39-45. doi: 10.1016/j.tips.2006.11.001.

[11] Hu SS, Mackie K. Distribution of the endocannabinoid system in the central nervous system. Handb Exp Pharmacol. 2015;231:59-93. doi: 10.1007/978-3-319-20825-1_3.

[12] Gerdeman G, Lovinger DM. CB1 cannabinoid receptor inhibits synaptic release of glutamate in rat dorsolateral striatum. J Neurophysiol. 2001;85(1):468-71. doi: 10.1016/j.bbr.2014.05.029.

[13] Kofalvi A, Rodrigues RJ, Ledent C, Mackie K, Vizi ES, Cunha RA, et al. Involvement of cannabinoid receptors in the regulation of neurotransmitter release in the rodent striatum: a combined immunochemical and pharmacological analysis. J Neurosci. 2005;25(11):2874-84. doi: 10.1523/JNEUROSCI.4232-04.2005.

[14] Herkenham M, Lynn AB, de Costa BR, Richfield EK. Neuronal localization of cannabinoid receptors in the basal ganglia of the rat. Brain Res. 1991;547(2):267-74. doi: 10.1001/archpsyc.58.4.334.

[15] Tsou K, Brown S, Sanudo-Pena MC, Mackie K, Walker JM. Immunohistochemical distribution of cannabinoid CB1 receptors in the rat central nervous system. Neuroscience. 1998;83(2):393-411. doi: 10.1016/S0306-4522(97)00436-3.

[16] Mailleux P, Vanderhaeghen JJ. Localization of cannabinoid receptor in the human developing and adult basal ganglia. Higher levels in the striatonigral neurons. Neurosci Lett. 1992;148(1-2):173-6. doi: 10.1016/0304-3940(92)90832-R.

[17] Gong JP, Onaivi ES, Ishiguro H, Liu QR, Tagliaferro PA, Brusco A, et al. Cannabinoid CB2 receptors: immunohistochemical localization in rat brain. Brain Res. 2006;1071(1):10-23. doi: 10.1016/j.brainres.2005.11.035.

[18] Onaivi ES, Ishiguro H, Gong JP, Patel S, Perchuk A, Meozzi PA, et al. Discovery of the presence and functional expression of cannabinoid CB2 receptors in brain. Ann N Y Acad Sci. 2006;1074:514-36. doi: 10.1196/annals.1369.052.

[19] Onaivi ES, Ishiguro H, Gu S, Liu QR. CNS effects of CB2 cannabinoid receptors: beyond neuro-immuno-cannabinoid activity. J Psychopharmacol. 2012;26(1):92-103. doi: 10.1177/0269881111400652.

[20] Mezey E, Toth ZE, Cortright DN, Arzubi MK, Krause JE, Elde R, et al. Distribution of mRNA for vanilloid receptor subtype 1 (VR1), and VR1-like immunoreactivity, in the central nervous system of the rat and human. Proc Natl Acad Sci U S A. 2000;97(7):3655-60. doi: 10.1073/pnas.060496197.

[21] Micale V, Cristino L, Tamburella A, Petrosino S, Leggio GM, Drago F, et al. Anxiolytic effects in mice of a dual blocker of fatty acid amide hydrolase and transient recep-

tor potential vanilloid type-1 channels. Neuropsychopharmacology. 2009;34(3): 593-606. doi: 10.1038/npp.2008.98.

[22] Egertova M, Simon GM, Cravatt BF, Elphick MR. Localization of N-acyl phosphatidylethanolamine phospholipase D (NAPE-PLD) expression in mouse brain: a new perspective on N-acylethanolamines as neural signaling molecules. J Comp Neurol. 2008;506(4):604-15. doi: 10.1002/cne.21568.

[23] Egertova M, Cravatt BF, Elphick MR. Comparative analysis of fatty acid amide hydrolase and cb(1) cannabinoid receptor expression in the mouse brain: evidence of a widespread role for fatty acid amide hydrolase in regulation of endocannabinoid signaling. Neuroscience. 2003;119(2):481-96. doi: 10.1016/S0306-4522(03)00145-3.

[24] Yoshida T, Fukaya M, Uchigashima M, Miura E, Kamiya H, Kano M, et al. Localization of diacylglycerol lipase-alpha around postsynaptic spine suggests close proximity between production site of an endocannabinoid, 2-arachidonoyl-glycerol, and presynaptic cannabinoid CB1 receptor. J Neurosci. 2006;26(18):4740-51. doi: 10.1523/JNEUROSCI.0054-06.2006.

[25] Morera-Herreras T, Miguelez C, Aristieta A, Ruiz-Ortega JA, Ugedo L. Endocannabinoid modulation of dopaminergic motor circuits. Front Pharmacol. 2012;3:110. doi: 10.3389/fphar.2012.00110.

[26] Lastres-Becker I, Cebeira M, de Ceballos ML, Zeng BY, Jenner P, Ramos JA, et al. Increased cannabinoid CB1 receptor binding and activation of GTP-binding proteins in the basal ganglia of patients with Parkinson's syndrome and of MPTP-treated marmosets. Eur J Neurosci. 2001;14(11):1827-32. doi: 10.1046/j.0953-816x.2001.01812.x.

[27] Pisani V, Moschella V, Bari M, Fezza F, Galati S, Bernardi G, et al. Dynamic changes of anandamide in the cerebrospinal fluid of Parkinson's disease patients. Mov Disord. 2010;25(7):920-4. doi: 10.1002/mds.23014.

[28] Pisani A, Fezza F, Galati S, Battista N, Napolitano S, Finazzi-Agro A, et al. High endogenous cannabinoid levels in the cerebrospinal fluid of untreated Parkinson's disease patients. Ann Neurol. 2005;57(5):777-9. doi: 10.1002/ana.20462.

[29] Glass M, Faull RL, Dragunow M. Loss of cannabinoid receptors in the substantia nigra in Huntington's disease. Neuroscience. 1993;56(3):523-7. doi: 10.1016/0306-4522(93)90352-G.

[30] Glass M, Dragunow M, Faull RL. The pattern of neurodegeneration in Huntington's disease: a comparative study of cannabinoid, dopamine, adenosine and GABA(A) receptor alterations in the human basal ganglia in Huntington's disease. Neuroscience. 2000;97(3):505-19. doi: 10.1016/S0306-4522(00)00008-7.

[31] Richfield EK, Herkenham M. Selective vulnerability in Huntington's disease: preferential loss of cannabinoid receptors in lateral globus pallidus. Ann Neurol. 1994;36(4): 577-84. doi: 10.1002/ana.410360406.

[32] Davis WM, Moreton JE, King WT, Pace HB. Marihuana on locomotor activity: biphasic effect and tolerance development. Res Commun Chem Pathol Pharmacol. 1972;3(1): 29-35. doi: 10.1016/j.neures.2011.07.1163.

[33] Dewey WL. Cannabinoid pharmacology. Pharmacol Rev. 1986;38(2):151-78. doi: 10.1016/0378-8741(87)90061-4.

[34] Consroe P. Brain cannabinoid systems as targets for the therapy of neurological disorders. Neurobiol Dis. 1998;5(6 Pt B):534-51. doi: 10.1006/nbdi.1998.0220.

[35] Volkow ND, Wang GJ, Telang F, Fowler JS, Alexoff D, Logan J, et al. Decreased dopamine brain reactivity in marijuana abusers is associated with negative emotionality and addiction severity. Proc Natl Acad Sci U S A. 2014;111(30):E3149-56. doi: 10.1073/pnas.1411228111.

[36] Prescott WR, Gold LH, Martin BR. Evidence for separate neuronal mechanisms for the discriminative stimulus and catalepsy induced by delta 9-THC in the rat. Psychopharmacology (Berl). 1992;107(1):117-24. doi: 10.3389/fphar.2012.00110.

[37] Pertwee RG. Pharmacological, physiological and clinical implications of the discovery of cannabinoid receptors. Biochem Soc Trans. 1998;26(2):267-72. doi: 10.1042/bst0260267.

[38] Sulcova E, Mechoulam R, Fride E. Biphasic effects of anandamide. Pharmacol Biochem Behav. 1998;59(2):347-52. doi: 10.1016/S0091-3057(97)00422-X.

[39] Sanudo-Pena MC, Romero J, Seale GE, Fernandez-Ruiz JJ, Walker JM. Activational role of cannabinoids on movement. Eur J Pharmacol. 2000;391(3):269-74. doi: 10.1016/S0014-2999(00)00044-3.

[40] Jarbe TU, Andrzejewski ME, DiPatrizio NV. Interactions between the CB1 receptor agonist Delta 9-THC and the CB1 receptor antagonist SR-141716 in rats: open-field revisited. Pharmacol Biochem Behav. 2002;73(4):911-9. doi: 10.1016/S0091-3057(02)00938-3.

[41] Navarro M, Fernandez-Ruiz JJ, de Miguel R, Hernandez ML, Cebeira M, Ramos JA. An acute dose of delta 9-tetrahydrocannabinol affects behavioral and neurochemical indices of mesolimbic dopaminergic activity. Behav Brain Res. 1993;57(1):37-46. doi: 10.1016/0166-4328(93)90059-Y.

[42] Navarro M, Rubio P, de Fonseca FR. Behavioural consequences of maternal exposure to natural cannabinoids in rats. Psychopharmacology (Berl). 1995;122(1):1-14. doi: 10.1016/j.bbr.2013.09.022.

[43] Romero J, Garcia-Palomero E, Lin SY, Ramos JA, Makriyannis A, Fernandez-Ruiz JJ. Extrapyramidal effects of methanandamide, an analog of anandamide, the endogenous CB1 receptor ligand. Life Sci. 1996;58(15):1249-57. doi: 10.1016/j.neures.2011.07.1163.

[44] Katsidoni V, Kastellakis A, Panagis G. Biphasic effects of Delta9-tetrahydrocannabinol on brain stimulation reward and motor activity. Int J Neuropsychopharmacol. 2013;16(10):2273-84. doi: 10.1017/S1461145713000709.

[45] Taffe MA, Creehan KM, Vandewater SA. Cannabidiol fails to reverse hypothermia or locomotor suppression induced by Delta(9) -tetrahydrocannabinol in Sprague-Dawley rats. Br J Pharmacol. 2015;172(7):1783-91. doi: 10.1111/bph.13024.

[46] Wickens AP, Pertwee RG. delta 9-Tetrahydrocannabinol and anandamide enhance the ability of muscimol to induce catalepsy in the globus pallidus of rats. Eur J Pharmacol. 1993;250(1):205-8. doi: 10.1016/0014-2999(93)90646-Y.

[47] Gorriti MA, Rodriguez de Fonseca F, Navarro M, Palomo T. Chronic (-)-delta9-tetrahydrocannabinol treatment induces sensitization to the psychomotor effects of amphetamine in rats. Eur J Pharmacol. 1999;365(2-3):133-42. doi: 10.1159/000317059.

[48] McLaughlin PJ, Delevan CE, Carnicom S, Robinson JK, Brener J. Fine motor control in rats is disrupted by delta-9-tetrahydrocannabinol. Pharmacol Biochem Behav. 2000;66(4):803-9. doi: 10.1016/S0091-3057(00)00281-1.

[49] McPartland JM, Duncan M, Di Marzo V, Pertwee RG. Are cannabidiol and Delta(9) -tetrahydrocannabivarin negative modulators of the endocannabinoid system? A systematic review. Br J Pharmacol. 2015;172(3):737-53. doi: 10.1111/bph.12944.

[50] Karniol IG, Carlini EA. Pharmacological interaction between cannabidiol and delta 9-tetrahydrocannabinol. Psychopharmacologia. 1973;33(1):53-70. doi: 10.1007/BF00428793.

[51] Formukong EA, Evans AT, Evans FJ. Inhibition of the cataleptic effect of tetrahydrocannabinol by other constituents of Cannabis sativa L. J Pharm Pharmacol. 1988;40(2):132-4. doi: 10.1111/j.2042-7158.1988.tb05198.

[52] Gomes FV, Del Bel EA, Guimaraes FS. Cannabidiol attenuates catalepsy induced by distinct pharmacological mechanisms via 5-HT1A receptor activation in mice. Prog Neuropsychopharmacol Biol Psychiatry. 2013;46:43-7. doi: 10.1016/j.pnpbp.2013.06.005.

[53] Hayakawa K, Mishima K, Hazekawa M, Sano K, Irie K, Orito K, et al. Cannabidiol potentiates pharmacological effects of Delta(9)-tetrahydrocannabinol via CB(1) receptor-dependent mechanism. Brain Res. 2008;1188:157-64. doi: 10.1016/j.brainres.2007.09.090.

[54] Hiltunen AJ, Jarbe TU, Wangdahl K. Cannabinol and cannabidiol in combination: temperature, open-field activity, and vocalization. Pharmacol Biochem Behav. 1988;30(3):675-8. doi: 10.1016/S0304-3940(03)00569-X.

[55] Espejo-Porras F, Fernandez-Ruiz J, Pertwee RG, Mechoulam R, Garcia C. Motor effects of the non-psychotropic phytocannabinoid cannabidiol that are mediated by 5-HT1A

receptors. Neuropharmacology. 2013;75:155-63. doi: 10.1016/j.neuropharm.2013.07.024.

[56] Arevalo C, de Miguel R, Hernandez-Tristan R. Cannabinoid effects on anxiety-related behaviours and hypothalamic neurotransmitters. Pharmacol Biochem Behav. 2001;70(1):123-31. doi: 10.1097/FBP.0000000000000154.

[57] Drews E, Schneider M, Koch M. Effects of the cannabinoid receptor agonist WIN 55,212-2 on operant behavior and locomotor activity in rats. Pharmacol Biochem Behav. 2005;80(1):145-50. doi: 10.1016/j.pbb.2004.10.023.

[58] Marcellino D, Carriba P, Filip M, Borgkvist A, Frankowska M, Bellido I, et al. Antagonistic cannabinoid CB1/dopamine D2 receptor interactions in striatal CB1/D2 heteromers. A combined neurochemical and behavioral analysis. Neuropharmacology. 2008;54(5):815-23. doi: 10.1016/j.neuropharm.2007.12.011.

[59] Robinson L, Goonawardena AV, Pertwee RG, Hampson RE, Riedel G. The synthetic cannabinoid HU210 induces spatial memory deficits and suppresses hippocampal firing rate in rats. Br J Pharmacol. 2007;151(5):688-700. doi: 10.1038/sj.bjp.0707273.

[60] Vlachou S, Stamatopoulou F, Nomikos GG, Panagis G. Enhancement of endocannabinoid neurotransmission through CB1 cannabinoid receptors counteracts the reinforcing and psychostimulant effects of cocaine. Int J Neuropsychopharmacol. 2008;11(7):905-23. doi: 10.1017/S1461145708008717.

[61] Polissidis A, Chouliara O, Galanopoulos A, Rentesi G, Dosi M, Hyphantis T, et al. Individual differences in the effects of cannabinoids on motor activity, dopaminergic activity and DARPP-32 phosphorylation in distinct regions of the brain. Int J Neuropsychopharmacol. 2010;13(9):1175-91. doi: 10.1017/S1461145709991003.

[62] Rodriguez de Fonseca F, Martin Calderon JL, Mechoulam R, Navarro M. Repeated stimulation of D1 dopamine receptors enhances (-)-11-hydroxy-delta 8-tetrahydrocannabinol-dimethyl-heptyl-induced catalepsy in male rats. Neuroreport. 1994;5(7):761-5. doi: 10.1097/00001756-199403000-00006.

[63] Andersson M, Usiello A, Borgkvist A, Pozzi L, Dominguez C, Fienberg AA, et al. Cannabinoid action depends on phosphorylation of dopamine- and cAMP-regulated phosphoprotein of 32 kDa at the protein kinase A site in striatal projection neurons. J Neurosci. 2005;25(37):8432-8. doi: 10.1523/JNEUROSCI.1289-05.2005.

[64] Rinaldi-Carmona M, Barth F, Heaulme M, Shire D, Calandra B, Congy C, et al. SR141716A, a potent and selective antagonist of the brain cannabinoid receptor. FEBS Lett. 1994;350(2-3):240-4. doi: 10.1016/0014-5793(94)00773-X.

[65] Anderson JJ, Kask AM, Chase TN. Effects of cannabinoid receptor stimulation and blockade on catalepsy produced by dopamine receptor antagonists. Eur J Pharmacol. 1996;295(2-3):163-8. doi: 10.1016/0014-2999(95)00661-3.

[66] Carriba P, Ortiz O, Patkar K, Justinova Z, Stroik J, Themann A, et al. Striatal adenosine A2A and cannabinoid CB1 receptors form functional heteromeric complexes that

mediate the motor effects of cannabinoids. Neuropsychopharmacology. 2007;32(11): 2249-59. doi: 10.1038/sj.npp.1301375.

[67] Ferreira SG, Goncalves FQ, Marques JM, Tome AR, Rodrigues RJ, Nunes-Correia I, et al. Presynaptic adenosine A2A receptors dampen cannabinoid CB1 receptor-mediated inhibition of corticostriatal glutamatergic transmission. Br J Pharmacol. 2015;172(4): 1074-86. doi: 10.1111/bph.12970.

[68] Chiodi V, Ferrante A, Ferraro L, Potenza RL, Armida M, Beggiato S, et al. Striatal adenosine-cannabinoid receptor interactions in rats overexpressing adenosine A receptors. J Neurochem. 2015. doi: 10.1111/jnc.13421.

[69] Pertwee RG. Elevating endocannabinoid levels: pharmacological strategies and potential therapeutic applications. Proc Nutr Soc. 2014;73(1):96-105. doi: 10.1017/S0029665113003649.

[70] de Lago E, Fernandez-Ruiz J, Ortega-Gutierrez S, Viso A, Lopez-Rodriguez ML, Ramos JA. UCM707, a potent and selective inhibitor of endocannabinoid uptake, potentiates hypokinetic and antinociceptive effects of anandamide. Eur J Pharmacol. 2002;449(1-2): 99-103. doi: 10.1111/j.1472-8206.2008.00626.

[71] Gonzalez S, Romero J, de Miguel R, Lastres-Becker I, Villanua MA, Makriyannis A, et al. Extrapyramidal and neuroendocrine effects of AM404, an inhibitor of the carrier-mediated transport of anandamide. Life Sci. 1999;65(3):327-36. doi: 10.3389/fphar.2012.00110.

[72] Giuffrida A, Rodriguez de Fonseca F, Nava F, Loubet-Lescoulie P, Piomelli D. Elevated circulating levels of anandamide after administration of the transport inhibitor, AM404. Eur J Pharmacol. 2000;408(2):161-8. doi: 10.1016/j.ejphar.2014.03.010.

[73] Zygmunt PM, Chuang H, Movahed P, Julius D, Hogestatt ED. The anandamide transport inhibitor AM404 activates vanilloid receptors. Eur J Pharmacol. 2000;396(1): 39-42. doi: 10.1016/S0014-2999(00)00207-7.

[74] Jayamanne A, Greenwood R, Mitchell VA, Aslan S, Piomelli D, Vaughan CW. Actions of the FAAH inhibitor URB597 in neuropathic and inflammatory chronic pain models. Br J Pharmacol. 2006;147(3):281-8. doi: 10.1038/sj.bjp.0706510.

[75] Long JZ, Nomura DK, Vann RE, Walentiny DM, Booker L, Jin X, et al. Dual blockade of FAAH and MAGL identifies behavioral processes regulated by endocannabinoid crosstalk in vivo. Proc Natl Acad Sci U S A. 2009;106(48):20270-5. doi: 10.1073/pnas.0909411106.

[76] Li GL, Winter H, Arends R, Jay GW, Le V, Young T, et al. Assessment of the pharmacology and tolerability of PF-04457845, an irreversible inhibitor of fatty acid amide hydrolase-1, in healthy subjects. Br J Clin Pharmacol. 2012;73(5):706-16. doi: 10.1111/j.1365-2125.2011.04137.x.

[77] Long JZ, Li W, Booker L, Burston JJ, Kinsey SG, Schlosburg JE, et al. Selective blockade of 2-arachidonoylglycerol hydrolysis produces cannabinoid behavioral effects. Nat Chem Biol. 2009;5(1):37-44. doi: 10.1038/nchembio.129.

[78] Ignatowska-Jankowska B, Wilkerson JL, Mustafa M, Abdullah R, Niphakis M, Wiley JL, et al. Selective monoacylglycerol lipase inhibitors: antinociceptive versus cannabimimetic effects in mice. J Pharmacol Exp Ther. 2015;353(2):424-32. doi: 10.1124/jpet.114.222315.

[79] Ramesh D, Gamage TF, Vanuytsel T, Owens RA, Abdullah RA, Niphakis MJ, et al. Dual inhibition of endocannabinoid catabolic enzymes produces enhanced antiwithdrawal effects in morphine-dependent mice. Neuropsychopharmacology. 2013;38(6):1039-49. doi: 10.1038/npp.2012.269.

[80] Souilhac J, Poncelet M, Rinaldi-Carmona M, Le Fur G, Soubrie P. Intrastriatal injection of cannabinoid receptor agonists induced turning behavior in mice. Pharmacol Biochem Behav. 1995;51(1):3-7. doi: 10.1016/0091-3057(94)00396-Z.

[81] Di Marzo V, Lastres-Becker I, Bisogno T, De Petrocellis L, Milone A, Davis JB, et al. Hypolocomotor effects in rats of capsaicin and two long chain capsaicin homologues. Eur J Pharmacol. 2001;420(2-3):123-31. doi: 10.1016/S0014-2999(01)01012-3.

[82] Compton DR, Aceto MD, Lowe J, Martin BR. In vivo characterization of a specific cannabinoid receptor antagonist (SR141716A): inhibition of delta 9-tetrahydrocannabinol-induced responses and apparent agonist activity. J Pharmacol Exp Ther. 1996;277(2):586-94. doi: 10.1124/jpet.111.187815.

[83] Bass CE, Griffin G, Grier M, Mahadevan A, Razdan RK, Martin BR. SR-141716A-induced stimulation of locomotor activity. A structure-activity relationship study. Pharmacol Biochem Behav. 2002;74(1):31-40. doi: 10.1016/S0091-3057(02)00945-0.

[84] Navarro M, Hernandez E, Munoz RM, del Arco I, Villanua MA, Carrera MR, et al. Acute administration of the CB1 cannabinoid receptor antagonist SR 141716A induces anxiety-like responses in the rat. Neuroreport. 1997;8(2):491-6. doi: 10.1097/00001756-199701200-00023.

[85] Thiemann G, van der Stelt M, Petrosino S, Molleman A, Di Marzo V, Hasenohrl RU. The role of the CB1 cannabinoid receptor and its endogenous ligands, anandamide and 2-arachidonoylglycerol, in amphetamine-induced behavioural sensitization. Behav Brain Res. 2008;187(2):289-96. doi: 10.1016/j.bbr.2007.09.022.

[86] Zimmer A, Zimmer AM, Hohmann AG, Herkenham M, Bonner TI. Increased mortality, hypoactivity, and hypoalgesia in cannabinoid CB1 receptor knockout mice. Proc Natl Acad Sci U S A. 1999;96(10):5780-5. doi: 10.1073/pnas.96.10.5780.

[87] Ledent C, Valverde O, Cossu G, Petitet F, Aubert JF, Beslot F, et al. Unresponsiveness to cannabinoids and reduced addictive effects of opiates in CB1 receptor knockout mice. Science. 1999;283(5400):401-4. doi: 10.1126/science.283.5400.401.

[88] Corbille AG, Valjent E, Marsicano G, Ledent C, Lutz B, Herve D, et al. Role of cannabinoid type 1 receptors in locomotor activity and striatal signaling in response to psychostimulants. J Neurosci. 2007;27(26):6937-47. doi: 10.1523/JNEUROSCI.3936-06.2007.

[89] Thiemann G, Di Marzo V, Molleman A, Hasenohrl RU. The CB(1) cannabinoid receptor antagonist AM251 attenuates amphetamine-induced behavioural sensitization while causing monoamine changes in nucleus accumbens and hippocampus. Pharmacol Biochem Behav. 2008;89(3):384-91. doi: 10.1016/j.pbb.2008.01.010.

[90] Starowicz K, Nigam S, Di Marzo V. Biochemistry and pharmacology of endovanilloids. Pharmacol Ther. 2007;114(1):13-33. doi: 10.1016/j.pharmthera.2007.01.005.

[91] Lang AE, Lozano AM. Parkinson's disease. First of two parts. N Engl J Med. 1998;339(15):1044-53. doi: 10.1056/NEJM199810083391506.

[92] Lang AE, Lozano AM. Parkinson's disease. Second of two parts. N Engl J Med. 1998;339(16):1130-43. doi: 10.1056/NEJM199810153391607.

[93] Kish SJ, Shannak K, Hornykiewicz O. Uneven pattern of dopamine loss in the striatum of patients with idiopathic Parkinson's disease. Pathophysiologic and clinical implications. N Engl J Med. 1988;318(14):876-80. doi: 10.1056/NEJM198804073181402.

[94] Papa SM. The cannabinoid system in Parkinson's disease: multiple targets to motor effects. Exp Neurol. 2008;211(2):334-8. doi: 10.1016/j.expneurol.2008.03.009.

[95] van der Stelt M, Fox SH, Hill M, Crossman AR, Petrosino S, Di Marzo V, et al. A role for endocannabinoids in the generation of parkinsonism and levodopa-induced dyskinesia in MPTP-lesioned non-human primate models of Parkinson's disease. FASEB J. 2005;19(9):1140-2. doi: 10.1096/fj.04-3010fje.

[96] Di Marzo V, Hill MP, Bisogno T, Crossman AR, Brotchie JM. Enhanced levels of endogenous cannabinoids in the globus pallidus are associated with a reduction in movement in an animal model of Parkinson's disease. FASEB J. 2000;14(10):1432-8. doi: 10.1096/fj.14.10.1432.

[97] Gubellini P, Picconi B, Bari M, Battista N, Calabresi P, Centonze D, et al. Experimental parkinsonism alters endocannabinoid degradation: implications for striatal glutamatergic transmission. J Neurosci. 2002;22(16):6900-7. doi: 20026732.

[98] Silverdale MA, McGuire S, McInnes A, Crossman AR, Brotchie JM. Striatal cannabinoid CB1 receptor mRNA expression is decreased in the reserpine-treated rat model of Parkinson's disease. Exp Neurol. 2001;169(2):400-6. doi: 10.1006/exnr.2001.7649.

[99] Mounsey RB, Mustafa S, Robinson L, Ross RA, Riedel G, Pertwee RG, et al. Increasing levels of the endocannabinoid 2-AG is neuroprotective in the 1-methyl-4-phenyl-1,2,3,6-tetrahydropyridine mouse model of Parkinson's disease. Exp Neurol. 2015;273:36-44. doi: 10.1016/j.expneurol.2015.07.024.

[100] Esposito E, Impellizzeri D, Mazzon E, Paterniti I, Cuzzocrea S. Neuroprotective activities of palmitoylethanolamide in an animal model of Parkinson's disease. PLoS One. 2012;7(8):e41880. doi: 10.1371/journal.pone.0041880.

[101] Van Laere K, Casteels C, Lunskens S, Goffin K, Grachev ID, Bormans G, et al. Regional changes in type 1 cannabinoid receptor availability in Parkinson's disease in vivo. Neurobiol Aging. 2012;33(3):620 e1-8. doi: 10.1016/j.neurobiolaging.2011.02.009.

[102] Hurley MJ, Mash DC, Jenner P. Expression of cannabinoid CB1 receptor mRNA in basal ganglia of normal and parkinsonian human brain. J Neural Transm (Vienna). 2003;110(11):1279-88. doi: 10.1007/s00702-003-0033-7.

[103] Farkas S, Nagy K, Jia Z, Harkany T, Palkovits M, Donohou SR, et al. The decrease of dopamine D(2)/D(3) receptor densities in the putamen and nucleus caudatus goes parallel with maintained levels of CB(1) cannabinoid receptors in Parkinson's disease: a preliminary autoradiographic study with the selective dopamine D(2)/D(3) antagonist [(3)H]raclopride and the novel CB(1) inverse agonist [(1)(2)(5)I]SD7015. Brain Res Bull. 2012;87(6):504-10. doi: 10.1016/j.brainresbull.2012.02.012.

[104] Zeng BY, Dass B, Owen A, Rose S, Cannizzaro C, Tel BC, et al. Chronic L-DOPA treatment increases striatal cannabinoid CB1 receptor mRNA expression in 6-hydroxydopamine-lesioned rats. Neurosci Lett. 1999;276(2):71-4. doi: 10.1016/S0304-3940(99)00762-4.

[105] Romero J, Berrendero F, Perez-Rosado A, Manzanares J, Rojo A, Fernandez-Ruiz JJ, et al. Unilateral 6-hydroxydopamine lesions of nigrostriatal dopaminergic neurons increased CB1 receptor mRNA levels in the caudate-putamen. Life Sci. 2000;66(6): 485-94. doi: 10.1016/S0024320599006189.

[106] Madeo G, Schirinzi T, Maltese M, Martella G, Rapino C, Fezza F, et al. Dopamine-dependent CB1 receptor dysfunction at corticostriatal synapses in homozygous PINK1 knockout mice. Neuropharmacology. 2016;101:460-70. doi:10.1016/j.neuropharm.2015.10.021.

[107] Concannon RM, Okine BN, Finn DP, Dowd E. Differential upregulation of the cannabinoid CB(2) receptor in neurotoxic and inflammation-driven rat models of Parkinson's disease. Exp Neurol. 2015;269:133-41. doi: 10.1016/j.expneurol.2015.04.007.

[108] Razavinasab M, Shamsizadeh A, Shabani M, Nazeri M, Allahtavakoli M, Asadi-Shekaari M, et al. Pharmacological blockade of TRPV1 receptors modulates the effects of 6-OHDA on motor and cognitive functions in a rat model of Parkinson's disease. Fundam Clin Pharmacol. 2013;27(6):632-40. doi: 10.1111/fcp.12015.

[109] Morgese MG, Cassano T, Cuomo V, Giuffrida A. Anti-dyskinetic effects of cannabinoids in a rat model of Parkinson's disease: role of CB(1) and TRPV1 receptors. Exp Neurol. 2007;208(1):110-9. doi: 10.1016/j.expneurol.2007.07.021.

[110] Pringsheim T, Wiltshire K, Day L, Dykeman J, Steeves T, Jette N. The incidence and prevalence of Huntington's disease: a systematic review and meta-analysis. Mov Disord. 2012;27(9):1083-91. doi: 10.1002/mds.25075.

[111] A novel gene containing a trinucleotide repeat that is expanded and unstable on Huntington's disease chromosomes. The Huntington's Disease Collaborative Research Group. Cell. 1993;72(6):971-83. doi: 10.1016/0092-8674(93)90585-E.

[112] Reiner A, Albin RL, Anderson KD, D'Amato CJ, Penney JB, Young AB. Differential loss of striatal projection neurons in Huntington disease. Proc Natl Acad Sci U S A. 1988;85(15):5733-7. doi: 10.1073/pnas.85.15.5733.

[113] Heinsen H, Strik M, Bauer M, Luther K, Ulmar G, Gangnus D, et al. Cortical and striatal neurone number in Huntington's disease. Acta Neuropathol. 1994;88(4):320-33. doi: 10.1007/BF00310376.

[114] Hedreen JC, Peyser CE, Folstein SE, Ross CA. Neuronal loss in layers V and VI of cerebral cortex in Huntington's disease. Neurosci Lett. 1991;133(2):257-61. doi: 10.1016/0304-3940(91)90583-F.

[115] Walker FO. Huntington's disease. Lancet. 2007;369(9557):218-28. doi: 10.1016/S0140-6736(07)60111-1.

[116] Sagredo O, Pazos MR, Valdeolivas S, Fernandez-Ruiz J. Cannabinoids: novel medicines for the treatment of Huntington's disease. Recent Pat CNS Drug Discov. 2012;7(1):41-8. doi: 10.2174/157488912798842278.

[117] Berardelli A, Noth J, Thompson PD, Bollen EL, Curra A, Deuschl G, et al. Pathophysiology of chorea and bradykinesia in Huntington's disease. Mov Disord. 1999;14(3):398-403. doi: 0.1002/1531-8257(199905)14:3<398::AID-MDS1003>3.0.CO;2-F.

[118] Allen KL, Waldvogel HJ, Glass M, Faull RL. Cannabinoid (CB(1)), GABA(A) and GABA(B) receptor subunit changes in the globus pallidus in Huntington's disease. J Chem Neuroanat. 2009;37(4):266-81. doi: 10.1016/S0891-0618(09)00020-9.

[119] Blazquez C, Chiarlone A, Sagredo O, Aguado T, Pazos MR, Resel E, et al. Loss of striatal type 1 cannabinoid receptors is a key pathogenic factor in Huntington's disease. Brain. 2011;134(Pt 1):119-36. doi: 10.1093/brain/awq278.

[120] Battista N, Bari M, Tarditi A, Mariotti C, Bachoud-Levi AC, Zuccato C, et al. Severe deficiency of the fatty acid amide hydrolase (FAAH) activity segregates with the Huntington's disease mutation in peripheral lymphocytes. Neurobiol Dis. 2007;27(1):108-16. doi: 10.1016/j.nbd.2007.04.012.

[121] Dowie MJ, Bradshaw HB, Howard ML, Nicholson LF, Faull RL, Hannan AJ, et al. Altered CB1 receptor and endocannabinoid levels precede motor symptom onset in a transgenic mouse model of Huntington's disease. Neuroscience. 2009;163(1):456-65. doi: 10.1016/j.neuroscience.2009.06.014.

[122] Bisogno T, Martire A, Petrosino S, Popoli P, Di Marzo V. Symptom-related changes of endocannabinoid and palmitoylethanolamide levels in brain areas of R6/2 mice, a transgenic model of Huntington's disease. Neurochem Int. 2008;52(1-2):307-13. doi: 10.1016/j.neuint.2007.06.031.

[123] Bari M, Battista N, Valenza M, Mastrangelo N, Malaponti M, Catanzaro G, et al. In vitro and in vivo models of Huntington's disease show alterations in the endocannabinoid system. FEBS J. 2013;280(14):3376-88. doi: 10.1111/febs.12329.

[124] Lastres-Becker I, Fezza F, Cebeira M, Bisogno T, Ramos JA, Milone A, et al. Changes in endocannabinoid transmission in the basal ganglia in a rat model of Huntington's disease. Neuroreport. 2001;12(10):2125-9. doi: 10.1097/00001756-200107200-00017.

[125] Horne EA, Coy J, Swinney K, Fung S, Cherry AE, Marrs WR, et al. Downregulation of cannabinoid receptor 1 from neuropeptide Y interneurons in the basal ganglia of patients with Huntington's disease and mouse models. Eur J Neurosci. 2013;37(3): 429-40. doi: 10.1111/ejn.12045.

[126] Van Laere K, Casteels C, Dhollander I, Goffin K, Grachev I, Bormans G, et al. Widespread decrease of type 1 cannabinoid receptor availability in Huntington disease in vivo. J Nucl Med. 2010;51(9):1413-7. doi: 10.2967/jnumed.110.077156.

[127] Denovan-Wright EM, Robertson HA. Cannabinoid receptor messenger RNA levels decrease in a subset of neurons of the lateral striatum, cortex and hippocampus of transgenic Huntington's disease mice. Neuroscience. 2000;98(4):705-13. doi: 10.1016/S0306-4522(00)00157-3.

[128] Lastres-Becker I, Berrendero F, Lucas JJ, Martin-Aparicio E, Yamamoto A, Ramos JA, et al. Loss of mRNA levels, binding and activation of GTP-binding proteins for cannabinoid CB1 receptors in the basal ganglia of a transgenic model of Huntington's disease. Brain Res. 2002;929(2):236-42. doi: 10.1016/S0006-8993(01)03403-5.

[129] Chiodi V, Uchigashima M, Beggiato S, Ferrante A, Armida M, Martire A, et al. Unbalance of CB1 receptors expressed in GABAergic and glutamatergic neurons in a transgenic mouse model of Huntington's disease. Neurobiol Dis. 2012;45(3):983-91. doi: 10.1016/j.nbd.2011.12.017.

[130] Lastres-Becker I, Hansen HH, Berrendero F, De Miguel R, Perez-Rosado A, Manzanares J, et al. Alleviation of motor hyperactivity and neurochemical deficits by endocannabinoid uptake inhibition in a rat model of Huntington's disease. Synapse. 2002;44(1):23-35. doi: 10.1002/syn.10054.

[131] Page KJ, Besret L, Jain M, Monaghan EM, Dunnett SB, Everitt BJ. Effects of systemic 3-nitropropionic acid-induced lesions of the dorsal striatum on cannabinoid and mu-opioid receptor binding in the basal ganglia. Exp Brain Res. 2000;130(2):142-50. doi: 10.1007/s002210050016.

[132] Ooms M, Rietjens R, Rangarajan JR, Vunckx K, Valdeolivas S, Maes F, et al. Early decrease of type 1 cannabinoid receptor binding and phosphodiesterase 10A activity

in vivo in R6/2 Huntington mice. Neurobiol Aging. 2014;35(12):2858-69. doi: 10.1016/j.neurobiolaging.2014.06.010.

[133] Casteels C, Vandeputte C, Rangarajan JR, Dresselaers T, Riess O, Bormans G, et al. Metabolic and type 1 cannabinoid receptor imaging of a transgenic rat model in the early phase of Huntington disease. Exp Neurol. 2011;229(2):440-9. doi: 10.1016/j.expneurol.2011.03.014.

[134] Chiarlone A, Bellocchio L, Blazquez C, Resel E, Soria-Gomez E, Cannich A, et al. A restricted population of CB1 cannabinoid receptors with neuroprotective activity. Proc Natl Acad Sci U S A. 2014;111(22):8257-62. doi: 10.1073/pnas.1400988111.

[135] Mievis S, Blum D, Ledent C. Worsening of Huntington disease phenotype in CB1 receptor knockout mice. Neurobiol Dis. 2011;42(3):524-9. doi: 10.1016/j.nbd.2011.03.006.

[136] Naydenov AV, Sepers MD, Swinney K, Raymond LA, Palmiter RD, Stella N. Genetic rescue of CB1 receptors on medium spiny neurons prevents loss of excitatory striatal synapses but not motor impairment in HD mice. Neurobiol Dis. 2014;71:140-50. doi: 10.1016/j.nbd.2014.08.009.

[137] Palazuelos J, Aguado T, Pazos MR, Julien B, Carrasco C, Resel E, et al. Microglial CB2 cannabinoid receptors are neuroprotective in Huntington's disease excitotoxicity. Brain. 2009;132(Pt 11):3152-64. doi: 10.1093/brain/awp239.

[138] Dowie MJ, Grimsey NL, Hoffman T, Faull RL, Glass M. Cannabinoid receptor CB2 is expressed on vascular cells, but not astroglial cells in the post-mortem human Huntington's disease brain. J Chem Neuroanat. 2014;59-60:62-71. doi: 10.1016/j.jchemneu.2014.06.004.

[139] Sagredo O, Gonzalez S, Aroyo I, Pazos MR, Benito C, Lastres-Becker I, et al. Cannabinoid CB2 receptor agonists protect the striatum against malonate toxicity: relevance for Huntington's disease. Glia. 2009;57(11):1154-67. doi: 10.1002/glia.20838.

[140] Bouchard J, Truong J, Bouchard K, Dunkelberger D, Desrayaud S, Moussaoui S, et al. Cannabinoid receptor 2 signaling in peripheral immune cells modulates disease onset and severity in mouse models of Huntington's disease. J Neurosci. 2012;32(50):18259-68. doi: 10.1523/JNEUROSCI.4008-12.2012.

[141] Carlsson A. Treatment of Parkinson's with L-D OPA. The early discovery phase, and a comment on current problems. J Neural Transm (Vienna). 2002;109(5-6):777-87. doi: 10.1007/s007020200064.

[142] Anderson LA, Anderson JJ, Chase TN, Walters JR. The cannabinoid agonists WIN 55,212-2 and CP 55,940 attenuate rotational behavior induced by a dopamine D1 but not a D2 agonist in rats with unilateral lesions of the nigrostriatal pathway. Brain Res. 1995;691(1-2):106-14. doi: 10.1016/0006-8993(95)00645-7.

[143] Maneuf YP, Crossman AR, Brotchie JM. The cannabinoid receptor agonist WIN 55,212-2 reduces D2, but not D1, dopamine receptor-mediated alleviation of akinesia

in the reserpine-treated rat model of Parkinson's disease. Exp Neurol. 1997;148(1): 265-70. doi: 10.1006/exnr.1997.6645.

[144] Brotchie JM. Adjuncts to dopamine replacement: a pragmatic approach to reducing the problem of dyskinesia in Parkinson's disease. Mov Disord. 1998;13(6):871-6. doi: 10.1002/mds.870130603.

[145] Sanudo-Pena MC, Patrick SL, Khen S, Patrick RL, Tsou K, Walker JM. Cannabinoid effects in basal ganglia in a rat model of Parkinson's disease. Neurosci Lett. 1998;248(3): 171-4. doi: 10.1016/S0304-3940(98)00368-1.

[146] Sanudo-Pena MC, Tsou K, Walker JM. Motor actions of cannabinoids in the basal ganglia output nuclei. Life Sci. 1999;65(6-7):703-13. doi: 10.1016/S0024-3205(99)00293-3.

[147] Fernandez-Espejo E, Caraballo I, de Fonseca FR, El Banoua F, Ferrer B, Flores JA, et al. Cannabinoid CB1 antagonists possess antiparkinsonian efficacy only in rats with very severe nigral lesion in experimental parkinsonism. Neurobiol Dis. 2005;18(3):591-601. doi: 10.1016/j.nbd.2004.10.015.

[148] Gonzalez S, Scorticati C, Garcia-Arencibia M, de Miguel R, Ramos JA, Fernandez-Ruiz J. Effects of rimonabant, a selective cannabinoid CB1 receptor antagonist, in a rat model of Parkinson's disease. Brain Res. 2006;1073-1074:209-19. doi: 10.1016/j.brainres. 2005.12.014.

[149] Kelsey JE, Harris O, Cassin J. The CB(1) antagonist rimonabant is adjunctively therapeutic as well as monotherapeutic in an animal model of Parkinson's disease. Behav Brain Res. 2009;203(2):304-7. doi: 10.1016/j.bbr.2009.04.035.

[150] Garcia-Arencibia M, Ferraro L, Tanganelli S, Fernandez-Ruiz J. Enhanced striatal glutamate release after the administration of rimonabant to 6-hydroxydopamine-lesioned rats. Neurosci Lett. 2008;438(1):10-3. doi: 10.1016/j.neulet.2008.04.041.

[151] de Lago E, de Miguel R, Lastres-Becker I, Ramos JA, Fernandez-Ruiz J. Involvement of vanilloid-like receptors in the effects of anandamide on motor behavior and nigrostriatal dopaminergic activity: in vivo and in vitro evidence. Brain Res. 2004;1007(1-2): 152-9. doi: 10.1016/j.brainres.2004.02.016.

[152] Ferrer B, Asbrock N, Kathuria S, Piomelli D, Giuffrida A. Effects of levodopa on endocannabinoid levels in rat basal ganglia: implications for the treatment of levodopa-induced dyskinesias. Eur J Neurosci. 2003;18(6):1607-14. doi: 10.1046/j. 1460-9568.2003.02896.

[153] Martinez A, Macheda T, Morgese MG, Trabace L, Giuffrida A. The cannabinoid agonist WIN55212-2 decreases L-DOPA-induced PKA activation and dyskinetic behavior in 6-OHDA-treated rats. Neurosci Res. 2012;72(3):236-42. doi: 10.1016/j.neures.2011.12.006.

[154] Fox SH, Henry B, Hill M, Crossman A, Brotchie J. Stimulation of cannabinoid receptors reduces levodopa-induced dyskinesia in the MPTP-lesioned nonhuman primate model of Parkinson's disease. Mov Disord. 2002;17(6):1180-7. doi: 10.1002/mds.10289.

[155] Sieradzan KA, Fox SH, Hill M, Dick JP, Crossman AR, Brotchie JM. Cannabinoids reduce levodopa-induced dyskinesia in Parkinson's disease: a pilot study. Neurology. 2001;57(11):2108-11. doi: org/10.1212/WNL.57.11.2108.

[156] Venderova K, Ruzicka E, Vorisek V, Visnovsky P. Survey on cannabis use in Parkinson's disease: subjective improvement of motor symptoms. Mov Disord. 2004;19(9): 1102-6. doi: 10.1002/mds.20111.

[157] Zuardi AW, Crippa JA, Hallak JE, Pinto JP, Chagas MH, Rodrigues GG, et al. Cannabidiol for the treatment of psychosis in Parkinson's disease. J Psychopharmacol. 2009;23(8):979-83. doi: 10.1177/0269881108096519.

[158] Carroll CB, Bain PG, Teare L, Liu X, Joint C, Wroath C, et al. Cannabis for dyskinesia in Parkinson disease: a randomized double-blind crossover study. Neurology. 2004;63(7):1245-50. doi: 10.1212/01.WNL.0000140288.48796.8E.

[159] Mesnage V, Houeto JL, Bonnet AM, Clavier I, Arnulf I, Cattelin F, et al. Neurokinin B, neurotensin, and cannabinoid receptor antagonists and Parkinson disease. Clin Neuropharmacol. 2004;27(3):108-10. doi: 10.1097/00002826-200405000-00003.

[160] Lastres-Becker I, Molina-Holgado F, Ramos JA, Mechoulam R, Fernandez-Ruiz J. Cannabinoids provide neuroprotection against 6-hydroxydopamine toxicity in vivo and in vitro: relevance to Parkinson's disease. Neurobiol Dis. 2005;19(1-2):96-107. doi: 10.1016/j.nbd.2004.11.009.

[161] Price DA, Martinez AA, Seillier A, Koek W, Acosta Y, Fernandez E, et al. WIN55,212-2, a cannabinoid receptor agonist, protects against nigrostriatal cell loss in the 1-methyl-4-phenyl-1,2,3,6-tetrahydropyridine mouse model of Parkinson's disease. Eur J Neurosci. 2009;29(11):2177-86. doi: 10.1111/j.1460-9568.2009.06764.x.

[162] Chung YC, Bok E, Huh SH, Park JY, Yoon SH, Kim SR, et al. Cannabinoid receptor type 1 protects nigrostriatal dopaminergic neurons against MPTP neurotoxicity by inhibiting microglial activation. J Immunol. 2011;187(12):6508-17. doi: 10.4049/jimmunol.1102435.

[163] Garcia-Arencibia M, Gonzalez S, de Lago E, Ramos JA, Mechoulam R, Fernandez-Ruiz J. Evaluation of the neuroprotective effect of cannabinoids in a rat model of Parkinson's disease: importance of antioxidant and cannabinoid receptor-independent properties. Brain Res. 2007;1134(1):162-70. doi: 10.1016/j.brainres.2006.11.063.

[164] Carroll CB, Zeissler ML, Hanemann CO, Zajicek JP. Delta(9)-tetrahydrocannabinol (Delta(9)-THC) exerts a direct neuroprotective effect in a human cell culture model of Parkinson's disease. Neuropathol Appl Neurobiol. 2012;38(6):535-47. doi: 10.1111/j. 1365-2990.2011.01248.x.

[165] Garcia C, Palomo-Garo C, Garcia-Arencibia M, Ramos J, Pertwee R, Fernandez-Ruiz J. Symptom-relieving and neuroprotective effects of the phytocannabinoid Delta(9)-

THCV in animal models of Parkinson's disease. Br J Pharmacol. 2011;163(7):1495-506. doi: 10.1111/j.1476-5381.2011.01278.x.

[166] Chagas MH, Zuardi AW, Tumas V, Pena-Pereira MA, Sobreira ET, Bergamaschi MM, et al. Effects of cannabidiol in the treatment of patients with Parkinson's disease: an exploratory double-blind trial. J Psychopharmacol. 2014;28(11):1088-98. doi: 10.1177/0269881114550355.

[167] Jimenez-Del-Rio M, Daza-Restrepo A, Velez-Pardo C. The cannabinoid CP55,940 prolongs survival and improves locomotor activity in Drosophila melanogaster against paraquat: implications in Parkinson's disease. Neurosci Res. 2008;61(4):404-11. doi: 10.1016/j.neures.2008.04.011.

[168] McGeer PL, Itagaki S, Boyes BE, McGeer EG. Reactive microglia are positive for HLA-DR in the substantia nigra of Parkinson's and Alzheimer's disease brains. Neurology. 1988;38(8):1285-91. doi: 10.3389/fncel.2015.00084.

[169] Mogi M, Harada M, Kondo T, Riederer P, Inagaki H, Minami M, et al. Interleukin-1 beta, interleukin-6, epidermal growth factor and transforming growth factor-alpha are elevated in the brain from parkinsonian patients. Neurosci Lett. 1994;180(2):147-50. doi: 10.1016/0304-3940(94)90508-8.

[170] Mogi M, Harada M, Kondo T, Riederer P, Nagatsu T. Brain beta 2-microglobulin levels are elevated in the striatum in Parkinson's disease. J Neural Transm Park Dis Dement Sect. 1995;9(1):87-92. doi: 10.1523/JNEUROSCI.3447-06.2006.

[171] Muller T, Blum-Degen D, Przuntek H, Kuhn W. Interleukin-6 levels in cerebrospinal fluid inversely correlate to severity of Parkinson's disease. Acta Neurol Scand. 1998;98(2):142-4. doi: 10.1111/j.1600-0404.1998.tb01736.x.

[172] Sagredo O, Garcia-Arencibia M, de Lago E, Finetti S, Decio A, Fernandez-Ruiz J. Cannabinoids and neuroprotection in basal ganglia disorders. Mol Neurobiol. 2007;36(1):82-91. doi: 10.1007/s12035-007-0004-3.

[173] Fernandez-Ruiz J. Cannabinoids in neurodegeneration and neuroprotection. In: Mechoulam R, editor. Cannabinoids and Therapeutics. Berlin 2005. p.79-109. doi: 10.1007/3-7643-7358-X_5.

[174] Benito C, Tolon RM, Pazos MR, Nunez E, Castillo AI, Romero J. Cannabinoid CB2 receptors in human brain inflammation. Br J Pharmacol. 2008;153(2):277-85. doi: 10.1038/sj.bjp.0707505.

[175] Little JP, Villanueva EB, Klegeris A. Therapeutic potential of cannabinoids in the treatment of neuroinflammation associated with Parkinson's disease. Mini Rev Med Chem. 2011;11(7):582-90. doi: 10.2174/138955711795906905.

[176] Ternianov A, Perez-Ortiz JM, Solesio ME, Garcia-Gutierrez MS, Ortega-Alvaro A, Navarrete F, et al. Overexpression of CB2 cannabinoid receptors results in neuroprotection against behavioral and neurochemical alterations induced by intracaudate

administration of 6-hydroxydopamine. Neurobiol Aging. 2012;33(2):421 e1-16. doi: 10.1016/j.neurobiolaging.2010.09.012.

[177] Marchalant Y, Brothers HM, Norman GJ, Karelina K, DeVries AC, Wenk GL. Cannabinoids attenuate the effects of aging upon neuroinflammation and neurogenesis. Neurobiol Dis. 2009;34(2):300-7. doi: 10.1016/j.nbd.2009.01.014.

[178] Chung ES, Bok E, Chung YC, Baik HH, Jin BK. Cannabinoids prevent lipopolysaccharide-induced neurodegeneration in the rat substantia nigra in vivo through inhibition of microglial activation and NADPH oxidase. Brain Res. 2012;1451:110-6. doi: 10.1016/j.brainres.2012.02.058.

[179] Pidgeon C, Rickards H. The pathophysiology and pharmacological treatment of Huntington disease. Behav Neurol. 2013;26(4):245-53. doi: 10.3233/BEN-2012-120267.

[180] Fernandez-Ruiz J, Romero J, Ramos JA. Endocannabinoids and Neurodegenerative Disorders: Parkinson's Disease, Huntington's Chorea, Alzheimer's Disease, and Others. Handb Exp Pharmacol. 2015;231:233-59. doi: 10.1007/978-3-319-20825-1_8.

[181] Kluger B, Triolo P, Jones W, Jankovic J. The therapeutic potential of cannabinoids for movement disorders. Mov Disord. 2015;30(3):313-27. doi: 10.1002/mds.26142.

[182] de Lago E, Fernandez-Ruiz J, Ortega-Gutierrez S, Cabranes A, Pryce G, Baker D, et al. UCM707, an inhibitor of the anandamide uptake, behaves as a symptom control agent in models of Huntington's disease and multiple sclerosis, but fails to delay/arrest the progression of different motor-related disorders. Eur Neuropsychopharmacol. 2006;16(1):7-18. doi: 10.1016/j.euroneuro.2005.06.001.

[183] de Lago E, Urbani P, Ramos JA, Di Marzo V, Fernandez-Ruiz J. Arvanil, a hybrid endocannabinoid and vanilloid compound, behaves as an antihyperkinetic agent in a rat model of Huntington's disease. Brain Res. 2005;1050(1-2):210-6. doi: 10.1016/j.brainres.2005.05.024.

[184] Lastres-Becker I, de Miguel R, De Petrocellis L, Makriyannis A, Di Marzo V, Fernandez-Ruiz J. Compounds acting at the endocannabinoid and/or endovanilloid systems reduce hyperkinesia in a rat model of Huntington's disease. J Neurochem. 2003;84(5): 1097-109. doi: 10.1046/j.1471-4159.2003.01595.x.

[185] Pietropaolo S, Bellocchio L, Ruiz-Calvo A, Cabanas M, Du Z, Guzman M, et al. Chronic cannabinoid receptor stimulation selectively prevents motor impairments in a mouse model of Huntington's disease. Neuropharmacology. 2015;89:368-74. doi: 10.1016/j.neuropharm.2014.07.021.

[186] Curtis A, Rickards H. Nabilone could treat chorea and irritability in Huntington's disease. J Neuropsychiatry Clin Neurosci. 2006;18(4):553-4. doi: 10.1176/appi.neuropsych.18.4.553.

[187] Curtis A, Mitchell I, Patel S, Ives N, Rickards H. A pilot study using nabilone for symptomatic treatment in Huntington's disease. Mov Disord. 2009;24(15):2254-9. doi: 10.1002/mds.22809.

[188] Consroe P, Laguna J, Allender J, Snider S, Stern L, Sandyk R, et al. Controlled clinical trial of cannabidiol in Huntington's disease. Pharmacol Biochem Behav. 1991;40(3): 701-8. doi: 0091-3057(91)90386-G.

[189] Muller-Vahl KR, Schneider U, Emrich HM. Nabilone increases choreatic movements in Huntington's disease. Mov Disord. 1999;14(6):1038-40. doi: 10.1002/1531-8257(199911)14:63.0.CO;2-7.

[190] Fernandez-Ruiz J. The endocannabinoid system as a target for the treatment of motor dysfunction. Br J Pharmacol. 2009;156(7):1029-40. doi: 10.1111/j.1476-5381.2008.00088.x.

[191] Blazquez C, Chiarlone A, Bellocchio L, Resel E, Pruunsild P, Garcia-Rincon D, et al. The CB(1) cannabinoid receptor signals striatal neuroprotection via a PI3K/Akt/mTORC1/ BDNF pathway. Cell Death Differ. 2015;22(10):1618-29. doi: 10.1038/cdd.2015.11.

[192] Demuth DG, Molleman A. Cannabinoid signalling. Life Sci. 2006;78(6):549-63. doi: 10.1016/j.lfs.2005.05.055.

[193] Monory K, Massa F, Egertova M, Eder M, Blaudzun H, Westenbroek R, et al. The endocannabinoid system controls key epileptogenic circuits in the hippocampus. Neuron. 2006;51(4):455-66. doi: 10.1016/j.neuron.2006.07.006.

[194] Foldy C, Neu A, Jones MV, Soltesz I. Presynaptic, activity-dependent modulation of cannabinoid type 1 receptor-mediated inhibition of GABA release. J Neurosci. 2006;26(5):1465-9. doi: 10.1523/JNEUROSCI.4587-05.2006.

[195] Randall MD, Harris D, Kendall DA, Ralevic V. Cardiovascular effects of cannabinoids. Pharmacol Ther. 2002;95(2):191-202. doi: 10.1016/S0163-7258(02)00258-9.

[196] Marsicano G, Moosmann B, Hermann H, Lutz B, Behl C. Neuroprotective properties of cannabinoids against oxidative stress: role of the cannabinoid receptor CB1. J Neurochem. 2002;80(3):448-56. doi: 10.1046/j.0022-3042.2001.00716.x.

[197] Sagredo O, Ramos JA, Decio A, Mechoulam R, Fernandez-Ruiz J. Cannabidiol reduced the striatal atrophy caused 3-nitropropionic acid in vivo by mechanisms independent of the activation of cannabinoid, vanilloid TRPV1 and adenosine A2A receptors. Eur J Neurosci. 2007;26(4):843-51. doi: 10.1111/j.1460-9568.2007.05717.x.

[198] Scotter EL, Goodfellow CE, Graham ES, Dragunow M, Glass M. Neuroprotective potential of CB1 receptor agonists in an in vitro model of Huntington's disease. Br J Pharmacol. 2010;160(3):747-61. doi: 10.1111/j.1476-5381.2010.00773.x.

[199] Laprairie RB, Bagher AM, Kelly ME, Denovan-Wright EM. Biased Type 1 Cannabinoid Receptor Signalling Influences Neuronal Viability in a Cell Culture Model of Huntington Disease. Mol Pharmacol. 2015. doi: 10.1124/mol.115.101980.

[200] Pintor A, Tebano MT, Martire A, Grieco R, Galluzzo M, Scattoni ML, et al. The cannabinoid receptor agonist WIN 55,212-2 attenuates the effects induced by quinolinic acid in the rat striatum. Neuropharmacology. 2006;51(5):1004-12. doi: 10.1016/j.neuropharm.2006.06.013.

[201] van Dellen A, Blakemore C, Deacon R, York D, Hannan AJ. Delaying the onset of Huntington's in mice. Nature. 2000;404(6779):721-2. doi: 10.1038/35008142.

[202] Glass M, van Dellen A, Blakemore C, Hannan AJ, Faull RL. Delayed onset of Huntington's disease in mice in an enriched environment correlates with delayed loss of cannabinoid CB1 receptors. Neuroscience. 2004;123(1):207-12. doi: 10.1016/S0306-4522(03)00595-5.

[203] Dowie MJ, Howard ML, Nicholson LF, Faull RL, Hannan AJ, Glass M. Behavioural and molecular consequences of chronic cannabinoid treatment in Huntington's disease transgenic mice. Neuroscience. 2010;170(1):324-36. doi: 10.1016/j.neuroscience.2010.06.056.

[204] Fernandez-Ruiz J, Garcia C, Sagredo O, Gomez-Ruiz M, de Lago E. The endocannabinoid system as a target for the treatment of neuronal damage. Expert Opin Ther Targets. 2010;14(4):387-404. doi: 10.1517/14728221003709792.

[205] Sagredo O, Pazos MR, Satta V, Ramos JA, Pertwee RG, Fernandez-Ruiz J. Neuroprotective effects of phytocannabinoid-based medicines in experimental models of Huntington's disease. J Neurosci Res. 2011;89(9):1509-18. doi: 10.1002/jnr.22682.

[206] Valdeolivas S, Satta V, Pertwee RG, Fernandez-Ruiz J, Sagredo O. Sativex-like combination of phytocannabinoids is neuroprotective in malonate-lesioned rats, an inflammatory model of Huntington's disease: role of CB1 and CB2 receptors. ACS Chem Neurosci. 2012;3(5):400-6. doi: 10.1021/cn200114w.

[207] Stella N. Cannabinoid signaling in glial cells. Glia. 2004;48(4):267-77. doi: 10.1002/glia.20084.

[208] Walter L, Stella N. Cannabinoids and neuroinflammation. Br J Pharmacol. 2004;141(5):775-85. doi: 10.1038/sj.bjp.0705667.

[209] Smith SR, Terminelli C, Denhardt G. Effects of cannabinoid receptor agonist and antagonist ligands on production of inflammatory cytokines and anti-inflammatory interleukin-10 in endotoxemic mice. J Pharmacol Exp Ther. 2000;293(1):136-50. doi: 10734163.

[210] Molina-Holgado F, Pinteaux E, Moore JD, Molina-Holgado E, Guaza C, Gibson RM, et al. Endogenous interleukin-1 receptor antagonist mediates anti-inflammatory and neuroprotective actions of cannabinoids in neurons and glia. J Neurosci. 2003;23(16):6470-4. doi: 12878687.

Chapter 5

Therapeutic Potential of Nonpsychoactive Cannabinoids by Targeting at Glycine Receptors

Li Zhang

Additional information is available at the end of the chapter

http://dx.doi.org/10.5772/63360

Abstract

The glycine receptors (GlyRs) have been identified as major inhibitory neurotransmission receptors in the brain since the mid of last century. Unfortunately, no therapeutic agent has been developed from targeting these receptors. Accumulating evidence has suggested that GlyRs are one primary target for exogenous and endogenous cannabinoids in the central nervous system. Cannabinoids enhance the function of GlyRs in various neurons in the brain. However, this line of research has been largely ignored since little is known about the molecular mechanism and behavioral implication of cannabinoid modulation of GlyRs. Recent studies using various experimental approaches have explored molecular insights into cannabinoid-GlyR interaction and shed light on the molecular basis of nonpsychoactive cannabinoid modulation of GlyRs. Emerging evidence has suggested that cannabinoid modulation of GlyRs can contribute to some of the cannabis-induced therapeutic effects. In this chapter, I discuss recent development in studies of mechanism and therapeutic potential of cannabinoid modulation of GlyR subunits. This research direction shows considerable promise toward the development of novel therapeutic agents acting at defined modulatory sites of GlyRs in the treatment of various chronic pain, neuromotor disorders, and other GlyR deficiency diseases.

Keywords: glycine, receptor, cannabinoid, pain, nonpsychoactive, therapeutics, action of mechanism

Abbreviations

AEA, anandamide; THC, Δ^9-tetrahydrocannabinol; CBD, cannabidiol; GABA, γ-aminobutyric acid; I_{Gly}, glycine-activated current; TM, transmembrane domain; VTA, ventral tegmental area

1. Molecular composition and tissue distribution

Glycine receptors (GlyRs) belong to the Cys-loop ligand-gated ion channel (LGIC) family, a group of membrane ion channel receptors including γ-aminobutyric acid type A ($GABA_A$), neuronal nicotinic acetylcholine (nACh), $5\text{-}HT_3$, and GlyRs. These receptors are critical for fast synaptic neurotransmission in the central nervous system. GlyRs are known to predominantly mediate fast synaptic inhibitory neurotransmission in the spinal cord and brain stem [1]. To date, four GlyRs subunits have been identified in humans including three α subunits (α1–3) and one β subunit [1]. The α subunits share a high degree of homology in the amino acid sequence (>90%), especially in the large extracellular domain that bears agonist- and antagonist-binding sites. This has posted a challenge to the development of selective ligands for specific GlyR subunits. Two very recent studies have resolved crystal structures of GlyRα1 and α3 subunits with high level of resolution (3.0 A) [2, 3]. These studies have detailed the molecular insights of GlyR-agonist/antagonist interaction and channel-gating dynamics.

It is well established that GlyR β subunits are expressed at postsynaptic sites where they can assemble with the α subunit to form heteromeric functional channels [4]. A cytoskeleton protein, gephyrin, plays a critical role in targeting heteromeric GlyRs at postsynaptic sites. While the GlyRs represent the primary inhibitory neurotransmission in spinal cord, the role of GlyRs in most supraspinal areas has been less clear [5, 6]. Although the β subunit mRNA is relatively abundant in all brain areas at the adult stage, the β subunit protein expression in many brain regions appears very low for an unknown mechanism [5]. Coincidently, glycinergic synaptic transmission in all brain areas except the spinal cord and brain stem are nearly absent at the adult stage [1]. While the α2 subunit represents the dominant form of GlyRs at early development stage, it gives way to the α1 subunit after postnatal stage [7, 8]. The α1β subunits are found to serve as the dominant functional form of GlyRs in the spinal cord and brain stem at the adult stage [9]. The biological switch between the α1 and α2 subunits occurs at a time point of ~postnatal 16–20 days [6, 10]. This timing is consistent with a shift from GABAergic to glycinergic transmission representing the maturity of brain stem and spinal inhibitory systems [6, 10]. In some brain areas such as forebrain and hippocampus, however, the mRNA levels of the α2 subunit remain to be at the steady state from developmental to adult stage [11–15]. Distinct expression of GlyR subunits is consistent with their physiological and pathological roles. For instance, the α3 subunits are restrictively expressed in the superficial layers of the spinal cord dorsal horn, consistent with the involvement of their role in the regulation of nociceptive process [16]. On the other hand, the dominant expression of GlyRα1 subunits in spinal cord and brain stem motor neurons explains well how the functional deficiency in the α1 subunits can cause human hyperekplexia disease, a neuromotor disorder [17, 18].

2. Presynaptic and extrasynaptic GlyRs

While postsynaptic GlyRs have been the major interest of many previous and current studies [1], evidence has emerged to suggest that functional GlyRs are also located at presynaptic terminals and extrasynaptic sites in many brain areas [19–25].

2.1. Presynaptic receptors

Presynaptic GlyRs are first described in calyceal synapses in the medial nucleus of the trapezoid body (MNTB) in rat brainstem [19]. These receptors are thought to play an important role in the modulation of glutamate release [6, 10, 23, 26]. Presynaptic GlyRs have also been reported from studies of other brain areas such as spinal cord, ventral tegmental area (VTA), hippocampus and periaqueductal gray area (PAG), and brain stem hypoglossal nucleus [22, 24, 25, 27, 28].

Presynaptic GlyRs are believed to regulate releases of major neurotransmitters including GABA, DA, and glutamate. All three α [1–3] subunits have been identified to contribute to presynaptic glycinergic activity in different brain regions. While the $\alpha 2$ subunits mediate the facilitation of presynaptic GABAergic transmission in VTA at early development stage [20], the $\alpha 1$ subunits emerge and facilitate glutamate release at presynaptic sites of brain stem calyx in the postnatal stage [6, 26]. A very recent study has shown that the $\alpha 3$ subunits are involved in presynaptic glycine release in brain stem hypoglossal motor neurons [25].

Different from postsynaptic heteromeric GlyRs, presynaptic GlyRs are the likely homomeric α subunits [23, 27, 28]. There are a number of evidence to support this idea. First, the β subunit is always bound with postsynaptic cytoskeleton protein, gephyrin [4, 29]. Second, low concentrations of picrotoxin (PTX) that are found to preferentially inhibit homomeric α GlyRs in vitro selectively alter presynaptic GlyR functionality in the spinal cord and brainstem [23, 27, 30–33]. Finally, this idea is consistent with microscopic observation that the GlyRs at presynaptic terminals of calyceal synapses are composed of homomeric $\alpha 1$ subunits [23]. The presynaptic GlyRs have been the interest of recent research because they disinhibit GABA-mediated synaptic inhibition of VTA dopaminergic neurons [20, 34]. There is evidence suggesting that these receptors are involved in the reward mechanism of drugs of abuse [34].

Presynaptic GlyRs are a potential therapeutic target for the treatment of hyperekplexia disease [26]. A very recent study has shown that streptozotocin-induced diabetic nerve injury caused a decrease in the paw withdrawal latency to mechanical stimuli and reduced the mean frequency of glycinergic miniature inhibitory post-synaptic current (mIPSC) in spinal dorsal horn neurons [35]. This effect is selectively mediated through a presynaptic mechanism because there is no change in miniature inhibitory post-synaptic current rise, decay kinetics, and mean mIPSC amplitude following streptozotocin injection.

2.2. Extrasynaptic GlyRs

Extrasynaptically located GlyRs have been identified in many brain regions, including hippocampus, supraoptic nucleus, and prefrontal cortex (PFC) [13, 36–39]. Functional extrasynaptic GlyRs are likely α homomers because clustering and synaptic targeting of GlyR β subunit requires postsynaptic protein gephyrin [4]. The endogenous agonists of nonsynaptic GlyRs have been postulated to be glycine and taurine [37, 39–41]. While glycine is originated from either synaptic spillover or via release from glia [39, 42], taurine is released from glial cells where the synthesizing enzyme and the transporter for taurine are present [40, 43–45]. Taurine can be released in high levels in response to physiological and pathological conditions. For instance, taurine is released in response to hypotonic stimulus [46]. There is strong evidence to suggest that ethanol can promote the release of taurine in mesolimbic structure [47–49]. The biological role of tonic activation of extrasynaptic GlyRs remains elusive. Accumulating evidence has suggested that these extrasynaptic GlyRs are likely the target for ethanol modulation in vitro and in vivo [48, 50, 51].

Although our knowledge about presynaptic and extrasynaptic GlyRs is still limited, these receptors could represent emerging targets attractive for future mechanistic and therapeutic studies.

3. GlyR-related disease

3.1. GlyRs in chronic pain

The GlyRs mediate fast synaptic inhibitory neurotransmission and regulate pain formation at spinal level. The α3GlyRs are thought to be the key player involving in spinal antinociceptive process [16, 52].

3.1.1. α3GlyRs in inflammatory pain

α3GlyR knockout mice demonstrate a reduction in pain hypersensitivity in several lines of chronic pain models. Prostaglandin E_2 (PGE_2), which promotes central and peripheral pain sensitization, selectively inhibits α3GlyRs channel activity through the activation of receptor phosphorylation in vitro [16]. Consistent with this, PGE_2 inhibits the glycinergic inhibitory postsynaptic currents in spinal cord slices of wild type (WT), but not in α3GlyRs knockout mice [16]. These α3 knockout mice reduce thermal hyperalgesia induced by the intrathecal injection of PGE_2 [16, 52]. PGE_2 inhibition of the α3GlyRs is attributed to the mechanism of chronic inflammatory pain induced by the intra-plantar injection of complete Freund's adjuvant (CFA) [16, 52]. The α3GlyRs are not involved in all inflammatory pain animal models. While the α3GlyR knockout mice show reduced pain hypersensitivity to spinal PGE_2 injection and CFA- or zymosan-induced peripheral inflammation, these mice do not display altered pain hypersensitivity after the injection of capsaicin, carrageenan, kaolin/carrageenan, or monosodium iodoacetate, which produces rheumatoid and osteoarthritis [53]. A very recent study suggested that glucose at 5 mM can allosterically increase α3GlyR receptor activity, and this interaction between the α3 subunit and sugar may underlie some of the analgesic effects of glucose [54].

3.1.2. α3GlyRs in neuropathic pain

Similarly, the α3GlyRs are also found to play a selective role in some forms of neuropathic and visceral pain models. For instance, there is no significant difference in pain behaviors between α3GlyR knockout mice and wild-type littermates following partial sciatic nerve ligation and colorectal distension [53]. On the other hand, evidence is also available suggesting that these receptors are involved in some forms of neuropathic pain models. For instance, there is a substantial reduction in the frequency of GlyR-mediated mIPSC of lamina I neurons in rat diabetic neuropathic pain after treatment with streptozotocin in rats [35]. Intrathecal injection of glycine reverses streptozotocin-induced tactile pain hypersensitivity. Moreover, the intrathecal injection of α3GlyR siRNA can reduce the anti-allodynia effect of platelet-activating factor antagonists in three different nerve injury animal models including partial sciatic nerve ligation injury, streptozotocin-induced diabetic nerve injury, and infraorbital nerve injury [55]. Overall, these data indicate that the α3GlyRs are involved in the mechanism of neuropathic pain pathway.

The role of the α2GlyR subunit in antinociception is unclear. A previous study has reported that the mice lacking the α2 subunits showed prolonged mechanical hyperalgesia induced by the peripheral injection of zymosan [56]. The α2 subunits are unlikely to play a role in persistent neuropathic pain (partial sciatic nerve ligation) as the mice lacking either α2 subunit demonstrated a normal nociceptive behavior after spinal nerve injury [56]. So far, the α1GlyRs have not been reported to play any role in pain modulation [57].

Taken together, the α3GlyRs have been the interest of many research interest because of their unique role in nociceptive process and their therapeutic potential in the development of new anti-pain drugs [52, 58–60].

3.2. Alcohol use disorder

Several lines of studies have provided consistent evidence to suggest that GlyRs are one primary target that mediates alcohol-induced behaviors in the brain [61–65]. Activation of VTA GlyRs reduces GABAergic transmission and increases the activity of dopaminergic neurons originated from VTA [20, 34]. GlyRs in the nAc are involved in modulating both basal- and ethanol-induced dopamine output in the same brain region as local injection of strychnine can inhibit ethanol-induced DA release in nAc [48, 66]. There is strong evidence that extrasynaptic GlyRs are the candidate that, at least in part, mediates ethanol-induced dopamine elevation and reward system in nAc [49, 51, 67, 68]. These receptors are likely activated by taurine, which is released from glial cells upon exposure to ethanol [49]. Microinjection of glycine into the VTA reduced the intake of ethanol in rats chronically exposed to ethanol under the intermittent-access and continuous-access procedures and decreased lever-press responding for ethanol under an operant self-administration procedure [69]. VTA microinjection of strychnine completely reversed glycine inhibition of alcohol consumption behaviors, suggesting that GlyRs in the VTA may play a critical role in ethanol self-administration in animals [69]. Consistent with this idea, a recent study in α2- and α3GlyR knockout mice has shown that the depletion of the α2GlyRs decreased ethanol intake and preference in the 24-h two-bottle choice test, whereas the depletion of the α3GlyRs increased ethanol intake and preference in the 24-h intermittent access test [70]. It appears that these GlyR subunits are selectively involved in ethanol consumption behavior but not acute ethanol intoxication-induced behaviors such as motor incoordination, loss of righting reflex, and acoustic startle response [70]. By contrast, mice carrying knock-in mutations in the GlyR α1 subunit alter the behaviors induced by acute ethanol intoxication [71, 72]. Thus, the α2- and α3GlyR subunits are involved in the reward mechanism of chronic ethanol consumption, while α1GlyR subunits are attributed to acute alcohol intoxicating-induced behaviors.

3.3. Rare genetic disease: hyperekplexia

Human exaggerated startle disease, also known as hyperekplexia, is a rare genetic neurological disorder caused by deficiency in glycinergic neurotransmission [73]. Missense point mutations in the human GlyRs α1 subunit gene disrupt GlyRs function resulting in familial startle disease, an autosomal-dominant disorder [74, 75]. Although rare, this disease is often characterized by an exaggerated startle reaction to sudden, unexpected auditory and tactile stimuli. The most frequently occurring mutation causing human hyperekplexia is the R271Q/L mutation in the α1 subunit [75]. Mice carrying the R271Q mutation exhibit severe neuromotor defects that resemble human hyperekplexia disease [57]. Except for the mutations occurring in the GlyR α1 subunit, point mutations in the GlyR β subunit are also linked to recessive human hyperekplexia disease [76].

4. Cannabinoid interaction with GlyRs

4.1. Cannabinoid potentiation of GlyRs

4.1.1. Allosteric modulation

A previous study from our laboratory has shown first evidence that both exogenous and endogenous cannabinoids such as Δ^9-tetrahydrocannabinol (THC), the principle psychoactive component of marijuana, and endocannabinoid anandamide (AEA) potentiate the amplitude of glycine-activated current (I_{Gly}) in cells expressing homomeric α1 and heteromeric α1β GlyRs and in acutely isolated VTA neurons [77]. The modulation by cannabinoids is not dependent on CB1 receptors. This initial finding has been tested and supported by a number of studies [58, 78–82]. The EC_{50} values for the THC-induced potentiation are 73 nM for human α1GlyRs, 109 nM for human α1β GlyRs expressed in *Xenopus* oocytes, and 320 nM for native GlyRs in rat VTA neurons [83]. THC at low concentrations of 100 and 300 nM can significantly enhance I_{Gly} in HEK-293 cells expressing the α1 and α3 subunits [58]. This concentration range of THC has been found to induce psychotropic and antinociceptive effects in humans [84]. The concentrations of THC in human blood can peak as high as 800 nM for 15 min after a casual marijuana inhalation and stay at 100 nM for 60 min after the smoke. The potentiation of I_{Gly} by either exogenous or endogenous cannabinoids depends on the concentration of glycine [58, 78, 81–83]. Maximal potentiation of GlyRs induced by cannabinoids occurs at the lowest concentration of glycine. With increasing glycine concentrations, the cannabinoid potentiation decreases [83].

4.1.2. Subunit-specific modulation

Both endogenous and exogenous cannabinoids modulate GlyRs in a subunit-specific manner [58, 78, 81, 82]. AEA has been found to produce various effects on I_{Gly} in different neurons [82, 83, 85]. Among all three GlyRs α subunits ($\alpha1$, $\alpha2$, and $\alpha3$) expressed in HEK-293 cells, the $\alpha1$ subunit is most sensitive to AEA-induced potentiation [78, 81, 82]. In addition to AEA, other cannabinoids and cannabinoid-mimic lipids such as *N*-arachidonyl-glycine (NA-glycine) exhibit complex action (both potentiation and inhibition) of I_{Gly} in a subunit-specific manner [81]. NA-glycine potentiated the amplitude of I_{Gly} in HEK-293 cells expressing the $\alpha1$ subunits and inhibits the amplitude of I_{Gly} in HEK-293 cells expressing the $\alpha2$ and $\alpha3$ subunits [81]. Similarly, THC has been shown to potentiate GlyRs in a subunit-specific manner expressed in HEK-293 cells [58]. The most significant difference among the three subunits appears to be the efficacy of the THC potentiation [58]. For instance, the magnitudes of the THC (1-μM)-induced potentiation of I_{Gly} are 1156, 1127, and 232% in HEK-293 cells expressing the $\alpha1$, $\alpha3$, and $\alpha2$ subunits, respectively. It should be mentioned that heteromeric $\alpha1\beta1$ subunits are less sensitive than their counterpart homomeric $\alpha1$ receptors to THC-induced potentiation [58, 83]. This is also the case that DH-cannabidiol (CBD), a modified cannabidiol, selectively rescues the function of mutant homomeric $\alpha1$GlyR subunits [26].

4.2. Molecular mechanisms

4.2.1. Direct interaction and the site

The $\alpha1$, $\alpha2$, and $\alpha3$GlyR subunits are differentially sensitive to THC- and AEA-induced potentiation of I_{Gly} [58]. Molecular analysis has identified single amino acid residue, serine (S), in the TM3, the $\alpha1$ and $\alpha3$ subunits critically involved in cannabinoid-GlyR interaction [58, 82]. Substituting the serine (S) at 296 of the $\alpha1$ subunit and at 307 of the $\alpha3$ subunit with an alanine (A) converts the $\alpha1/\alpha3$ subunits from cannabinoid high-sensitive receptors to cannabinoid low-sensitivity receptors. This suggests that S296 is a molecular determinant of cannabinoid potentiation of GlyRs. This idea has gained support from an experiment involving nuclear magnetic resonance (NMR) chemical shift measurement [58]. THC selectively shifts the S296 residue in a concentration-dependent manner in the purified proteins of the full-length four TMs of the human $\alpha1$ subunit. This hypothesis is further tested by NMR titration and nuclear Overhauser effect spectroscopy (NOESY) analysis of the interaction between cannabidiol and purified $\alpha3$GlyR protein. The data from these experiments favor a direct interaction of cannabidiol with residue S296 of the GlyR $\alpha3$ subunit. The analysis of the $\alpha3$GlyR transmembrane (TM) domains indicates that S296 is located near the intracellular end of the TM3 helix. Direct interaction of CBD with $\alpha3$GlyR-TM protein is confirmed by the intermolecular NOESY cross-peaks between CBD and the protein. This finding also favors a protein conformational change at S296 in the presence of CBD.

Electrophysiological experiments using mutagenesis analysis indicate a hydrogen-bonding interaction between cannabinoid and S296 residue [58, 86]. Consistent with this idea, chemically the removal of both hydroxyl and oxygen groups from THC abolishes the efficacy of THC in potentiating GlyRs [58]. However, the compound with retaining oxygen group is still potent in potentiating GlyR function but demonstrates significantly reduced binding affinity to CB1 receptors.

4.2.2. A common molecular basis for endogenous and exogenous cannabinoids

It has been proposed that exogenous and endogenous cannabinoids potentiate GlyRs via a common molecular basis. This idea is based on the following evidence. First, the point mutation at the S296 residue in the TM3 is critical for both THC and AEA potentiation of the $\alpha1$ and $\alpha3$ subunits [58, 83, 86]. Second, the hydroxyl/oxygen groups are essential for AEA and THC potentiation of GlyRs. Third, the deletion of these groups results in reduction in the efficacy of AEA and THC potentiation. Finally, desoxy-AEA and didesoxy-THC are found to inhibit AEA- and THC-induced potentiation of GlyRs in a similar manner.

5. Therapeutic potential of glycinergic cannabinoids

5.1. Suppression of acute and chronic pain by targeting α3GlyRs

One popular medical benefit from the use of cannabis is its therapeutic relief of chronic pain. There is evidence showing that some of the THC-induced cellular and behavioral effects are independent of CB1 receptors.

5.1.1. α3GlyR dependent

A previous study has shown that the THC-induced analgesic effect in tail-flick reflex (TFR) test remained unchanged in CB1 and CB1-CB2 double-knockout mice, suggesting a different target that may mediate THC analgesia [87]. In view of this observation, we tested whether or not GlyRs are involved in the THC-induced analgesia in the TFR. Both THC and 5-desoxy-THC, a nonpsychoactive cannabinoid, produced a strong analgesic effect in TFR test, and this effect was completely abolished by the administration of strychnine. Cannabinoid-induced analgesic effect was completely absent in the α3GlyR knockout mice. By contrast, the analgesic effect induced by THC remains unchanged in both CB1 and α2GlyR subunit knockout mice [58]. The THC-induced hypothermia did not significantly differ between the α3GlyR knockout and wild-type mice. While 5-desoxy-THC is analgesic, it does not significantly affect locomotor activity and body temperature of mice. Collectively, these data have provided first evidence that α3GlyRs are the target that selectively mediates some of cannabinoid analgesic effects.

The α3GlyRs contribute to the mechanism of chronic inflammatory pain induced by the intra-plantar injection of complete Freund's adjuvant [16, 53]. Intrathecal injection of cannabidiol, the major nonpsychoactive component of cannabis, and DH-CBD, a chemically modified CBD, suppress pain hypersensitivity following CFA intra-plantar injection [52]. In addition, DH-CBD significantly attenuates both mechanical and heat-induced pain hypersensitivity following spinal sciatic nerve ligation [52]. Both DH-CBD- and CBD-induced analgesic effects in CFA-induced pain hypersensitivity were significantly reduced in mice lacking the $\alpha3$ subunits. On the other hand, CBD- and DH-CBD-induced analgesic effects remained unchanged in either CB1 or CB2 knockout mice as compared to their WT littermates.

http://dx.doi.org/10.5772/63360

5.1.2. A correlation between cannabinoid potentiation of I_{Gly} and cannabinoid analgesia

To explore the interrelationship between cannabinoid in vitro and in vivo effects, 11 synthetic cannabinoids structurally similar to CBD were collected and their structural and functional activity was evaluated. Overall, there is a strong correlation between the cannabinoid-induced potentiation of GlyRs and cannabinoid-induced analgesic effect in chronic inflammatory pain in mice. By contrast, there is no such interrelationship between cannabinoid-induced analgesia and cannabinoid-binding affinity for either CB1 or CB2 receptors. Neither cannabinoid-induced potentiation of GlyRs nor cannabinoid-induced analgesia is significantly correlated with cannabinoid-induced psychoactive effects such as hypothermia, hypolocomotion, and incoordination. Collectively, these data suggest that cannabinoids selectively target at α3GlyRs to produce some of the analgesic effects.

5.2. Rescue of hyperekplexia by targeting presynaptic α1GlyRs

Despite overwhelming evidence for functional deficiency of GlyRs in hyperekplexia disease, current therapeutic agents do not target GlyRs [88]. While postsynaptic GlyRs as α/β heteromers attract the most research attention, little is known about the role of presynaptic GlyRs, likely α homomers, in diseases. Therefore, two testable questions emerge. Can DH-CBD treat exaggerated startle response by restoring deficiency in GlyR function? What is the role of presynaptic α1GlyRs in hyperekplexia disease?

5.2.1. Cannabinoid restoration of exaggerated startle response

DH-CBD, in a concentration-dependent manner, rescued the functional deficiency caused by α1R271Q-mutant GlyRs expressed in HEK-293 cells in spinal neurons isolated from α1R271Q-mutant mice [26]. Intraperitoneal injection of DH-CBD at 10–50 mg/kg suppressed both acoustic noise and tactile-induced exaggerated reflex displayed in α1R271Q-mutant mice. Similarly, DH-CBD restored a hind feet-clenching behavior and exaggerated tremor when picked up by the tail demonstrated in these hyperekplexia mice. 9 hyperekplexic-mutant α1GlyRs are classified as cannabinoid-sensitive and -insensitive receptors based on their response to cannabinoid potentiation of I_{Gly} and rescue of startle behavior. A correlational analysis was conducted between DH-CBD potentiation of mutant GlyR function and DH-CBD therapeutic efficacy of 4 hyperekplexia-mutant α1GlyR knock-in mice. The efficacy of DH-CBD rescue of GlyR function is correlated with its restoration of exaggerated startle behaviors. This suggests that DH-CBD restoration of hyperekplexic-mutant receptors and mice appears to be a site/genotype-specific effect.

5.2.2. Therapeutic potential of presynaptic GlyRs

There is strong evidence to suggest that presynaptic GlyRs are a potential therapeutic target of dominant hyperekplexia disease [26]. First, hyperekplexic point mutations in the α1 subunits disrupted the function of homomers more significantly than that of heteromers when expressed in HEK-293 cells. Consistent with this, the hyperekplexic mutation was found to preferentially impair I_{Gly} recorded in presynaptic terminals but not that from postsynaptic sites of calyceal/MNTB synapses. Second, hyperekplexic-mutant homomers were more sensitive than heteromers to DH-CBD-induced rescue. Third, DH-CBD potentiated presynaptic homomeric α1GlyRs without significantly altering postsynaptic GlyR activity recorded in calyx slices isolated from hyperekplexic-mutant mice. In line with this observation, DH-CBD preferentially restored the diminished frequencies of Gly sIPSCs and mIPSCs, whereas DH-CBD did not significantly alter the amplitudes of Gly sIPSCs and mIPSCs in spinal cord slices from hyperekplexic-mutant mice. PTX at a concentration preferentially blocked DH-CBD rescue of functional deficiency of homomeric-mutant GlyRs but not their heteromeric counterparts. Finally, the observation that DH-CBD increased pre-pulse ratio (PPR) suggests an enhanced probability of glycine release in the spinal cord slice of adult hyperekplexic-mutant mice.

6. Summary

Recent progress as summarized in this chapter has indicated that GlyRs are the target that mediates some of the therapeutic effects of nonpsychoactive cannabinoids in the brain. The widespread medical use of cannabis has been so controversial because the plant can produce both therapeutic and unwanted effects. The cannabinoid-GlyRs interaction opens up a new avenue to separate cannabis-induced analgesic effects from cannabis-induced psychoactive effects [89]. For instance, a very recent study has successfully developed a strategy to discover and develop analgesic drugs based on NMR structure of the GlyR and the critical role of residue S296 in THC potentiation of GlyRs [60]. The therapeutic potential for nonpsychoactive cannabinoids by targeting GlyRs has been implied to hyperekplexia disease. Unlike $GABA_A$-acting agents that are plagued by various side effects [90], DH-CBD does not produce significant psychoactive or sedative effects even at high concentrations [58]. Finally, presynaptic GlyRs are proposed to be an emerging target for the pathological mechanism of hyperekplexia disease. This idea is consistent with recent research trend toward the roles of presynaptic and extrasynaptic GlyRs in various neurological disorders [25, 63, 66, 69, 91, 92]. Thus, like postsynaptic GlyRs, presynaptic and extrasynaptic GlyRs should emerge as therapeutic targets for nonpsychoactive cannabinoids in the treatment of various neurological diseases with GlyR deficiency.

Author details

Li Zhang

Address all correspondence to: lzhang@mail.nih.gov

Laboratory of Integrative Neuroscience, National Institute on Alcohol Abuse and Alcoholism, National Institutes of Health, Rockville, MA, USA

References

[1] Lynch JW. Native glycine receptor subtypes and their physiological roles. Neuropharmacology. 2009 Jan;56(1):303–9. PubMed PMID: 18721822.

[2] Du J, Lu W, Wu S, Cheng Y, Gouaux E. Glycine receptor mechanism elucidated by electron cryo-microscopy. Nature. 2015 Oct 8;526(7572):224–9. PubMed PMID: 26344198. Pubmed Central PMCID: 4659708.

[3] Huang X, Chen H, Michelsen K, Schneider S, Shaffer PL. Crystal structure of human glycine receptor-alpha3 bound to antagonist strychnine. Nature. 2015 Oct 8;526(7572): 277–80. PubMed PMID: 26416729.

[4] Meyer G, Kirsch J, Betz H, Langosch D. Identification of a gephyrin binding motif on the glycine receptor beta subunit. Neuron. 1995 Sep;15(3):563–72. PubMed PMID: 7546736.

[5] Weltzien F, Puller C, O'Sullivan GA, Paarmann I, Betz H. Distribution of the glycine receptor beta-subunit in the mouse CNS as revealed by a novel monoclonal antibody. J Comp Neurol. 2012 Dec 1;520(17):3962–81. PubMed PMID: 22592841.

[6] Turecek R, Trussell LO. Reciprocal developmental regulation of presynaptic ionotropic receptors. Proc Natl Acad Sci U S A. 2002 Oct 15;99(21):13884–9. PubMed PMID: 12370408. Pubmed Central PMCID: 129792.

[7] Becker CM, Hoch W, Betz H. Glycine receptor heterogeneity in rat spinal cord during postnatal development. EMBO J. 1988 Dec 1;7(12):3717–26. PubMed PMID: 2850172. Pubmed Central PMCID: 454946. Epub 1988/12/01. eng.

[8] Becker CM, Betz H, Schroder H. Expression of inhibitory glycine receptors in postnatal rat cerebral cortex. Brain Res. 1993 Mar 26;606(2):220–6. PubMed PMID: 8387859.

[9] Malosio ML, Marqueze-Pouey B, Kuhse J, Betz H. Widespread expression of glycine receptor subunit mRNAs in the adult and developing rat brain. EMBO J. 1991 Sep;10(9): 2401–9. PubMed PMID: 1651228.

[10] Awatramani GB, Turecek R, Trussell LO. Staggered development of GABAergic and glycinergic transmission in the MNTB. J Neurophysiol. 2005 Feb;93(2):819–28. PubMed PMID: 15456797.

[11] Betz H, Kuhse J, Schmieden V, Laube B, Kirsch J, Harvey RJ. Structure and functions of inhibitory and excitatory glycine receptors. Ann New York Acad Sci. 1999 Apr 30;868:667–76. PubMed PMID: 10414351.

[12] Jonsson S, Kerekes N, Hyytia P, Ericson M, Soderpalm B. Glycine receptor expression in the forebrain of male AA/ANA rats. Brain Res. 2009 Dec 11;1305 Suppl:S27–36. PubMed PMID: 19781529. Epub 2009/09/29. eng.

[13] Danglot L, Rostaing P, Triller A, Bessis A. Morphologically identified glycinergic synapses in the hippocampus. Mol Cell Neurosci. 2004 Dec;27(4):394–403. PubMed PMID: 15555918.

[14] Aroeira RI, Ribeiro JA, Sebastiao AM, Valente CA. Age-related changes of glycine receptor at the rat hippocampus: from the embryo to the adult. J Neurochem. 2011 Aug; 118(3):339–53. PubMed PMID: 21272003.

[15] Avila A, Vidal PM, Dear TN, Harvey RJ, Rigo JM, Nguyen L. Glycine receptor alpha2 subunit activation promotes cortical interneuron migration. Cell Reports. 2013 Aug 29;4(4):738–50. PubMed PMID: 23954789. Pubmed Central PMCID: 3763372.

[16] Harvey RJ, Depner UB, Wassle H, Ahmadi S, Heindl C, Reinold H, et al. GlyR alpha3: an essential target for spinal PGE2-mediated inflammatory pain sensitization. Science. 2004 May 7;304(5672):884–7. PubMed PMID: 15131310.

[17] Baer K, Waldvogel HJ, Faull RL, Rees MI. Localization of glycine receptors in the human forebrain, brainstem, and cervical spinal cord: an immunohistochemical review. Front Mol Neurosci. 2009;2:25. PubMed PMID: 19915682. Pubmed Central PMCID: 2776491.

[18] Bode A, Lynch JW. The impact of human hyperekplexia mutations on glycine receptor structure and function. Mol Brain. 2014;7:2. PubMed PMID: 24405574. Pubmed Central PMCID: 3895786.

[19] Turecek R, Trussell LO. Presynaptic glycine receptors enhance transmitter release at a mammalian central synapse. Nature. 2001 May 31;411(6837):587–90. PubMed PMID: 11385573.

[20] Ye JH, Wang F, Krnjevic K, Wang W, Xiong ZG, Zhang J. Presynaptic glycine receptors on GABAergic terminals facilitate discharge of dopaminergic neurons in ventral tegmental area. J Neurosci. 2004 Oct 13;24(41):8961–74. PubMed PMID: 15483115.

[21] Wang F, Xiao C, Ye JH. Taurine activates excitatory non-synaptic glycine receptors on dopamine neurones in ventral tegmental area of young rats. J Physiol. 2005 Jun 1;565(Pt 2):503–16. PubMed PMID: 15817633. Pubmed Central PMCID: 1464534.

[22] Lee EA, Cho JH, Choi IS, Nakamura M, Park HM, Lee JJ, et al. Presynaptic glycine receptors facilitate spontaneous glutamate release onto hilar neurons in the rat hippocampus. J Neurochem. 2009 Apr;109(1):275–86. PubMed PMID: 19200346.

[23] Hruskova B, Trojanova J, Kulik A, Kralikova M, Pysanenko K, Bures Z, et al. Differential distribution of glycine receptor subtypes at the rat calyx of held synapse. J Neurosci. 2012 Nov 21;32(47):17012–24. PubMed PMID: 23175852. Pubmed Central PMCID: 3531607.

[24] Choi KH, Nakamura M, Jang IS. Presynaptic glycine receptors increase GABAergic neurotransmission in rat periaqueductal gray neurons. Neural Plast. 2013;2013:954302. PubMed PMID: 24078885. Pubmed Central PMCID: 3773970.

[25] Kono Y, Hulsmann S. Presynaptic facilitation of glycinergic mIPSC is reduced in mice lacking alpha3 glycine receptor subunits. Neuroscience. 2016 Feb 3;320:1–7. PubMed PMID: 26851771.

[26] Xiong W, Chen SR, He L, Cheng K, Zhao YL, Chen H, et al. Presynaptic glycine receptors as a potential therapeutic target for hyperekplexia disease. Nat Neurosci. 2014 Feb; 17(2):232–9. PubMed PMID: 24390226. Pubmed Central PMCID: 4019963.

[27] Jeong H-J, Jang I-S, Moorhouse AJ, Akaike N. Activation of presynaptic glycine receptors facilitates glycine release from presynaptic terminals synapsing onto rat spinal sacral dorsal commissural nucleus neurons. J Physiol. 2003 July 15;550(2):373–83.

[28] Ye J-H, Wang F, Krnjevic K, Wang W, Xiong Z-G, Zhang J. Presynaptic glycine receptors on GABAergic terminals facilitate discharge of dopaminergic neurons in ventral tegmental area. J Neurosci.. 2004 October 13, 2004;24(41):8961–74.

[29] Griffon N, Buttner C, Nicke A, Kuhse J, Schmalzing G, Betz H. Molecular determinants of glycine receptor subunit assembly. EMBO J. 1999 Sep 1;18(17):4711–21. PubMed PMID: 10469650. Pubmed Central PMCID: 1171544.

[30] Pribilla I, Takagi T, Langosch D, Bormann J, Betz H. The atypical M2 segment of the beta subunit confers picrotoxinin resistance to inhibitory glycine receptor channels. EMBO J. 1992 Dec;11(12):4305–11. PubMed PMID: 1385113. Pubmed Central PMCID: 557003. Epub 1992/12/01. eng.

[31] Yang Z, Cromer BA, Harvey RJ, Parker MW, Lynch JW. A proposed structural basis for picrotoxinin and picrotin binding in the glycine receptor pore. J Neurochem. 2007 Oct;103(2):580–9. PubMed PMID: 17714449.

[32] Turecek R, Trussell LO. Presynaptic glycine receptors enhance transmitter release at a mammalian central synapse. Nature. 2001;411(6837):587.

[33] Deleuze C, Runquist M, Orcel H, Rabie A, Dayanithi G, Alonso G, et al. Structural difference between heteromeric somatic and homomeric axonal glycine receptors in the hypothalamo-neurohypophysial system. Neuroscience. 2005;135(2):475–83. PubMed PMID: 16125853. Epub 2005/08/30. eng.

[34] Guan YZ, Ye JH. Glycine blocks long-term potentiation of GABAergic synapses in the ventral tegmental area. Neuroscience. 2016 Mar 24;318:134–42. PubMed PMID: 26806277. Pubmed Central PMCID: 4753108.

[35] Chiu YC, Liao WT, Liu CK, Wu CH, Lin CR. Reduction of spinal glycine receptor-mediated miniature inhibitory postsynaptic currents in streptozotocin-induced diabetic neuropathic pain. Neurosci Lett. 2016 Jan 12;611:88–93. PubMed PMID: 26598022.

[36] Chattipakorn SC, McMahon LL. Pharmacological characterization of glycine-gated chloride currents recorded in rat hippocampal slices. J Neurophysiol. 2002 Mar;87(3): 1515–25. PubMed PMID: 11877523.

[37] Deleuze C, Alonso G, Lefevre IA, Duvoid-Guillou A, Hussy N. Extrasynaptic localization of glycine receptors in the rat supraoptic nucleus: further evidence for their involvement in glia-to-neuron communication. Neuroscience. 2005;133(1):175–83. PubMed PMID: 15893641.

[38] Karnani MM, Venner A, Jensen LT, Fugger L, Burdakov D. Direct and indirect control of orexin/hypocretin neurons by glycine receptors. J Physiol. 2011 Feb 1;589(Pt 3):639–51. PubMed PMID: 21135047. Pubmed Central PMCID: 3055548.

[39] Salling MC, Harrison NL. Strychnine-sensitive glycine receptors on pyramidal neurons in layers II/III of the mouse prefrontal cortex are tonically activated. J Neurophysiol. 2014 Sep 1;112(5):1169–78. PubMed PMID: 24872538. Pubmed Central PMCID: 4122733.

[40] Flint AC, Liu X, Kriegstein AR. Nonsynaptic glycine receptor activation during early neocortical development. Neuron. 1998 Jan;20(1):43–53. PubMed PMID: 9459441.

[41] Mangin JM, Baloul M, Prado De Carvalho L, Rogister B, Rigo JM, Legendre P. Kinetic properties of the alpha2 homo-oligomeric glycine receptor impairs a proper synaptic functioning. J Physiol. 2003 Dec 1;553(Pt 2):369–86. PubMed PMID: 12972628. Pubmed Central PMCID: 2343566.

[42] Sipila ST, Spoljaric A, Virtanen MA, Hiironniemi I, Kaila K. Glycine transporter-1 controls nonsynaptic inhibitory actions of glycine receptors in the neonatal rat hippocampus. J Neurosci. 2014 Jul 23;34(30):10003–9. PubMed PMID: 25057202.

[43] Almarghini K, Remy A, Tappaz M. Immunocytochemistry of the taurine biosynthesis enzyme, cysteine sulfinate decarboxylase, in the cerebellum: evidence for a glial localization. Neuroscience. 1991;43(1):111–9. PubMed PMID: 1922763.

[44] Hussy N, Bres V, Rochette M, Duvoid A, Alonso G, Dayanithi G, et al. Osmoregulation of vasopressin secretion via activation of neurohypophysial nerve terminals glycine receptors by glial taurine. J Neurosci. 2001 Sep 15;21(18):7110–6. PubMed PMID: 11549721.

[45] Choe KY, Olson JE, Bourque CW. Taurine release by astrocytes modulates osmosensitive glycine receptor tone and excitability in the adult supraoptic nucleus. J Neurosci. 2012 Sep 5;32(36):12518–27. PubMed PMID: 22956842.

[46] Deleuze C, Duvoid A, Hussy N. Properties and glial origin of osmotic-dependent release of taurine from the rat supraoptic nucleus. J Physiol. 1998 Mar 1;507 (Pt 2):463–71. PubMed PMID: 9518705. Pubmed Central PMCID: 2230788.

[47] Dahchour A, Quertemont E, De Witte P. Taurine increases in the nucleus accumbens microdialysate after acute ethanol administration to naive and chronically alcoholised rats. Brain Res. 1996 Sep 30;735(1):9–19. PubMed PMID: 8905164.

[48] Adermark L, Clarke RB, Olsson T, Hansson E, Soderpalm B, Ericson M. Implications for glycine receptors and astrocytes in ethanol-induced elevation of dopamine levels in the nucleus accumbens. Addict Biol. 2011 Jan;16(1):43–54. PubMed PMID: 20331561.

[49] Ericson M, Chau P, Adermark L, Soderpalm B. Rising taurine and ethanol concentrations in nucleus accumbens interact to produce the dopamine-activating effects of alcohol. Adv Exp Med. Biol. 2013;775:215–23. PubMed PMID: 23392937.

[50] Badanich KA, Mulholland PJ, Beckley JT, Trantham-Davidson H, Woodward JJ. Ethanol reduces neuronal excitability of lateral orbitofrontal cortex neurons via a glycine receptor dependent mechanism. Neuropsychopharmacology. 2013 Jun;38(7): 1176–88. PubMed PMID: 23314219. Pubmed Central PMCID: 3656360.

[51] Jonsson S, Adermark L, Ericson M, Soderpalm B. The involvement of accumbal glycine receptors in the dopamine-elevating effects of addictive drugs. Neuropharmacology. 2014 Jul;82:69–75. PubMed PMID: 24686030.

[52] Xiong W, Cui T, Cheng K, Yang F, Chen SR, Willenbring D, et al. Cannabinoids suppress inflammatory and neuropathic pain by targeting alpha3 glycine receptors. J Exp Med. 2012 Jun 4;209(6):1121–34. PubMed PMID: 22585736. Pubmed Central PMCID: 3371734.

[53] Harvey VL, Caley A, Muller UC, Harvey RJ, Dickenson AH. A selective role for alpha3 subunit glycine receptors in inflammatory pain. Front Mol Neurosci. 2009;2:14. PubMed PMID: 19915732. Pubmed Central PMCID: 2776487. Epub 2009/11/17. eng.

[54] Breitinger U, Breitinger HG. Augmentation of glycine receptor alpha3 currents suggests a mechanism for glucose-mediated analgesia. Neurosci Lett. 2016 Jan 26;612:110–5. PubMed PMID: 26656729.

[55] Motoyama N, Morita K, Kitayama T, Shiraishi S, Uezono Y, Nishimura F, et al. Pain-releasing action of platelet-activating factor (PAF) antagonists in neuropathic pain animal models and the mechanisms of action. Eur J Pain. 2013 Sep;17(8):1156–67. PubMed PMID: 23355413.

[56] Kallenborn-Gerhardt W, Lu R, Lorenz J, Gao W, Weiland J, Del Turco D, et al. Prolonged zymosan-induced inflammatory pain hypersensitivity in mice lacking glycine receptor alpha2. Behav Brain Res. 2012 Jan 1;226(1):106–11. PubMed PMID: 21924294.

[57] Becker L, von Wegerer J, Schenkel J, Zeilhofer HU, Swandulla D, Weiher H. Disease-specific human glycine receptor alpha1 subunit causes hyperekplexia phenotype and impaired glycine- and GABA(A)-receptor transmission in transgenic mice. J Neurosci. 2002 Apr 1;22(7):2505–12. PubMed PMID: 11923415.

[58] Xiong W, Cheng K, Cui T, Godlewski G, Rice KC, Xu Y, et al. Cannabinoid potentiation of glycine receptors contributes to cannabis-induced analgesia. Nat Chem Biol. 2011 May;7(5):296–303. PubMed PMID: 21460829. Pubmed Central PMCID: 3388539.

[59] Zhang JY, Gong N, Huang JL, Guo LC, Wang YX. Gelsemine, a principal alkaloid from Gelsemium sempervirens Ait., exhibits potent and specific antinociception in chronic

pain by acting at spinal alpha3 glycine receptors. Pain. 2013 Nov;154(11):2452–62. PubMed PMID: 23886522.

[60] Wells MM, Tillman TS, Mowrey DD, Sun T, Xu Y, Tang P. Ensemble-based virtual screening for cannabinoid-like potentiators of the human glycine receptor alpha1 for the treatment of pain. J Med Chem. 2015 Apr 9;58(7):2958–66. PubMed PMID: 25790278. Pubmed Central PMCID: 4414066.

[61] Molander A, Soderpalm B. Accumbal strychnine-sensitive glycine receptors: an access point for ethanol to the brain reward system. Alcohol Clin Exp Res. 2005 Jan;29(1):27–37. PubMed PMID: 15654288.

[62] Molander A, Soderpalm B. Glycine receptors regulate dopamine release in the rat nucleus accumbens. Alcohol Clin Exp Res. 2005 Jan;29(1):17–26. PubMed PMID: 15654287.

[63] Chau P, Hoifodt-Lido H, Lof E, Soderpalm B, Ericson M. Glycine receptors in the nucleus accumbens involved in the ethanol intake-reducing effect of acamprosate. Alcohol Clin Exp Res. 2009 Jan;34(1):39–45. PubMed PMID: 19860809. Epub 2009/10/29. eng.

[64] Adermark L, Clarke RB, Olsson T, Hansson E, Soderpalm B, Ericson M. Implications for glycine receptors and astrocytes in ethanol-induced elevation of dopamine levels in the nucleus accumbens. Addict Biol. 2010 Jan;16(1):43–54. PubMed PMID: 20331561. Epub 2010/03/25. eng.

[65] Li J, Nie H, Bian W, Dave V, Janak PH, Ye JH. Microinjection of glycine into the ventral tegmental area selectively decreases ethanol consumption. J Pharmacol Exp Ther. Epub 2012 Jan 11. Apr;341(1):196–204. doi: 10.1124/jpet.111.190058.

[66] Adermark L, Clarke RB, Soderpalm B, Ericson M. Ethanol-induced modulation of synaptic output from the dorsolateral striatum in rat is regulated by cholinergic interneurons. Neurochem Int. 2011 May;58(6):693–9. PubMed PMID: 21333709.

[67] Clarke RB, Adermark L, Chau P, Soderpalm B, Ericson M. Increase in nucleus accumbens dopamine levels following local ethanol administration is not mediated by acetaldehyde. Alcohol Alcohol. 2014 Sep–Oct;49(5):498–504. PubMed PMID: 25063803.

[68] Clarke RB, Soderpalm B, Lotfi A, Ericson M, Adermark L. Involvement of inhibitory receptors in modulating dopamine signaling and synaptic activity following acute ethanol exposure in striatal subregions. Alcohol Clin Exp Res. 2015 Dec;39(12):2364–74. PubMed PMID: 26614538.

[69] Li J, Nie H, Bian W, Dave V, Janak PH, Ye JH. Microinjection of glycine into the ventral tegmental area selectively decreases ethanol consumption. J Pharmacol Exp Ther. 2012 Apr;341(1):196–204. PubMed PMID: 22238211. Pubmed Central PMCID: 3310696.

[70] Blednov YA, Benavidez JM, Black M, Leiter CR, Osterndorff-Kahanek E, Harris RA. Glycine receptors containing alpha2 or alpha3 subunits regulate specific ethanol-

mediated behaviors. J Pharmacol Exp Ther. 2015 Apr;353(1):181–91. PubMed PMID: 25678534. Pubmed Central PMCID: 4366753.

[71] Blednov YA, Benavidez JM, Homanics GE, Harris RA. Behavioral characterization of knockin mice with mutations M287L and Q266I in the glycine receptor alpha1 subunit. J PharmacolExp Ther. 2012 Feb;340(2):317–29. PubMed PMID: 22037202. Pubmed Central PMCID: 3263963.

[72] Aguayo LG, Castro P, Mariqueo T, Munoz B, Xiong W, Zhang L, et al. Altered sedative effects of ethanol in mice with alpha1 glycine receptor subunits that are insensitive to Gbetagamma modulation. Neuropsychopharmacology. 2014 Oct;39(11):2538–48. PubMed PMID: 24801766. Pubmed Central PMCID: 4207329.

[73] Davies JS, Chung SK, Thomas RH, Robinson A, Hammond CL, Mullins JG, et al. The glycinergic system in human startle disease: a genetic screening approach. Front Mol Neurosci. 2010;3:8. PubMed PMID: 20407582. Pubmed Central PMCID: 2854534.

[74] Shiang R, Ryan SG, Zhu YZ, Hahn AF, O'Connell P, Wasmuth JJ. Mutations in the alpha 1 subunit of the inhibitory glycine receptor cause the dominant neurologic disorder, hyperekplexia. Nat Genet. 1993 Dec;5(4):351–8. PubMed PMID: 8298642.

[75] Harvey RJ, Topf M, Harvey K, Rees MI. The genetics of hyperekplexia: more than startle! Trends Genet. 2008 Sep;24(9):439–47. PubMed PMID: 18707791. Epub 2008/08/19. eng.

[76] James VM, Bode A, Chung SK, Gill JL, Nielsen M, Cowan FM, et al. Novel missense mutations in the glycine receptor beta subunit gene (GLRB) in startle disease. Neurobiol Dis. 2013 Apr;52:137–49. PubMed PMID: 23238346. Pubmed Central PMCID: 3581774.

[77] Hejazi N, Zhou C, Oz M, Sun H, Ye JH, Zhang L. {Delta}9-tetrahydrocannabinol and endogenous cannabinoid anandamide directly potentiate the function of glycine receptors. Mol Pharmacol. 2006 Mar;69(3):991–7. PubMed PMID: 16332990.

[78] Yang Z, Aubrey KR, Alroy I, Harvey RJ, Vandenberg RJ, Lynch JW. Subunit-specific modulation of glycine receptors by cannabinoids and N-arachidonyl-glycine. Biochem Pharmacol. 2008 Oct 15;76(8):1014–23. PubMed PMID: 18755158. Epub 2008/08/30. eng.

[79] Ahrens J, Demir R, Leuwer M, de la Roche J, Krampfl K, Foadi N, et al. The nonpsychotropic cannabinoid cannabidiol modulates and directly activates alpha-1 and alpha-1-Beta glycine receptor function. Pharmacology. 2009;83(4):217–22. PubMed PMID: 19204413.

[80] Delaney AJ, Esmaeili A, Sedlak PL, Lynch JW, Sah P. Differential expression of glycine receptor subunits in the rat basolateral and central amygdala. Neurosci Lett. 2009 Jan 22;469(2):237–42. PubMed PMID: 19995593. Epub 2009/12/10. eng.

[81] Yevenes GE, Zeilhofer HU. Molecular sites for the positive allosteric modulation of glycine receptors by endocannabinoids. PloS One. 2011;6(8):e23886. PubMed PMID: 21901142. Pubmed Central PMCID: 3162021.

[82] Xiong W1, Wu X, Li F, Cheng K, Rice KC, Lovinger DM, Zhang L. A common molecular basis for exogenous and endogenous cannabinoid potentiation of glycine receptors. J Neurosci. 2012; Sep 12;32(37):12979.

[83] Hejazi N, Zhou C, Oz M, Sun H, Ye JH, Zhang L. Delta9-tetrahydrocannabinol and endogenous cannabinoid anandamide directly potentiate the function of glycine receptors. Mol Pharmacol. 2006 Mar;69(3):991–7. PubMed PMID: 16332990.

[84] Huestis MA, Cone EJ. Relationship of Delta 9-tetrahydrocannabinol concentrations in oral fluid and plasma after controlled administration of smoked cannabis. J Anal Toxicol. 2004 Sep;28(6):394–9. PubMed PMID: 15516285.

[85] Lozovaya N, Yatsenko N, Beketov A, Tsintsadze T, Burnashev N. Glycine receptors in CNS neurons as a target for nonretrograde action of cannabinoids. J Neurosci. 2005 Aug 17;25(33):7499–506. PubMed PMID: 16107637.

[86] Xiong W, Wu X, Li F, Cheng K, Rice KC, Lovinger DM, et al. A common molecular basis for exogenous and endogenous cannabinoid potentiation of glycine receptors. J Neurosci. 2012 Apr 11;32(15):5200–8. PubMed PMID: 22496565. Pubmed Central PMCID: 3334839.

[87] Zimmer A, Zimmer AM, Hohmann AG, Herkenham M, Bonner TI. Increased mortality, hypoactivity, and hypoalgesia in cannabinoid CB1 receptor knockout mice. Proc Natl Acad Sci U S A. 1999 May 11;96(10):5780–5. PubMed PMID: 10318961. Pubmed Central PMCID: 21937.

[88] Bakker MJ, van Dijk JG, van den Maagdenberg AM, Tijssen MA. Startle syndromes. Lancet Neurol. 2006 Jun;5(6):513–24. PubMed PMID: 16713923. Epub 2006/05/23. eng.

[89] Christie MJ, Vaughan CW. Receptors: cannabis medicine without a high. Nat Chem Biol. 2011 May;7(5):249–50. PubMed PMID: 21502945. Epub 2011/04/20. eng.

[90] Ashton H. Guidelines for the rational use of benzodiazepines. When and what to use. Drugs. 1994 Jul;48(1):25–40. PubMed PMID: 7525193. Epub 1994/07/01. eng.

[91] Ye JH, Tao L, Ren J, Schaefer R, Krnjevic K, Liu PL, et al. Ethanol potentiation of glycine-induced responses in dissociated neurons of rat ventral tegmental area. Journal Pharmacol Exp Ther. 2001 Jan;296(1):77–83. PubMed PMID: 11123365.

[92] Sebe JY, Eggers ED, Berger AJ. Differential effects of ethanol on GABA(A) and glycine receptor-mediated synaptic currents in brain stem motoneurons. J Neurophysiol. 2003 Aug;90(2):870–5. PubMed PMID: 12702707.

Chapter 6

Dietary Omega-6/Omega-3 and Endocannabinoids: Implications for Brain Health and Diseases

Clémentine Bosch-Bouju and Sophie Layé

Additional information is available at the end of the chapter

http://dx.doi.org/10.5772/62498

Abstract

Omega-3 (ω-3) and omega-6 (ω-6) are polyunsaturated fatty acids (PUFAs) that play critical role in human health and have to be provided by food. In the brain, PUFAs are also precursors of endocannabinoids. The aim of this chapter is to review the existing literature on how dietary PUFAs impact on the endocannabinoid system in the brain and what are the consequences for brain function and dysfunction. In this chapter, we will first describe how PUFAs enter the brain, what are their metabolism processes and roles in brain function. We will describe the pathways from PUFAs to endocannabinoid production. Then, we will review the literature on how dietary ω-6/ω-3 ratio impacts the endocannabinoid system, in terms of endocannabinoid levels, proteins and endocannabinoid-dependent synaptic plasticity. In the next part, we will describe what we know about the interactions between PUFAs and endocannabinoids in neurological and neuropsychiatric disorders. Finally, we will conclude on the possible implications of the interactions between dietary PUFAs and endocannabinoids in the normal and pathological brain. In particular, we will discuss how dietary PUFAs, as homeostatic regulators of endocannabinoids, can constitute interesting therapeutic strategies for the prevention and/or treatment of neurological disorders with endocannabinoids impairment.

Keywords: brain, polyunsaturated fatty acids, endocannabinoids, omega-3, synaptic plasticity

1. Introduction

Polyunsaturated fatty acids (PUFAs) are essential constituents of plasma membranes and depending on their chemical structure, PUFAs are of the n-3 or the n-6 family and are commonly called ω-3 or ω-6, respectively. In addition, PUFAs are precursors of an almost infinite variety of metabolites, and endocannabinoids are part of them. In particular, anandamide and 2-arachidonoylglycerol (2-AG), the two major endocannabinoids in the brain, are directly derived from arachidonic acid (ARA), the more abundant ω-6 PUFA in the brain. Interestingly, other endocannabinoids are derived from ω-3 PUFA, but their role in the brain remains elusive.

Amount of ω-3 and ω-6 PUFAs provided by food has direct consequences on their bioavailability and it has been established that the ideal ratio in the diet is of about 5:1 of ω-6:ω-3 PUFAs precursors. However, our modern diet is hugely unbalanced with an estimated average ratio of 20:1 [1]. The dietary deficit in ω-3 PUFAs has been associated with numerous diseases, and it becomes evident that imbalance of ω-3/ω-6 PUFAs in the brain is linked to several neurological and neuropsychiatric disorders [2, 3].

One possible mechanism for the involvement of dietary PUFAs in brain health is its role in modulating the endocannabinoid system. Indeed, bioavailability of ω-6 and ω-3 PUFAs modulates brain endocannabinoids: an increase in dietary ω-6 PUFAs is associated with increased levels of anandamide and 2-AG [4–6]. In this context, our group recently demonstrated that developmental ω-3 PUFA deficiency in mice abolishes the endocannabinoid-dependent synaptic plasticity and associated signaling pathways [7, 8]. This was the first evidence that a change in dietary precursors can have a strong impact on the outcome of the endocannabinoid system. Endocannabinoids are thus in a unique position to link food lipids and synaptic activity and our working hypothesis is that the effects of dietary ω-6/ω-3 PUFAs on brain function are mediated by their modulatory actions on the endocannabinoid system.

In this chapter, PUFAs entry in the brain and metabolism linking PUFAs to endocannabinoids production will be described. Then, how dietary ω-6/ω-3 PUFAs impact on the functioning of endocannabinoid system will be reviewed. In the third part, what is known about the interactions between PUFAs and endocannabinoids in neurological and neuropsychiatric disorders will be described. Finally, we will conclude on the possible implications of the interactions between PUFAs and endocannabinoids in the brain.

2. PUFAs in the brain: metabolism and function

2.1. Entry of PUFAs in the brain and metabolism

The main PUFAs present in the brain are arachidonic acid (ARA, 20:4n-6) and docosahexaenoic acid (DHA, 22:6n-3). These two long-chain PUFAs can be directly provided by food, or metabolized from dietary precursors in the liver (**Figure 1**). Blood ARA and DHA enter the brain, probably by a free diffusion across the cell membranes of the blood–brain barrier, even active transporters may exist [3, 9–12] (**Figure 1**). Once in the brain, active processes preserve ARA and DHA in high concentrations and degrade or recycle the other types of PUFAs [13]. Some evidence also suggest active transporters with specificity for some PUFAs to regulate the levels of each PUFA in the brain [14–18].

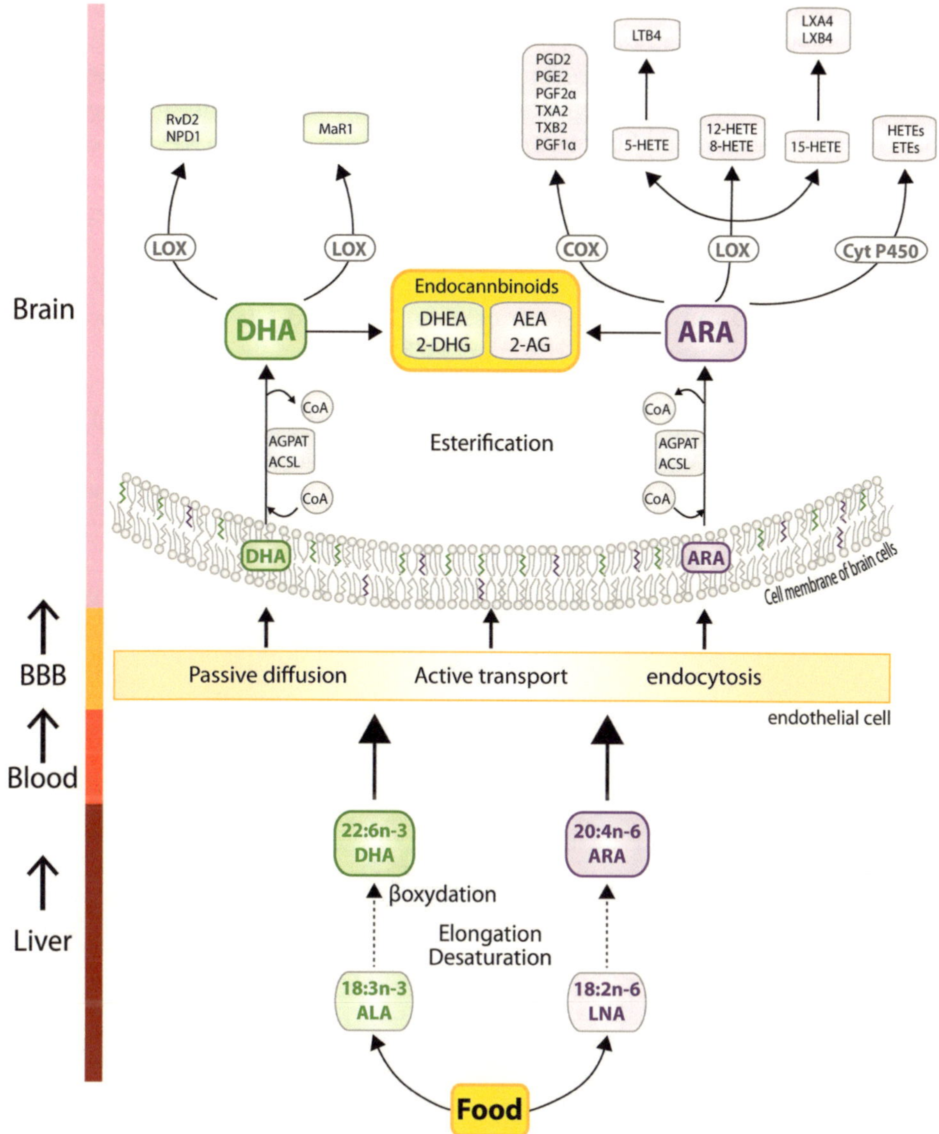

Figure 1. From PUFAs synthesis to PUFAs derivates in the brain. Precursors of ω-6 and ω-3 fatty acids are provided by food (bottom). They are metabolized in the liver into more unsaturated and elongated fatty acids (long-chain PUFAs) through successive elongation and desaturation. Long chain PUFAs, ARA (20:4n-6) and DHA (22:6n-3), then enter the brain *via* the blood and the blood–brain barrier (BBB), successively. Delivery into the brain can be made through free diffusion, active transport with specific transporters, or *via* endocytosis into the BBB endothelial cells. Once in the brain, PUFAs are esterified in phospholipids of cell membranes. When released from the membrane they are metabolized in endocannabinoids or in multiple derivates with COX, LOX and Cytochrome P450 enzymes. ALA (18:3n-3), alpha linoleic acid; LNA (18:2n-6), linolenic acid; AGPAT, 1-acylglycerol-3-phosphate-O-acyltransferase; ACSL, long-chain-fatty-acid-CoA synthase; RvD2, resolving D2; NPD1, neuroprotectin D1; Mar1, maresin 1; PGD2, prostaglandin D2; PGE2, prostaglandin E2; PGF2a, prostaglandin F2a; TXA2, thromboxane A2; TXB2, thromboxane B2; PGF1a, prostaglandin F1a; LTB4, leukotriene B4; HETE, hydroxyeicosatetraenoic acid; LXA4, lipoxin A4; LXB4, lipoxin B4; ETE, ecosatetraenoic acid.

PUFAs are constituent of plasma membranes and they accumulate into brain cells phospholipids predominantly during brain development [19]. This means that the PUFA composition of membranes in the brain is predominantly determined during cerebral development, which raises the importance of adequate ARA and DHA dietary supply during perinatal periods. At adult age, ARA and DHA supply in the brain is mainly to recycle existing pools used for PUFA metabolites and it is estimated that in humans half-life of ARA is five months, compared to two years for DHA [20]. Accordingly, it has been estimated that the brain needs 18 mg/day of ARA and 4 mg/day of DHA. Even if the developmental period is crucial for PUFAs accretion in brain membranes and therefore composition, changes in the diet or in the metabolism of PUFAs can alter the ratio between ARA and DHA at adulthood. This is particularly true in some neurological disorders such as depression, schizophrenia, Alzheimer disease or Parkinson's disease [3, 21], where the organism is not able to buffer PUFAs concentrations. In regard to the endocannabinoid system, dietary PUFAs levels have profound consequences because PUFAs are the precursors of brain endocannabinoids (**Figure 2**). In animal models fed three to four months with a diet deficient in ω-3 PUFAs, the amount of DHA in the brain is reduced by 30% [7, 8, 22–26], with a consequence on endocannabinoid system (see part 3b and **Figure 3**).

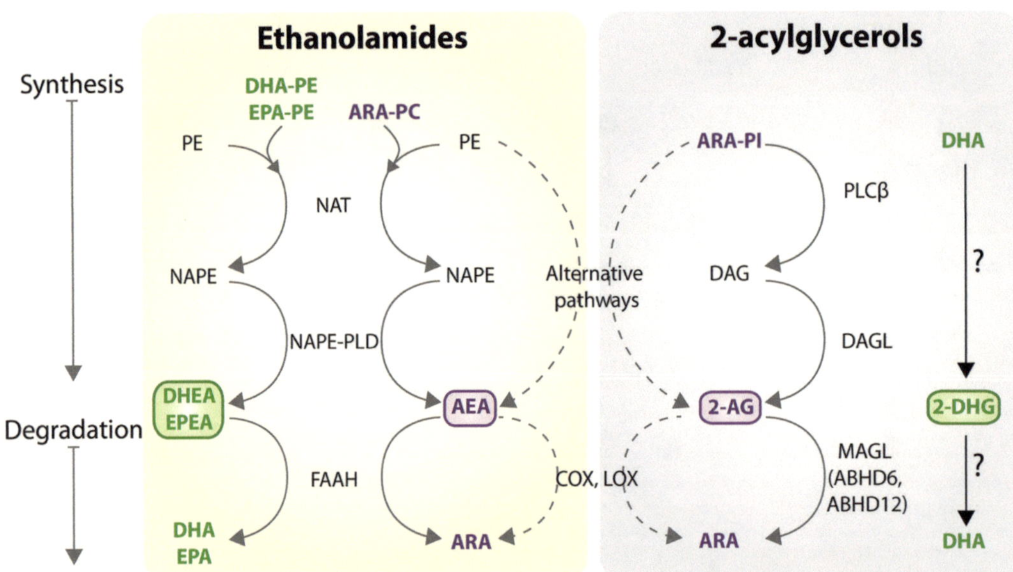

Figure 2. Metabolic pathways of the two families of endocannabinoids, ethanolamides and 2-acylglycerols. Ethanolamides are produced from PUFAs by an enzymatic pathway involving NAT and NAPE-PLD. FAAH is the main enzyme responsible for ethanolamides degradation. 2-acylglycerols are produced from PUFAs by a successive action of PLCβ and DAGL. MAGL is the main enzyme of 2-acylglycerols degradation, but ABHD6 and ABHD12 are also important degradation enzymes. For both families of endocannabinoids, alternative production pathways exist, but their characteristics and importance remain to be established. COX and LOX are other enzymes able to degrade endocannabinoids, by oxydation of their PUFA part. Synthesis and degradation pathway for 2-DHG remain mostly unknown. PE, phosphatidylethanolamine; PI, phosphatidylinositol. For 2-DHG, '?' indicates that no data exists in the literature about its metabolic pathway.

http://dx.doi.org/10.5772/62498

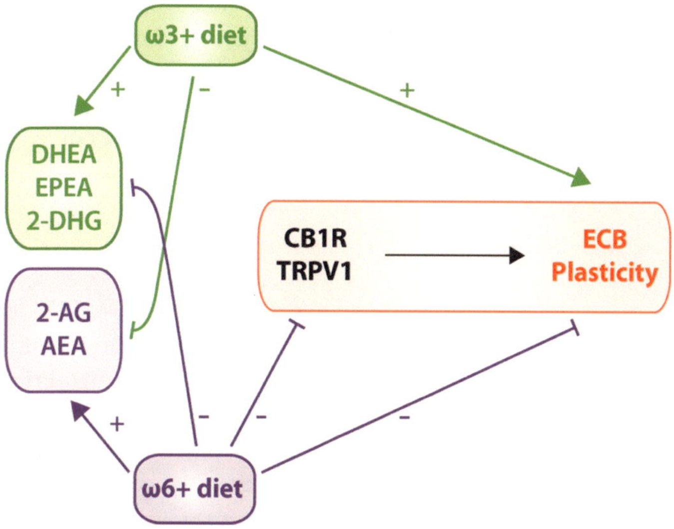

Figure 3. Effects of dietary PUFAs on endocannabinoid-dependent plasticity. In the brain of rodents fed with a diet rich in ω-6 PUFAs, 2-AG and AEA levels are increased, while ω-3-derived endocannabinoids (DHEA, EPEA and 2-DHG) are decreased. In addition, ω-6 rich diet impairs endocannabinoid plasticity and CB1 receptor (CB1R) activity. Conversely, a diet rich in ω-3 and especially DHA and/or EPA, increases levels of ω-3-derived endocannabinoids and decreases levels of 2-AG and AEA. An ω-3 rich diet positively impacts on synaptic plasticity, but the precise mechanisms remain to be determined.

Once into the brain PUFAs do not stay free in the medium, they are immediately esterified to phospholipids by specific enzymes (Figure 1). When associated to phospholipids, PUFAs play important role in the structure of membranes, by determining its curveting and flexibility [27, 28]. More importantly, PUFAs can be released by phospholipase enzymes to be metabolized by cyclooxygenase (COX) / lipoxygenase (LOX) pathways in a huge variety of derivates [3, 29–31] (**Figure 1**). These derivates are mainly involved in neuroinflammatory processes and the classical picture is that derivates from ω-6 PUFAs, in particular ARA, are pro-inflammatory whereas ω-3 PUFAs derivates, mainly EPA (ecosapentaenoic acid) and DHA, are anti-inflammatory and pro-resolutive factors. The main enzymes involved in these processes are COX, LOX and cytochrome P450 [3, 29–31]. In the brain, it is still unclear whether neurons and/or glial cells are the main cellular type involved in the production of PUFA derivates with pro or anti-inflammatory activities. Apart of inflammatory derivates, PUFAs are also precursors of endocannabinoids and this is the object of the present review (see part 2c).

2.2. Functions of PUFAs in the brain

2.2.1. Synaptic effects of PUFAs

There are various means by which PUFAs can influence synaptic function. First, as structural elements of plasma membranes, PUFAs can modulate the dynamic of membranes [27, 28, 32] and thus the functionality and traffic of transmembrane and membrane-associated proteins. These proteins are very numerous at both pre- and post-synapses (receptors, transporters, ion channels ...) and are essential for the function of the synapse. Second, PUFAs and/or their derivates are agonists of receptors with synaptic functions. This mode of action of PUFAs is very complex and hardly understood, therefore still being an intense research topic [3]. Third, PUFAs are precursors of endocannabinoids, which are lipid mediators with essential functions in neurotransmission and synaptic plasticity [33]. This will be largely developed in parts 3 and 4.

2.2.2. *Role of PUFAs in neurogenesis and neuroprotection*

DHA has positive effects on neuronal survival and neurogenesis [34, 35]. However, underlying mechanisms remain poorly understood. Interestingly, it has been recently discovered that synaptamide, an endocannabinoid derivate of DHA, play an important role in cellular growing and differentiation in the brain during development [36]. Neuroprotectin D1 (NPD1) is another derivate from DHA that protects against neuronal death by triggering the synthesis of anti-apoptotic proteins [37, 38]. It is also known that DHA stimulates neuronal survival by inducing the synthesis of BDNF (brain-derived neurotrophic factor) [39]. These positive effects could explain the potential benefit of DHA supplementation in neurodegenerative disorders [21, 40], but this needs to be further explored.

2.2.3. *Role of PUFAs in neuroinflammation*

As previously mentioned, PUFAs are precursors of an infinite variety of derivates, preferentially pro-inflammatory for ARA derivates and anti-inflammatory for DHA and EPA derivates (**Figure 1**). As a consequence, a diet rich in DHA in humans is associated with a decreased risk of developing neurological disorders with an inflammatory component, such as Alzheimer's disease or depression [41–43]. In animal models, our laboratory demonstrated that neuroinflammatory processes are over-activated in the brain of mice fed a diet deficient for ω-3 PUFAs [26, 44]. Conversely, ω-3 PUFA brain enrichment protects against deleterious effects of inflammation on cognitive performances [24, 45, 46]

3. PUFAs are precursors of endocannabinoids

Endocannabinoids are defined as endogenous lipids able to activate CB1 or CB2 cannabinoid receptors. The two major endocannabinoids described in the organism are 2-AG and anandamide (AEA). They are part of two families of endocannabinoids, 2-acylglycerols for 2-AG, and ethanolamides for AEA (**Figure 2**), but all species in these families are not ligand of cannabinoid receptors. AEA and 2-AG are the two species with the highest affinity for CB1 and CB2, and their role in neuronal plasticity has been thoroughly demonstrated [33, 47]. These two canonical endocannabinoids are derived from the ω-6 PUFA ARA and most of studies have focused on these endocannabinoids. However, more and more studies are highlighting the role of ω-3-derived endocannabinoids. These species are agonists of CB1 and CB2 receptors, but their role in neuroplasticity is yet to be unraveled.

http://dx.doi.org/10.5772/62498

Briefly, there is a two-step process to form endocannabinoids from phospholipids. Endocannabinoids are made on-demand and they are rapidly degraded, back into PUFAs or oxydized into active metabolites. Interestingly, degradation enzymes are more numerous and more active than production enzymes of endocannabinoids, suggesting that endocannabinoids are highly regulated and never stay for long at the synapse [48]. This may be explained by the fast desensitization of CB1 receptor. Endocannabinoid system thus appears as a highly dynamic and regulated system.

Here, we will describe the canonical pathways for endocannabinoids production and degradation at the synapse. However, these canonical are still under debate, especially because the importance of secondary pathways is unknown [49].

3.1. 2-AG metabolism

The first step of 2-AG formation is the hydrolysis by a phospholipase C (PLC) enzyme of a phosphatidylinositol (PI) containing an ARA PUFA. In postsynaptic neurons, it is mainly the PLCβ that is involved in this process because it is activated by $G_{q/11}$-coupled receptors, such as group I metabotropic glutamate receptors or acetylcholine receptors [48, 50–52]. The product of this reaction is ARA-containing diacylglycerol (DAG). This DAG is then the substrate of a DAG-lipase enzyme (DAGL) that hydrolyzes the DAG into 2-AG (removal of the acyl group) (**Figure 2**). DAGL enzyme has two isoforms, DAGLα and DAGLβ and it is likely that DAGLα is the main enzyme responsible for the formation of 2-AG in the brain. Indeed, DAGLα is spatially close to PLCβ, and DAGLα-deficient but not DAGLβ-deficient mice display a strong reduction in 2-AG brain levels [53, 54].

Once it is formed, 2-AG exerts its action by targeting CB1 receptors on presynaptic neurons or CB2 receptors on glial cells surrounding the synapse (microglia and astrocyte). 2-AG is thus a retrograde messenger that is released from the post-synapse into the synaptic cleft. The question of an active transporter for 2-AG has been densely investigated but up to now, there is no identified transporter for 2-AG [55]. The most likely hypothesis at present is that DAGL enzyme is responsible for release of 2-AG in the synaptic cleft.

Once 2-AG binds to CB1 and/or CB2 receptors, it is rapidly processed for degradation by the enzyme MAGL (monoacylglycerol lipase) (**Figure 2**). The MAGL enzyme is present in postsynaptic astro-glial compartments [56–58] and it hydrolyzes 2-AG to form ARA and glycerol. There is some redundancy in degradation enzymes for 2-AG because ABHD6 (Abhydrolase domain containe protein 6) and ABHD12 can also hydrolyze 2-AG [48, 56]. Degradation of 2-AG can also be performed by its oxygenation with COX and LOX enzymes, which produces PUFA derivates with bioactive functions [59–61] (**Figure 2**).

3.2. AEA metabolism

Metabolism of AEA follows a similar process as 2-AG. First, the N-acyltransferase enzyme (NAT) uses the ARA of a phosphatidylcholine (PC) and a phosphatidylethanolamine (PE) to form a N-acyl-phosphatidylethanolamine product (NAPE) (**Figure 2**). Anandamide production is triggered by calcium entry into the cell, since the NAT enzyme is activated by calcium [62]. Sources of calcium can be diverse, mainly NMDA receptor and voltage-gated calcium channels, or alternatively release from intracellular stores. Interestingly this calcium-dependent NAT remains molecularly uncharacterized [48], which reflects the gaps in the literature that exist concerning the endocannabinoid system. The NAPE formed is then hydrolyzed in AEA by a NAPE-phospholipase D enzyme (NAPE-PLD) (**Figure 2**). Here again, this enzyme is not well characterized and many questions remain about its activity, regulation and localization [48].

Transport of AEA is better characterized than 2-AG transport, but it is still largely under debate. A FLAT transporter (fatty acid amide hydrolase-like anandamide transporter) has been discovered recently for intracellular transport of AEA [63], but a study published one year later contradicts its putative role [64]. It is thus too soon to conclude clearly on this point [49, 55]. In addition, recent studies revealed that the preferred target of AEA in the brain may be postsynaptic TRPV1 (transient receptor potential vallinoid 1) channels and not necessarily presynaptic receptors. It is thus possible that AEA does not need to travel the synaptic cleft but may act directly by travelling through the plasma membrane to activate intracellular postsynaptic TRPV1 receptors. TRPV channels are vallinoid receptors involved in nociception that are primarily activated by capsaicin [65–67]. In the brain, AEA appears as a potent agonist of TRPV1 and its role in endocannabinoid-dependent synaptic plasticity has been demonstrated [33, 68–70].

The main enzyme responsible for degradation of AEA is FAAH (fatty acid amide hydrolase) which produces an ethanolamine and an ARA PUFA (**Figure 2**). FAAH is situated in the intracellular compartment and is bound to membranes, which can modulate the access of AEA to its degradation enzyme [71]. Drugs targeting the FAAH enzyme have been extensively studied for the treatment of endocannabinoids-related disorders, such as anxiety, depression, inflammation or neuropathic pain [72]. However, pharmaceutics are struggling to find a compound with high efficiency and low side effects, which may be due to chronic effects of FAAH inhibition that differ from acute effects [73, 74] (**Figure 2**).

Contrarily to 2-AG, there is no known other enzyme for degradation of AEA, except COX and LOX enzymes that can oxygenate the ARA group of AEA to form bioactive derivates of ARA [59–61].

3.3. Alternative production pathways

One of the reasons for the complexity of the endocannabinoid system and its study is the existence of multiple alternative enzymatic pathways. Transgenic mice constitute a good tool to investigate the redundancy of a protein. Mice deficient for DAGLα have a strong decrease in 2-AG levels, while mice deficient for MAGL display very high levels of 2-AG [48, 53, 75]. This suggests that redundancy for 2-AG synthesis and degradation is not the majority. Conversely, mice deficient for NAPE-PLD have elevated levels of NAPE, but there is almost no change in AEA levels [48, 76, 77]. This suggests that NAPE-PLD is the main pathway to hydrolyze NAPE but that robust redundant mechanisms do exist to form AEA. However, these secondary mechanisms have not yet been discovered. Apart from these studies, other pathways have been described to form and degrade endocannabinoids [49]. For example, 2-

http://dx.doi.org/10.5772/62498

AG can be formed by hydrolysis of lyso-PI by phospholipase 1 enzyme [48]. However, the physiological significance of these secondary pathways has yet to be unraveled.

3.4. Endocannabinoids derived from ω-3 PUFAs

In the brain, 2-AG and AEA are the canonical endocannabinoids but other bioactive lipids derived from ω-3 PUFAs are ligand of CB1 and CB2 receptors. The two main ω-3 PUFAs described in the literature are ethanolamides derived from DHA, called DHEA (N-Docosahexaenoyl ethanolamine), and from EPA, called EPEA (N-Eicosapentaenoyl ethanolamine). Endocannabinoids EPEA and DHEA are present in the brain in concentrations about two fold higher compared to AEA [78], but their binding affinity for CB1 and CB2 receptors is probably lower [79, 80]. EPEA and DHEA share the exact same pathways of production as AEA, except that NAT enzyme uses respectively the EPA or the DHA group of a phosphatidylethanolamine to form the NAPE product (**Figure 2**). The ω-3-derived endocannabinoids also follow the degradation pathways of AEA, with FAAH as the main degradation enzyme, and there is the possibility for DHEA and EPEA to be oxidized by COX and LOX enzymes (**Figure 2**).

As discussed in parts 4 and 5, dietary ω-6/ω-3 ratio directly modulates the proportion of ethanolamides derived from ω-6 and ω-3, but the role of ω-3 derived endocannabinoids remains elusive. One issue that faces researchers to study the role of ω-3-derived endocannabinoids is that they share exactly the same enzymatic pathways as AEA. It is thus currently not possible to precisely target their synthesis or degradation.

So far, the role of DHEA has been demonstrated in neuronal development and synaptogenesis [36, 81, 82], but its effect is likely independent of activation of cannabinoid receptors. It exists other ethanolamides derived from monounsaturated fatty acids (such as N-oleoyl amide derived from oleic acid). They don't bind to CB1 or CB2 receptors, but they can have cannabimimetic activities. It has been suggested that these ethanolamides could serve as 'entourage molecules' to modulate the signaling of AEA [59]. Finally the ω-3 derived endocannabinoid 2-docosahexanoylglycerol (2-DHG) is sometimes evoked in the literature [83, 84], but there is a crucial lack of data about the enzymatic pathways and the binding affinity of this bioactive lipid (**Figure 2**).

4. Impact of dietary ω-6/ω-3 on the endocannabinoid system

4.1. What do we know from research at the periphery

At the periphery, endocannabinoids receptors are mostly present in adipose tissue, immune system, musculoskeletal system, gonads and cardiovascular system. All of these compartments are also regulated by dietary PUFAs. Because PUFAs are precursors of endocannabinoids, the effect of dietary PUFAs on endocannabinoids in these compartments has been relatively well documented [85–92]. Consistently, it appears that increasing dietary ω-6 PUFAs does increase levels of ARA-derived endocannabinoids in the organism (**Figure 3**). Conversely, diets enriched in ω-3 decreases ARA-derived endocannabinoids (AEA and 2-AG) while it increases levels of endocannabinoids derived from ω-3 PUFAs, namely DHEA and EPEA (**Figure 3**). However, studies have rarely investigated the functional consequences of this link between dietary PUFAs and levels of endocannabinoids. There is a strong hypothesis that beneficial effects of ω-3 supplementation pass through an effect on the endocannabinoid system, but it has never been directly tested.

In details, the impact of dietary PUFA on endocannabinoids has been investigated in the context of obesity. Indeed, activation of CB1 receptors in adipose tissue increases food intake and increases the creation of new adipocytes [93]. Endocannabinoids are thus a target to treat obesity [94]. Rimonabant, an antagonist of CB1 receptors, has been used in overweighed patients to reduce their food intake, with very positive results. However, strong side effects on mood for some patients lead to the withdrawal of rimonabant from the market. In this context, dietary PUFAs appeared as homeostatic regulators of endocannabinoids [95], encouraging researchers to investigate the effect of ω-3 rich diet on obesity. It has been shown that a diet rich in ω-3 leads to weight loss, in parallel to a decrease of AEA and 2-AG [88, 93]. Interestingly, a high fat diet rich in ω-3 does not induce weight gain, while a low fat diet rich in ω-6 increases weight gain [89, 90, 96]. These evidence suggest that dietary PUFAs act on fat formation and thus on weight gain *via* the endocannabinoid system. This hypothesis has been reinforced by a study showing that blockade of CB1 receptor (with rimonabant) blocks weight gain induced by high fat diet [96]. However, evidence remains indirect and we can hardly conclude that the endocannabinoid system is the only pathway by which dietary PUFAs influence weight gain and adipose tissue formation.

Inflammation is another component of obesity that can be modulated by endocannabinoids and PUFAs. Endocannabinoids are homeostatic regulator of the immune system and their oxydized metabolites (directly derived from PUFAs) can have a direct role in inflammation [97]. In parallel, the role of PUFAs on inflammation is well documented [98, 99]. Globally, we can summarize that ω-6 PUFAs, such as ARA, are metabolized in pro-inflammatory derivates while ω-3 PUFAs, such as DHA and EPA, are metabolized in anti-inflammatory and pro-resolution derivates [3, 29–31]. PUFAs play thus a central role in the immune response of the organism. However, very little is known about the interactions between PUFAs and endocannabinoids in the peripheral immune system.

Concerning the musculoskeletal compartment, evidence exists for a correlation between dietary ω-6/ω-3 ratio and levels of ARA- and ω-3-derived endocannabinoids [91, 100, 101]. More interestingly, addition of free ω-3 in the culture medium of osteoblastes changes the level of proteins of the endocannabinoid system: CB2 receptors and NAPE-PLD [101]. Moreover, a diet enriched with DHA for 2 to 4 months increases expression of CB1 and CB2 receptors in muscles, and it favors glucose uptake by the muscle and not by the adipose tissue [91]. It thus appears that in the musculoskeletal system, dietary PUFAs could affect not only endocannabinoid levels, but also the regulation of the proteins of the endocannabinoid system.

In the field of cardiovascular health, it is recognized that both endocannabinoids and ω-3 PUFAs have beneficial effects [102, 103], but the link between endocannabinoids and PUFAs has never been investigated to our knowledge. Of note, we found one review paper suggesting that ω-3-derived endocannabinoids could be beneficial for heart function [102], but this hypothesis remain to be tested.

Finally, there is an emerging role of endocannabinoids in gonadic function and more largely in the control of fertility [104–106]. Endocannabinoids and associated receptors are present in female and male gonads and they play a role of fertility signal in the reproduction cycle. In addition, endocannabinoids can regulate gonadic hormones [106]. As a consequence, an aberrant endocannabinoid signaling impairs fertility at all stages [104]. In parallel, PUFAs also play important role in fertility and especially in function of spermatozoa. Indeed, testis and sperm are very rich in DHA and the high concentration of PUFAs —DHA in particular— is necessary for optimal motility and thus fertility of germ cells [92, 107, 108]. It is suggested that PUFAs are necessary to sperm function due to their role in membrane fluidity, however, the hypothesis that PUFAs play a role in sperm fertility *via* their endocannabinoids metabolites has not yet been explored clearly.

Generally, we can conclude from these studies that modulating dietary PUFAs inevitably modulates levels of endocannabinoids in the organism. In addition, it often emerges from these studies the idea that it exists 'good endocannabinoids' and 'bad endocannabinoids'. In this concept, ARA-derived endocannabinoids need to be down-regulated in pathological states (obesity, inflammation, etc.), and a diet rich in ω-3 decreases the levels of ARA-derived endocannabinoids (the 'bad' one), in favor to ω-3-derived endocannabinoids (the 'good' one). This appealing hypothesis needs to be studied because the presence of ω-3-derived endocannabinoids in the organism is known, but their function remains to be fully investigated.

4.2. Impact of dietary ω-6/ω3 PUFAs on endocannabinoid levels in the brain

Similar to studies at the periphery, dietary ω-6 PUFAs increases levels of 2-AG and AEA in the brain (is this where levels are increased?), while dietary ω-3 PUFAs increases levels of ω-3-derived endocannabinoids (**Figure 3**). Specifically in the brain, a first study in 2001 compared diets with or without PUFAs on ethanolamides, without distinguishing ω-3 and ω-6 [4]. In this study, three weeks of diet deficient for PUFAs was enough to reduce levels of ethanolamides in piglet brains. Interestingly, levels of ethanolamides were strongly affected in brainstem, cerebellum, visual cortex and striatum, while they were unaffected in visual cortex and hippocampus. Two years later, another study focused on ω-3 PUFAs content of the diet and its impact on 2-AG in mouse brain [5]. In this study, analysis was done on mice fed with one or the other diet for two generations. As expected, brain levels of 2-AG were increased by a diet rich in ω-6 and they were decreased by a diet rich in ω-3. More interestingly, DHA brain levels were modified by the diet, while ARA, the precursor of 2-AG remained perfectly stable. Indeed, consistently in the literature, ARA levels are hardly modified by PUFAs content of the diet, while DHA brain levels are easily correlated to dietary ω-6/ω-3. This suggests that ARA levels in the brain are highly controlled to maintain homeostasis and increase in 2-AG and AEA following ω-6 rich diet could be one way of buffering ARA concentrations. More recently, a dietary experiment has been conducted on rats with only one week of diet at adult age and no difference has been found compared to the control diet [6]. Another study with two weeks of DHA-rich diet showed increased levels of DHEA and decreased levels of AEA, without changes on 2-AG levels [78].

These studies confirm that dietary PUFAs modulate levels of endocannabinoids in the brain, as well as in the periphery. However, the function of the endocannabinoid system in the brain depends also on the ability of the signaling machinery to trigger the appropriate production of endocannabinoids, on the functionality of the receptors, and on the function of degradation enzymes.

4.3. Impact of dietary ω-6/ω3 PUFAs on proteins of the endocannabinoid system

Very little is known about modifications of the endocannabinoid system in the brain due to dietary PUFAs. A recent study examined the impact of ω-3 deficient diet on enzymes implicated in the metabolism of PUFAs, but not concerning directly the endocannabinoid system [22]. In this study, 15 weeks of ω-3 deficient diet modified the levels of phospholipases A2 and COX enzymes, to favor degradation of ARA and reduce the metabolism of DHA. This suggests that imbalanced PUFAs content in the diet are compensated by enzymatic processes in the brain, but the question remains open for enzymes of the endocannabinoid system. One study reported that DHA supplementation increases levels of CB1 and TRPV1, in terms of mRNA expression and protein levels [109] (**Figure 3**). Recently, our laboratory demonstrated that a dietary ω-3 deficiency from gestation induces a desensitization of the CB1 receptor [7, 8] (**Figure 3**). We hypothesize that this is due to high levels of 2-AG and AEA produced by developmental ω-3 deficiency, but this remains to be fully investigated. Our results have been reinforced by a recent study showing that a diet with 5% krill oil (rich in EPA and DHA) given for six weeks to adult mice enhanced the activity of CB1 receptor [110]. It is known that the CB1 receptor can be easily desensitized and internalized by its ligand [111]. This has been particularly studied in the context of chronic cannabinoid consumption to decipher the mechanisms of addiction. Mechanisms of desensitization and downregulation are not totally elucidated but they probably involve phosphorylation of the receptor and transcription of immediate early genes [112, 113]. Interestingly, CB1 receptors do not desensitize at the same rate, depending on the brain structure [113]. Studies on the role of dietary PUFAs on CB1 receptors demonstrate that dietary PUFAs can constitute another powerful mechanism for regulation of the functionality of the CB1 receptor.

4.4. Impact of dietary ω-6/ω-3 PUFAs on endocannabinoid-dependent synaptic plasticity

In the brain, synaptic plasticity is the main measurable outcome of the functionality of the endocannabinoid system. Indeed, endocannabinoids act to reduce the synaptic efficacy, at very short, medium, or long periods of time, depending on the signaling pathways that trigger endocannabinoid production. As we described above, endocannabinoids are produced on-demand *via* activation of specific enzymes depending on the endocannabinoid produced [33]. Released endocannabinoids then activate receptors, which leads to a decrease of efficacy of the synaptic transmission [33]. Importantly, endocannabinoids are rapidly degraded and released PUFAs are re-esterified at the membrane, to precisely regulate duration of endocannabinoid action [27]. This general principle of action of endocannabinoid at the synapse is

http://dx.doi.org/10.5772/62498

developed in a wide variety of mechanisms, depending on the structure and the triggering event, and it induces plasticity phenomenon lasting for seconds to hours [33, 56, 114] but always in the direction of a decrease of synaptic efficacy. Very recent studies suggest that endocannabinoids can also act to increase synaptic efficacy [115, 116], but mechanisms remain unclear so it can be an indirect consequence of an endocannabinoid activation.

Some studies have investigated the link between dietary PUFAs and synaptic plasticity [44, 82, 117, 118]. It appears that ω-3 PUFA dietary deficiency impairs glutamatergic synaptic transmission and plasticity [44, 82, 117, 119, 120], whereas DHA-rich diet can prevent loss of synaptic plasticity induced by prenatal ethanol exposure [118] (**Figure 3**). Apart from these studies, only one study from our laboratory precisely investigated the impact of dietary PUFAs on the endocannabinoid-dependent synaptic plasticity [7]. This study demonstrated that developmental dietary ω-3 PUFA deficiency abolishes the endocannabinoid-dependent synaptic plasticity in the prefrontal cortex and in the nucleus accumbens [7]. This is the first evidence that a change in dietary precursors can have a strong impact on the outcome of the endocannabinoid system. Following this study, we investigated the impact of developmental dietary ω-3 PUFA deficiency on endocannabinoid-dependent synaptic plasticity in the hippocampus. We demonstrated that ω-3 PUFA deficiency strongly impaired the endocannabinoid-dependent heterosynaptic plasticity at GABAergic synapses, which prevents the induction of plasticity at glutamatergic synapses (Thomazeau, Bosch-Bouju, Manzoni and Layé, article accepted at Cerebral Cortex). Conversely, another ongoing study from our team shows that ω-3 PUFA-rich diet maintains endocannabinoid-dependent Hebbian plasticity in the nucleus accumbens following a chronic social defeat stress. Mechanistically, it is still unclear how dietary PUFAs impact on endocannabinoid plasticity. As evoked above, dietary PUFAs can change levels of endocannabinoids. This could impact on the endocannabinoid system and notably on the CB1 receptor that easily desensitizes. Along with this hypothesis, we demonstrated in our recent study that the loss of plasticity following ω-3 PUFA deficiency was due to a loss of functionality of the CB1 receptor, by its uncoupling from the Gi protein [7, 8] (**Figure 3**).

Other hypotheses need to be explored to better understand the impact of dietary PUFAs on endocannabinoid plasticity. Notably, it is suggested that endocannabinoid signaling is sensitive to the lipid environment, namely, the levels of lipid rafts in the membrane [121–123]. Lipid rafts are high density domains rich in sphingolipids and cholesterol [124]. It has been proposed that synapses are especially enriched in lipid rafts and that these microdomains are necessary to maintain synapses and allow protein trafficking [125]. At the opposite of lipid rafts are DHA-rich domains; they are thin, 'leaky', dynamic and flexible [126]. This is notably due to the high flexibility of DHA. High density lipid rafts and low-density DHA-domains are competing permanently. It is suggested that lipid rafts are initially small nanodomains that organize together to form bigger domains, of the microscale. In this configuration, the organization of lipid rafts would be controlled by DHA, which aggregates nanodomains together or conversely disrupt large lipid rafts [126–128]. We can thus hypothesize that dietary PUFAs modulate the endocannabinoid plasticity in the brain by playing on the fine structure of plasma membranes.

5. Dietary ω-6/ω-3 PUFAs and the endocannabinoid system: implication for neurological disorders

Studying the impact of dietary PUFAs on brain endocannabinoids is of interest in the context of brain disorders. It exists dense literature about the role of dietary PUFAs on brain health, and endocannabinoids are implicated in numerous brain diseases. However, the link between dietary PUFAs and endocannabinoids in the context of brain disorders has been only rarely investigated.

5.1. PUFAs / endocannabinoids interactions in mood and anxiety disorders

On one hand, dietary PUFAs appear to be determinant for the regulation of mood and anxiety disorders. In humans, the risk of developing depression is associated with low content of ω-3 in the diet [129], and patients with mood and/or anxiety disorders have lower levels of ω-3 in the blood and in the brain, compared to healthy subjects [3, 130–132] (**Figure 4**). Supplementation of food supply with ω-3 PUFAs constitutes thus an interesting strategy for the prevention and treatment of mood and anxiety disorders, in particular because of the low side effects expected compared to pharmacological agents. Several trials have been conducted in this context, however, meta-analyses reported mitigated outcomes so far [129, 133]. Some trials showed no convincing effect while others demonstrated that ω-3 supplementation for 8-12 weeks have significant positive effects, notably because it improves the efficiency of antidepressants and thus increases the proportion of remission [134]. The lack of clear effect of ω-3 supplementation to treat mood and anxiety disorders in humans can be explained by the complexity of neuropsychiatric disorders and the heterogeneity of methods in the different studies. As an example, a recent study highlighted the positive effect of EPA treatment in patients suffering from major depression homogenized on the basis of their inflammatory status [43]. The clinical studies are corroborated by preclinical studies. Dietary ω-3 deficiency in rodents induces strong anxiety- and depressive-like behaviors [7–9, 135–137]. Conversely, ω-3 supplementation given beforehand a protocol of acute or chronic stress plays a protective role against anxiety- and depressive-like behaviors [136, 138, 139].

On the other hand, the role of endocannabinoids system in the regulation of mood and anxiety disorders has recently raised much interest in preclinical studies. The first evidence came from behavioral studies showing that mice lacking the gene for CB1 receptor display strong depressive and anxiety-like behaviors, which can be reproduced in control mice with CB1 receptor antagonists [140, 141]. Inversely, depressive- and anxiety-like behaviors induced by acute or chronic stress are associated with alteration of AEA and 2-AG levels [142, 143], CB1 receptor desensitization [144, 145] and impairment of endocannabinoid-dependent synaptic plasticity [144, 146, 147]. Recently, we conducted a study in this context demonstrating that a chronic social defeat stress in mice totally abolished spike-timing endocannabinoid-dependent synaptic plasticity. In humans, it is established that patients suffering from mood and anxiety disorders have lower levels of endocannabinoids in blood [148]. Even if cannabis has been used for decades as a self-medication to dampen stress and anxiety, only few clinical studies so far have tried enhancement of endocannabinoid signaling as a potential therapeu-

http://dx.doi.org/10.5772/62498

tics to treat mood and anxiety disorders [149, 150]. This may be due to the potential side effects of directly targeting the endocannabinoid system, and in this context dietary PUFAs, as homeostatic regulators of endocannabinoids [95], could constitute a very interesting and promising therapeutic candidate to target the endocannabinoid system.

From these studies, it thus appears that both dietary PUFAs and endocannabinoids play a role in mood and anxiety disorders and the link between both has been made only in our laboratory in preclinical studies. We demonstrated that an ω-3 deficient diet from the first gestational stage greatly impairs endocannabinoid signaling, which is associated to anxiety and depressive-like behaviors in mice [7, 136]. Currently, our ongoing studies tend to demonstrate that DHA-rich diet protects mice from deleterious effects of a chronic social defeat stress on anxiety- and depressive-like behaviors and on endocannabinoid-dependent synaptic plasticity. At long-term, we believe these studies will constitute a solid argument to investigate the effect of ω-3 supplementation to normalize endocannabinoid levels in patients suffering from anxiety or depressive disorders.

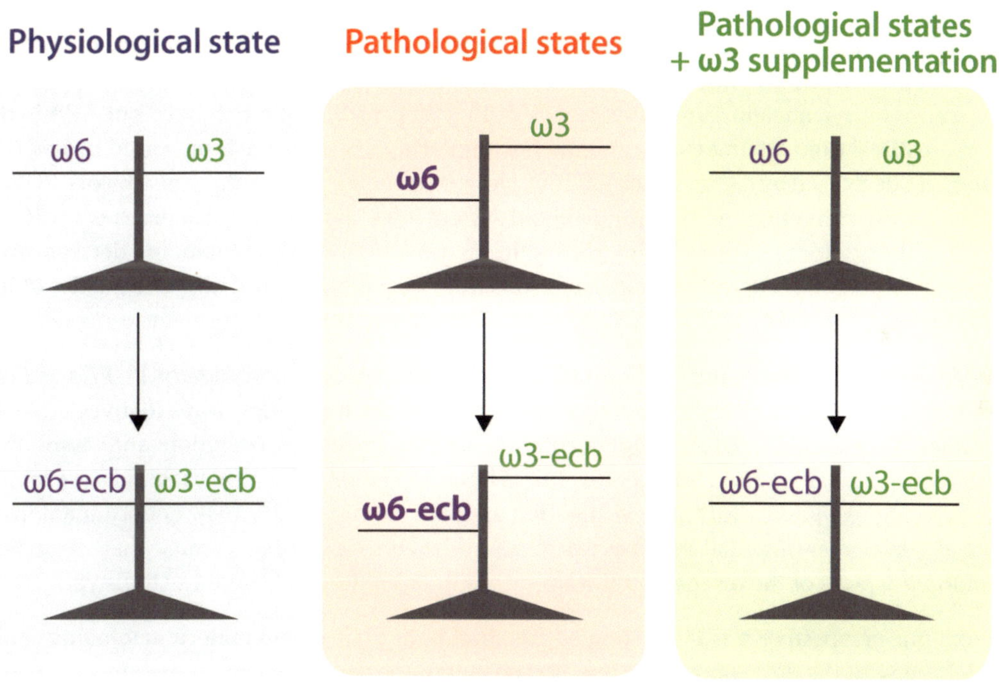

Figure 4. PUFA/endocannabinoid interactions in the pathological brain: an hypothesis. In the normal brain, (left panel), ω-6, ω-3 PUFAs and endocannabinoids derived from ω-6 and ω-3 are present in physiological concentrations. In pathological conditions (middle panel) such as mood disorders, autism, schizophrenia, neuropathic pain or neurodegenerative diseases, there is an imbalance between ω-6 and ω-3 in favor of ω-6, independently of the diet. This leads to an imbalance in brain endocannabinoids in favor of AEA and 2-AG which can potentially contribute to the physiopathology of the disease. Dietary supplementation with ω-3 PUFAs reduces ω-6/ω-3 imbalance induced by brain disorders (right panel). This normalization could normalize levels of endocannabinoids derived from ω-6 and ω-3 and contribute to prevent/treat the disorder.

In the investigation of the interactions between endocannabinoids and dietary PUFAs in mood and anxiety disorders, we also need to consider the HPA (hypothalamus-pituitary-adrenal) axis. Indeed, dietary PUFAs are powerful modulators of the HPA axis, and function of endocannabinoids is also tightly related to the HPA axis. Our studies demonstrated that variations in dietary ω-3 PUFAs impact on the HPA axis [136, 151]: mice fed with an ω-3 PUFA deficient diet exhibit higher levels of corticosterone while mice fed with a DHA rich diet display control levels of corticosterone, and these levels are not affected by social defeat stress. In parallel, interactions between endocannabinoids and the HPA axis are reciprocal. Studies have shown that glucocorticoids can activate the release of endocannabinoids, AEA and 2-AG [152]. Conversely, endocannabinoids act efficiently to regulate stress response, partly by modulating the glucocorticoid system [150, 153]. For future studies, it is thus crucial to consider the HPA axis as a potential intermediate between dietary PUFAs and endocannabinoids in the context of depressive and anxiety disorders.

5.2. PUFAs / endocannabinoids interactions in neurodegenerative diseases

In Parkinson's disease, endocannabinoids seem to play a protective role by decreasing the oxidative stress [154]. Similarly, ω-3 rich diet improves survival of dopaminergic neurons in rodent models of the disease with MPTP (1-méthyl-4-phényl-1,2,3,6-tétrahydropyridine) injections or α-synuclein transgenic mice [155–159] (**Figure 4**). In patients, levels of AEA in the cerebrospinal fluid are increased, and the risk for Parkinson's disease is increased by ω-6 rich diet, and decreased by ω-3 rich diet [42, 160]. However, clinical trials with either dietary PUFAs or with drugs targeting the endocannabinoid system have shown inconsistent results [154]. In this pathology too, it would be interesting to investigate if endocannabinoids derived from ω-3 are of potential interest to protect neurons from degeneration and improve quality of life of patients (**Figure 4**).

In Alzheimer's disease, implication of both endocannabinoids and dietary PUFAs are not central in the study of the physiopathology, still, there are interesting ways to investigate. In animal models, ω-3 PUFA supplementation clearly improves cognition and associated neurobiological markers [21, 45, 46, 161, 162] (**Figure 4**). However, clinical trials did not provide convincing results and further investigation are thus needed [3, 21, 163]. Endocannabinoids are also trialed as potential therapeutics to treat Alzheimer's disease, because they can act on multiple aspects of the disease, but no strong result has emerged from these trials yet.

From our perspective it is interesting to note that both PUFAs and endocannabinoids could interfere with the development of the disease by dampening neuroinflammation and oxidative stress. We thus believe these are the two neurobiological aspects of the disease that have to be studied to determine if dietary PUFAs can act *via* the endocannabinoid system to improve health of patients.

5.3. PUFAs / endocannabinoids interactions in physical pain

The role of endocannabinoids in neuropathic and physical pain has been clearly established [164, 165]. Indeed, endocannabinoids have the ability to lower the excitability of nociceptors and thus reduce the intensity of the nociceptive information [165]. A recent study interestingly demonstrated that ω-3 rich diet was able to reduce physical pain and that this relief was significantly correlated to an increase in DHEA and 2-DHG, the two DHA-derived endocannabinoids [84] (**Figure 4**). This reinforces the hypothesis that ω-3 dietary PUFAs favor 'good' endocannabinoids, derived from ω-3 PUFAs (**Figure 4**). As proposed by Piomelli et al., [165], the links between endocannabinoids and dietary PUFAs in the context of pain are probably related to inflammatory processes and this is another way to explore.

6. Perspectives: implications for future therapeutics of endocannabinoid modulation by dietary PUFAs

In 1996, a study demonstrated that lithium, a mood stabilizer used for bipolar disorders, decreases recycling of ARA, COX2 activity and levels of prostaglandins [166]. Similar effects have been reported with other mood stabilizers and antipsychotic molecules. Metabolism of ARA could thus serve as a marker for the development of new molecules for the treatment of mood and anxiety disorders.

As we mentioned above, supplementation with ω-3 PUFAs in the treatment of mood and anxiety disorders have provided mitigated results, but this could be due to the low turnover of PUFAs in the brain [20]. A possibility to bypass this issue would be to accelerate the bioavailability of PUFAs to the brain, by direct injection of free or esterified PUFAs into the brain. A preclinical study in rat demonstrated that an injection of DHA can reduce seizure score within one hour or one day, where three months are needed to reach the same result through the diet [167–169]. These promising results could be applied in the future to humans to reduce damages following stroke or reduce seizure events, but further investigations are needed before such clinical trials.

Another field that needs to be explored to our opinion is the role of dietary PUFAs on endocannabinoids during brain development. As mentioned in this chapter, PUFA accretion in the brain occurs largely during brain development and our laboratory published many articles on the effects of imbalanced dietary PUFA during development on the adult brain [3, 7, 26]. In parallel, increasing evidence highlights that endocannabinoid signaling is essential for brain wiring [170, 171]. Notably, endocannabinoids and CB1 receptors serve as guidance signals for axon cone growth [171]. The link between dietary PUFA and endocannabinoids is not yet clearly established, but it is very likely that effects of imbalanced PUFAs during development has strong consequences on the role of endocannabinoid as guidance molecules during brain wiring. This can have strong implication for brain disorders with developmental origin, such as schizophrenia.

In conclusion, dietary ω-6/ω-3 PUFAs appears as potent modulators and homeostatic regulators of endocannabinoids in the brain. The consequences of this modulation need to be investigated to understand its putative role in brain health and diseases (in particular those with endocannabinoid impairment) and develop future therapeutics to target the endocannabinoid system through dietary ω-6/ω-3 PUFAs. The most promising hypothesis that needs to be explored to our opinion is that dietary PUFAs could switch the system from 'bad' (ω-6-derived) endocannabinoids to 'good' (ω-3-derived) endocannabinoids.

Acknowledgements

This research was financially supported by INRA, Agence Nationale de la Recherche (ANR-MoodFood) and the Region Aquitaine. CBB had fellowships from the Agence Nationale de la Recherche and the European Agreenskills program (COFUND FP7-267196).

Author details

Clémentine Bosch-Bouju[1,2*] and Sophie Layé[1,2]

*Address all correspondence to: clementine.bosch@bordeaux.inra.fr

1 INRA, Nutrition and Integrative Neurobiology, UMR, Bordeaux, France

2 Bordeaux University, Nutrition and Integrative Neurobiology, UMR, Bordeaux, France

References

[1] Simopoulos AP, Leaf A, Salem N. Workshop statement on the essentiality of and recommended dietary intakes for Omega-6 and Omega-3 fatty acids. Prostaglandins Leukot Essent Fatty Acids. 2000;63: 119–121. doi: 10.1054/plef.2000.0176.

[2] Calon F, Cole G. Neuroprotective action of omega-3 polyunsaturated fatty acids against neurodegenerative diseases: evidence from animal studies. Prostaglandins Leukot Essent Fatty Acids. 2007;77: 287–293. doi: 10.1016/j.plefa.2007.10.019.

[3] Bazinet RP,Layé S. Polyunsaturated fatty acids and their metabolites in brain function and disease. Nat Rev Neurosci. 2014;15: 771–785. doi: 10.1038/nrn3820.

[4] Berger A, Crozier G, Bisogno T, Cavaliere P, Innis S, Di Marzo V. Anandamide and diet: inclusion of dietary arachidonate and docosahexaenoate leads to increased brain levels of the corresponding N-acylethanolamines in piglets. Proc Natl Acad Sci USA. 2001;98: 6402–6406. doi: 10.1073/pnas.101119098.

[5] Watanabe S, Doshi M, Hamazaki T. n-3 Polyunsaturated fatty acid (PUFA) deficiency elevates and n-3 PUFA enrichment reduces brain 2-arachidonoylglycerol level in mice. Prostaglandins Leukot Essent Fatty Acids. 2003;69: 51–59.

[6] Artmann A, Petersen G, Hellgren LI, Boberg J, Skonberg C, Nellemann C, et al. Influence of dietary fatty acids on endocannabinoid and N-acylethanolamine levels in

rat brain, liver and small intestine. Biochim Biophys Acta. 2008;1781: 200–212. doi: 10.1016/j.bbalip.2008.01.006.

[7] Lafourcade M, Larrieu T, Mato S, Duffaud A, Sepers M, Matias I, et al. Nutritional omega-3 deficiency abolishes endocannabinoid-mediated neuronal functions. Nat Neurosci. 2011;14: 345–350. doi: 10.1038/nn.2736.

[8] Larrieu T, Madore C, Joffre C, Layé S. Nutritional n-3 polyunsaturated fatty acids deficiency alters cannabinoid receptor signaling pathway in the brain and associated anxiety-like behavior in mice. J Physiol Biochem. 2012;68: 671–681. doi: 10.1007/s13105-012-0179-6.

[9] DeMar JC, Ma K, Bell JM, Igarashi M, Greenstein D, Rapoport SI. One generation of n-3 polyunsaturated fatty acid deprivation increases depression and aggression test scores in rats. J Lipid Res. 2006;47: 172–180. doi: 10.1194/jlr.M500362-JLR200.

[10] Ouellet M, Emond V, Chen CT, Julien C, Bourasset F, Oddo S, et al. Diffusion of docosahexaenoic and eicosapentaenoic acids through the blood-brain barrier: an in situ cerebral perfusion study. Neurochem Int. 2009;55: 476–482. doi: 10.1016/j.neuint.2009.04.018.

[11] Hamilton JA, Brunaldi K. A model for fatty acid transport into the brain. J Mol Neurosci. 2007;33: 12–17.

[12] Mitchell RW, Hatch GM. Fatty acid transport into the brain: of fatty acid fables and lipid tails. Prostaglandins Leukot Essent Fatty Acids. 2011;85: 293–302. doi: 10.1016/j.plefa.2011.04.007.

[13] Chen CT, Bazinet RP. β-oxidation and rapid metabolism, but not uptake regulate brain eicosapentaenoic acid levels. Prostaglandins Leukot Essent Fatty Acids. 2015;92: 33–40. doi: 10.1016/j.plefa.2014.05.007.

[14] Chen CT, Ma DWL, Kim JH, Mount HTJ, Bazinet RP. The low density lipoprotein receptor is not necessary for maintaining mouse brain polyunsaturated fatty acid concentrations. J Lipid Res. 2008;49: 147–152. doi: 10.1194/jlr.M700386-JLR200.

[15] Goldberg IJ, Eckel RH, Abumrad NA. Regulation of fatty acid uptake into tissues: lipoprotein lipase- and CD36-mediated pathways. J Lipid Res. 2009;50 (Suppl): S86–90. doi: 10.1194/jlr.R800085-JLR200.

[16] Song BJ, Elbert A, Rahman T, Orr SK, Chen CT, Febbraio M, et al. Genetic ablation of CD36 does not alter mouse brain polyunsaturated fatty acid concentrations. Lipids. 2010;45: 291–299. doi: 10.1007/s11745-010-3398-z.

[17] Rahman T, Taha AY, Song BJ, Orr SK, Liu Z, Chen CT, et al. The very low density lipoprotein receptor is not necessary for maintaining brain polyunsaturated fatty acid concentrations. Prostaglandins Leukot Essent Fatty Acids. 2010;82: 141–145. doi: 10.1016/j.plefa.2009.11.003.

[18] Nguyen H-B, Bagot RC, Diorio J, Wong TP, Meaney MJ. Maternal care differentially affects neuronal excitability and synaptic plasticity in the dorsal and ventral hippocampus. Neuropsychopharmacology. 2015;40: 1590–1599. doi: 10.1038/npp.2015.19.

[19] Innis SM. Dietary omega 3 fatty acids and the developing brain. Brain Res. 2008;1237: 35–43. doi: 10.1016/j.brainres.2008.08.078.

[20] Rapoport SI, Rao JS, Igarashi M. Brain metabolism of nutritionally essential polyunsaturated fatty acids depends on both the diet and the liver. Prostaglandins Leukot Essent Fatty Acids. 2007;77: 251–261. doi: 10.1016/j.plefa.2007.10.023.

[21] Joffre C, Nadjar A, Lebbadi M, Calon F, Laye S. n-3 LCPUFA improves cognition: the young, the old and the sick. Prostaglandins Leukot Essent Fatty Acids. 2014;91: 1–20. doi: 10.1016/j.plefa.2014.05.001.

[22] Rao JS, Ertley RN, DeMar JC, Rapoport SI, Bazinet RP, Lee H-J. Dietary n-3 PUFA deprivation alters expression of enzymes of the arachidonic and docosahexaenoic acid cascades in rat frontal cortex. Mol Psychiatry. 2007;12: 151–157. doi: 10.1038/sj.mp.4001887.

[23] Green JT, Liu Z, Bazinet RP. Brain phospholipid arachidonic acid half-lives are not altered following 15 weeks of N-3 polyunsaturated fatty acid adequate or deprived diet. J Lipid Res. 2010;51: 535–543. doi: 10.1194/jlr.M000786.

[24] Moranis A, Delpech J-C, De Smedt-Peyrusse V, Aubert A, Guesnet P, Lavialle M, et al. Long term adequate n-3 polyunsaturated fatty acid diet protects from depressive-like behavior but not from working memory disruption and brain cytokine expression in aged mice. Brain Behav Immun. 2012;26: 721–731. doi: 10.1016/j.bbi.2011.11.001.

[25] Igarashi M, Kim H-W, Chang L, Ma K, Rapoport SI. Dietary n-6 polyunsaturated fatty acid deprivation increases docosahexaenoic acid metabolism in rat brain. J Neurochem. 2012;120: 985–997. doi: 10.1111/j.1471-4159.2011.07597.x.

[26] Madore C, Nadjar A, Delpech J-C, Sere A, Aubert A, Portal C, et al. Nutritional n-3 PUFAs deficiency during perinatal periods alters brain innate immune system and neuronal plasticity-associated genes. Brain Behav Immun. 2014;41: 22–31. doi: 10.1016/j.bbi.2014.03.021.

[27] Piomelli D, Astarita G, Rapaka R. A neuroscientist's guide to lipidomics. Nat Rev Neurosci. 2007;8: 743–754. doi: 10.1038/nrn2233.

[28] Pinot M, Vanni S, Pagnotta S, Lacas-Gervais S, Payet L-A, Ferreira T, et al. Lipid cell biology. Polyunsaturated phospholipids facilitate membrane deformation and fission by endocytic proteins. Science. 2014;345: 693–697. doi: 10.1126/science.1255288.

[29] Chen C, Bazan NG. Lipid signaling: sleep, synaptic plasticity, and neuroprotection. Prostaglandins Other Lipid Mediat. 2005;77: 65–76. doi: 10.1016/j.prostaglandins.2005.07.001.

[30] Serhan CN. Pro-resolving lipid mediators are leads for resolution physiology. Nature. 2014;510: 92–101. doi: 10.1038/nature13479.

[31] Dennis EA, Norris PC. Eicosanoid storm in infection and inflammation. Nat Rev Immunol. 2015;15: 511–523. doi: 10.1038/nri3859.

[32] Salem N, Litman B, Kim HY, Gawrisch K. Mechanisms of action of docosahexaenoic acid in the nervous system. Lipids. 2001;36: 945–959.

[33] Castillo PE, Younts TJ, Chávez AE, Hashimotodani Y. Endocannabinoid signaling and synaptic function. Neuron. 2012;76: 70–81. doi: 10.1016/j.neuron.2012.09.020.

[34] Kim HY, Akbar M, Lau A, Edsall L. Inhibition of neuronal apoptosis by docosahexaenoic acid (22:6n-3). Role of phosphatidylserine in antiapoptotic effect. J Biol Chem. 2000;275: 35215–35223. doi: 10.1074/jbc.M004446200.

[35] Calderon F, Kim H-Y. Docosahexaenoic acid promotes neurite growth in hippocampal neurons. J Neurochem. 2004;90: 979–988. doi: 10.1111/j.1471-4159.2004.02520.x.

[36] Kim H-Y, Spector AA, Xiong Z-M. A synaptogenic amide N-docosahexaenoylethanolamide promotes hippocampal development. Prostaglandins Other Lipid Mediat. 2011;96: 114–120. doi: 10.1016/j.prostaglandins.2011.07.002.

[37] Lukiw WJ, Cui J-G, Marcheselli VL, Bodker M, Botkjaer A, Gotlinger K, et al. A role for docosahexaenoic acid-derived neuroprotectin D1 in neural cell survival and Alzheimer disease. J Clin Invest. 2005;115: 2774–2783. doi: 10.1172/JCI25420.

[38] Bazan NG. The docosanoid neuroprotectin D1 induces homeostatic regulation of neuroinflammation and cell survival. Prostaglandins Leukot Essent Fatty Acids. 2013;88: 127–129. doi: 10.1016/j.plefa.2012.08.008.

[39] Wu A, Ying Z, Gomez-Pinilla F. Dietary omega-3 fatty acids normalize BDNF levels, reduce oxidative damage, and counteract learning disability after traumatic brain injury in rats. J Neurotrauma. 2004;21: 1457–1467.

[40] Calon F. Omega-3 polyunsaturated fatty acids in Alzheimer's disease: key questions and partial answers. Curr Alzheimer Res. 2011;8: 470–478.

[41] Cunnane SC, Plourde M, Pifferi F, Bégin M, Féart C, Barberger-Gateau P. Fish, docosahexaenoic acid and Alzheimer's disease. Prog Lipid Res. 2009;48: 239–256. doi: 10.1016/j.plipres.2009.04.001.

[42] Kamel F, Goldman SM, Umbach DM, Chen H, Richardson G, Barber MR, et al. Dietary fat intake, pesticide use, and Parkinson's disease. Parkinsonism Relat Disord. 2014;20: 82–87. doi: 10.1016/j.parkreldis.2013.09.023.

[43] Rapaport MH, Nierenberg AA, Schettler PJ, Kinkead B, Cardoos A, Walker R, et al. Inflammation as a predictive biomarker for response to omega-3 fatty acids in major depressive disorder: a proof-of-concept study. Mol Psychiatry. 2016;21: 71–79. doi: 10.1038/mp.2015.22.

[44] Delpech J-C, Thomazeau A, Madore C, Bosch-Bouju C, Larrieu T, Lacabanne C, et al. Dietary n-3 PUFAs deficiency increases vulnerability to inflammation-induced spatial memory impairment. Neuropsychopharmacology. 2015;40: 2774–2787. doi: 10.1038/npp.2015.127.

[45] Labrousse VF, Nadjar A, Joffre C, Costes L, Aubert A, Grégoire S, et al. Short-term long chain omega3 diet protects from neuroinflammatory processes and memory impairment in aged mice. PLoS ONE. 2012;7: e36861. doi: 10.1371/journal.pone.0036861.

[46] Delpech J-C, Madore C, Joffre C, Aubert A, Kang JX, Nadjar A, et al. Transgenic increase in n-3/n-6 fatty acid ratio protects against cognitive deficits induced by an immune challenge through decrease of neuroinflammation. Neuropsychopharmacology. 2015;40: 525–536. doi: 10.1038/npp.2014.196.

[47] Heifets BD, Castillo PE. Endocannabinoid signaling and long-term synaptic plasticity. Annu Rev Physiol. 2009;71: 283–306. doi: 10.1146/annurev.physiol.010908.163149.

[48] Ueda N, Tsuboi K, Uyama T. Metabolism of endocannabinoids and related N-acylethanolamines: canonical and alternative pathways. FEBS J. 2013;280: 1874–1894. doi: 10.1111/febs.12152.

[49] Piomelli D. More surprises lying ahead. The endocannabinoids keep us guessing. Neuropharmacology. 2014;76 (Pt B): 228–234. doi: 10.1016/j.neuropharm.2013.07.026.

[50] Robbe D, Bockaert J, Manzoni OJ. Metabotropic glutamate receptor 2/3-dependent long-term depression in the nucleus accumbens is blocked in morphine withdrawn mice. Eur J Neurosci. 2002;16: 2231–2235.

[51] Robbe D, Alonso G, Chaumont S, Bockaert J, Manzoni OJ. Role of p/q-Ca2+ channels in metabotropic glutamate receptor 2/3-dependent presynaptic long-term depression at nucleus accumbens synapses. J Neurosci. 2002;22: 4346–4356. doi: 20026420.

[52] Fino E, Paille V, Cui Y, Morera-Herreras T, Deniau J-M, Venance L. Distinct coincidence detectors govern the corticostriatal spike timing-dependent plasticity. J Physiol (Lond). 2010;588: 3045–3062. doi: 10.1113/jphysiol.2010.188466.

[53] Tanimura A, Yamazaki M, Hashimotodani Y, Uchigashima M, Kawata S, Abe M, et al. The endocannabinoid 2-arachidonoylglycerol produced by diacylglycerol lipase alpha mediates retrograde suppression of synaptic transmission. Neuron. 2010;65: 320–327. doi: 10.1016/j.neuron.2010.01.021.

[54] Reisenberg M, Singh PK, Williams G, Doherty P. The diacylglycerol lipases: structure, regulation and roles in and beyond endocannabinoid signalling. Philos Trans R Soc Lond, B, Biol Sci. 2012;367: 3264–3275. doi: 10.1098/rstb.2011.0387.

[55] Nicolussi S, Gertsch J. Endocannabinoid transport revisited. Vitam Horm. 2015;98: 441–485. doi: 10.1016/bs.vh.2014.12.011.

[56] Ahn K, McKinney MK, Cravatt BF. Enzymatic pathways that regulate endocannabinoid signaling in the nervous system. Chem Rev. 2008;108: 1687–1707. doi: 10.1021/cr0782067.

[57] Ludányi A, Hu SS-J, Yamazaki M, Tanimura A, Piomelli D, Watanabe M, et al. Complementary synaptic distribution of enzymes responsible for synthesis and inactivation of the endocannabinoid 2-arachidonoylglycerol in the human hippocampus. Neuroscience. 2011;174: 50–63. doi: 10.1016/j.neuroscience.2010.10.062.

[58] Viader A, Blankman JL, Zhong P, Liu X, Schlosburg JE, Joslyn CM, et al. Metabolic Interplay between astrocytes and neurons regulates endocannabinoid action. Cell Rep. 2015;12: 798–808. doi: 10.1016/j.celrep.2015.06.075.

[59] Cascio MG. PUFA-derived endocannabinoids: an overview. Proc Nutr Soc. 2013;72: 451–459. doi: 10.1017/S0029665113003418.

[60] Alhouayek M, Muccioli GG. COX-2-derived endocannabinoid metabolites as novel inflammatory mediators. Trends Pharmacol Sci. 2014;35: 284–292. doi: 10.1016/j.tips.2014.03.001.

[61] Hermanson DJ, Gamble-George JC, Marnett LJ, Patel S. Substrate-selective COX-2 inhibition as a novel strategy for therapeutic endocannabinoid augmentation. Trends Pharmacol Sci. 2014;35: 358–367. doi: 10.1016/j.tips.2014.04.006.

[62] Astarita G, Ahmed F, Piomelli D. Identification of biosynthetic precursors for the endocannabinoid anandamide in the rat brain. J Lipid Res. 2008;49: 48–57. doi: 10.1194/jlr.M700354-JLR200.

[63] Fu J, Bottegoni G, Sasso O, Bertorelli R, Rocchia W, Masetti M, et al. A catalytically silent FAAH-1 variant drives anandamide transport in neurons. Nat Neurosci. 2012;15: 64–69. doi: 10.1038/nn.2986.

[64] Leung K, Elmes MW, Glaser ST, Deutsch DG, Kaczocha M. Role of FAAH-like anandamide transporter in anandamide inactivation. PLoS ONE. 2013;8: e79355. doi: 10.1371/journal.pone.0079355.

[65] Di Marzo V, De Petrocellis L. Why do cannabinoid receptors have more than one endogenous ligand? Philos Trans R Soc Lond B Biol Sci. 2012;367: 3216–3228. doi: 10.1098/rstb.2011.0382.

[66] Starowicz K, Nigam S, Di Marzo V. Biochemistry and pharmacology of endovanilloids. Pharmacol Ther. 2007;114: 13–33. doi: 10.1016/j.pharmthera.2007.01.005.

[67] Tóth A, Blumberg PM, Boczán J. Anandamide and the vanilloid receptor (TRPV1). Vitam Horm. 2009;81: 389–419. doi: 10.1016/S0083-6729(09)81015-7.

[68] Grueter BA, Brasnjo G, Malenka RC. Postsynaptic TRPV1 triggers cell type-specific long-term depression in the nucleus accumbens. Nat Neurosci. 2010;13: 1519–1525. doi: 10.1038/nn.2685.

[69] Chávez AE, Chiu CQ, Castillo PE. TRPV1 activation by endogenous anandamide triggers postsynaptic long-term depression in dentate gyrus. Nat Neurosci. 2010;13: 1511–1518. doi: 10.1038/nn.2684.

[70] Puente N, Cui Y, Lassalle O, Lafourcade M, Georges F, Venance L, et al. Polymodal activation of the endocannabinoid system in the extended amygdala. Nat Neurosci. 2011;14: 1542–1547. doi: 10.1038/nn.2974.

[71] Placzek EA, Okamoto Y, Ueda N, Barker EL. Membrane microdomains and metabolic pathways that define anandamide and 2-arachidonyl glycerol biosynthesis and breakdown. Neuropharmacology. 2008;55: 1095–1104. doi: 10.1016/j.neuropharm.2008.07.047.

[72] Petrosino S, Di Marzo V. FAAH and MAGL inhibitors: therapeutic opportunities from regulating endocannabinoid levels. Curr Opin Investig Drugs. 2010;11: 51–62.

[73] Fowler CJ. The potential of inhibitors of endocannabinoid metabolism for drug development: a critical review. Handb Exp Pharmacol. 2015;231: 95–128. doi: 10.1007/978-3-319-20825-1_4.

[74] Lodola A, Castelli R, Mor M, Rivara S. Fatty acid amide hydrolase inhibitors: a patent review (2009–2014). Expert Opin Ther Pat. 2015;25: 1247–1266. doi: 10.1517/13543776.2015.1067683.

[75] Gao Y, Vasilyev DV, Goncalves MB, Howell FV, Hobbs C, Reisenberg M, et al. Loss of retrograde endocannabinoid signaling and reduced adult neurogenesis in diacylglycerol lipase knock-out mice. J Neurosci. 2010;30: 2017–2024. doi: 10.1523/JNEUROSCI.5693-09.2010.

[76] Leung D, Saghatelian A, Simon GM, Cravatt BF. Inactivation of N-acyl phosphatidylethanolamine phospholipase D reveals multiple mechanisms for the biosynthesis of endocannabinoids. Biochemistry. 2006;45: 4720–4726. doi: 10.1021/bi060163l.

[77] Tsuboi K, Okamoto Y, Ikematsu N, Inoue M, Shimizu Y, Uyama T, et al. Enzymatic formation of N-acylethanolamines from N-acylethanolamine plasmalogen through N-acylphosphatidylethanolamine-hydrolyzing phospholipase D-dependent and -independent pathways. Biochim Biophys Acta. 2011;1811: 565–577. doi: 10.1016/j.bbalip.2011.07.009.

[78] Wood JT, Williams JS, Pandarinathan L, Janero DR, Lammi-Keefe CJ, Makriyannis A. Dietary docosahexaenoic acid supplementation alters select physiological endocannabinoid-system metabolites in brain and plasma. J Lipid Res. 2010;51: 1416–1423. doi: 10.1194/jlr.M002436.

[79] Sheskin T, Hanus L, Slager J, Vogel Z, Mechoulam R. Structural requirements for binding of anandamide-type compounds to the brain cannabinoid receptor. J Med Chem. 1997;40: 659–667. doi: 10.1021/jm960752x.

[80] Meijerink J, Balvers M, Witkamp R. N-Acyl amines of docosahexaenoic acid and other n-3 polyunsatured fatty acids—from fishy endocannabinoids to potential leads. Br J Pharmacol. 2013;169: 772–783. doi: 10.1111/bph.12030.

[81] Kim H-Y, Spector AA. Synaptamide, endocannabinoid-like derivative of docosahexaenoic acid with cannabinoid-independent function. Prostaglandins Leukot Essent Fatty Acids. 2013;88: 121–125. doi: 10.1016/j.plefa.2012.08.002.

[82] Cao D, Kevala K, Kim J, Moon H-S, Jun SB, Lovinger D, et al. Docosahexaenoic acid promotes hippocampal neuronal development and synaptic function. J Neurochem. 2009;111: 510–521. doi: 10.1111/j.1471-4159.2009.06335.x.

[83] Bisogno T, Delton-Vandenbroucke I, Milone A, Lagarde M, Di Marzo V. Biosynthesis and inactivation of N-arachidonoylethanolamine (anandamide) and N-docosahexaenoylethanolamine in bovine retina. Arch Biochem Biophys. 1999;370: 300–307. doi: 10.1006/abbi.1999.1410.

[84] Ramsden CE, Zamora D, Makriyannis A, Wood JT, Mann JD, Faurot KR, et al. Diet-induced changes in n-3- and n-6-derived endocannabinoids and reductions in headache pain and psychological distress. J Pain. 2015;16: 707–716. doi: 10.1016/j.jpain.2015.04.007.

[85] Piscitelli F, Carta G, Bisogno T, Murru E, Cordeddu L, Berge K, et al. Effect of dietary krill oil supplementation on the endocannabinoidome of metabolically relevant tissues from high-fat-fed mice. Nutr Metab (Lond). 2011;8: 51. doi: 10.1186/1743-7075-8-51.

[86] Balvers MGJ, Verhoeckx KCM, Bijlsma S, Rubingh CM, Meijerink J, Wortelboer HM, et al. Fish oil and inflammatory status alter the n-3 to n-6 balance of the endocannabinoid and oxylipin metabolomes in mouse plasma and tissues. Metabolomics. 2012;8: 1130–1147. doi: 10.1007/s11306-012-0421-9.

[87] Matias I, Carta G, Murru E, Petrosino S, Banni S, Di Marzo V. Effect of polyunsaturated fatty acids on endocannabinoid and N-acyl-ethanolamine levels in mouse adipocytes. Biochim Biophys Acta. 2008;1781: 52–60. doi: 10.1016/j.bbalip.2007.11.001.

[88] Batetta B, Griinari M, Carta G, Murru E, Ligresti A, Cordeddu L, et al. Endocannabinoids may mediate the ability of (n-3) fatty acids to reduce ectopic fat and inflammatory mediators in obese Zucker rats. J Nutr. 2009;139: 1495–1501. doi: 10.3945/jn.109.104844.

[89] Alvheim AR, Malde MK, Osei-Hyiaman D, Lin YH, Pawlosky RJ, Madsen L, et al. Dietary linoleic acid elevates endogenous 2-AG and anandamide and induces obesity. Obesity (Silver Spring). 2012;20: 1984–1994. doi: 10.1038/oby.2012.38.

[90] Alvheim AR, Torstensen BE, Lin YH, Lillefosse HH, Lock E-J, Madsen L, et al. Dietary linoleic acid elevates the endocannabinoids 2-AG and anandamide and promotes weight gain in mice fed a low fat diet. Lipids. 2014;49: 59–69. doi: 10.1007/s11745-013-3842-y.

[91] Kim J, Carlson ME, Kuchel GA, Newman JW, Watkins BA. Dietary DHA reduces downstream endocannabinoid and inflammatory gene expression and epididymal fat mass while improving aspects of glucose use in muscle in C57BL/6J mice. Int J Obes (Lond). 2016;40: 129–137. doi: 10.1038/ijo.2015.135.

[92] Yan L, Bai X, Fang Z, Che L, Xu S, Wu D. Effect of different dietary omega-3/omega-6 fatty acid ratios on reproduction in male rats. Lipids Health Dis. 2013;12: 33. doi: 10.1186/1476-511X-12-33.

[93] Banni S, Di Marzo V. Effect of dietary fat on endocannabinoids and related mediators: consequences on energy homeostasis, inflammation and mood. Mol Nutr Food Res. 2010;54: 82–92. doi: 10.1002/mnfr.200900516.

[94] Mazier W, Saucisse N, Gatta-Cherifi B, Cota D. The endocannabinoid system: pivotal orchestrator of obesity and metabolic disease. Trends Endocrinol Metab. 2015;26: 524–537. doi: 10.1016/j.tem.2015.07.007.

[95] McPartland JM, Guy GW, Di Marzo V. Care and feeding of the endocannabinoid system: a systematic review of potential clinical interventions that upregulate the endocannabinoid system. PLoS ONE. 2014;9: e89566. doi: 10.1371/journal.pone.0089566.

[96] Koolman AH, Bloks VW, Oosterveer MH, Jonas I, Kuipers F, Sauer PJJ, et al. Metabolic responses to long-term pharmacological inhibition of CB1-receptor activity in mice in relation to dietary fat composition. Int J Obes (Lond). 2010;34: 374–384. doi: 10.1038/ijo.2009.219.

[97] Chiurchiù V, Battistini L, Maccarrone M. Endocannabinoid signaling in innate and adaptive immunity. Immunology. 2015; doi: 10.1111/imm.12441.

[98] Marion-Letellier R, Savoye G, Ghosh S. Polyunsaturated fatty acids and inflammation. IUBMB Life. 2015;67: 659–667. doi: 10.1002/iub.1428.

[99] Masoodi M, Kuda O, Rossmeisl M, Flachs P, Kopecky J. Lipid signaling in adipose tissue: connecting inflammation & metabolism. Biochim Biophys Acta. 2015;1851: 503–518. doi: 10.1016/j.bbalip.2014.09.023.

[100] Watkins BA, Hutchins H, Li Y, Seifert MF. The endocannabinoid signaling system: a marriage of PUFA and musculoskeletal health. J Nutr Biochem. 2010;21: 1141–1152. doi: 10.1016/j.jnutbio.2010.04.011.

[101] Hutchins HL, Li Y, Hannon K, Watkins BA. Eicosapentaenoic acid decreases expression of anandamide synthesis enzyme and cannabinoid receptor 2 in osteoblast-like cells. J Nutr Biochem. 2011;22: 195–200. doi: 10.1016/j.jnutbio.2010.06.001.

[102] Wainwright CL, Michel L. Endocannabinoid system as a potential mechanism for n-3 long-chain polyunsaturated fatty acid mediated cardiovascular protection. Proc Nutr Soc. 2013;72: 460–469. doi: 10.1017/S0029665113003406.

[103] Endo J, Arita M. Cardioprotective mechanism of omega-3 polyunsaturated fatty acids. J Cardiol. 2016;67: 22–27. doi: 10.1016/j.jjcc.2015.08.002.

[104] Battista N, Meccariello R, Cobellis G, Fasano S, Di Tommaso M, Pirazzi V, et al. The role of endocannabinoids in gonadal function and fertility along the evolutionary axis. Mol Cell Endocrinol. 2012;355: 1–14. doi: 10.1016/j.mce.2012.01.014.

[105] Meccariello R, Battista N, Bradshaw HB, Wang H. Updates in reproduction coming from the endocannabinoid system. Int J Endocrinol. 2014;2014: 412354. doi: 10.1155/2014/412354.

[106] Bovolin P, Cottone E, Pomatto V, Fasano S, Pierantoni R, Cobellis G, et al. Endocannabinoids are involved in male vertebrate reproduction: regulatory mechanisms at central and gonadal level. Front Endocrinol (Lausanne). 2014;5: 54. doi: 10.3389/fendo.2014.00054.

[107] Vrablik TL, Watts JL. Polyunsaturated fatty acid derived signaling in reproduction and development: insights from Caenorhabditis elegans and Drosophila melanogaster. Mol Reprod Dev. 2013;80: 244–259. doi: 10.1002/mrd.22167.

[108] Björkgren I, Gylling H, Turunen H, Huhtaniemi I, Strauss L, Poutanen M, et al. Imbalanced lipid homeostasis in the conditional Dicer1 knockout mouse epididymis causes instability of the sperm membrane. FASEB J. 2015;29: 433–442. doi: 10.1096/fj.14-259382.

[109] Pan J-P, Zhang H-Q, Wei-Wang null, Guo Y-F, Na-Xiao null, Cao X-H, et al. Some subtypes of endocannabinoid/endovanilloid receptors mediate docosahexaenoic acid-induced enhanced spatial memory in rats. Brain Res. 2011;1412: 18–27. doi: 10.1016/j.brainres.2011.07.015.

[110] Yamada D, Takeo J, Koppensteiner P, Wada K, Sekiguchi M. Modulation of fear memory by dietary polyunsaturated fatty acids via cannabinoid receptors. Neuropsychopharmacology. 2014;39: 1852–1860. doi: 10.1038/npp.2014.32.

[111] Martini L, Waldhoer M, Pusch M, Kharazia V, Fong J, Lee JH, et al. Ligand-induced down-regulation of the cannabinoid 1 receptor is mediated by the G-protein-coupled receptor-associated sorting protein GASP1. FASEB J. 2007;21: 802–811. doi: 10.1096/fj.06-7132com.

[112] Stadel R, Ahn KH, Kendall DA. The cannabinoid type-1 receptor carboxyl-terminus, more than just a tail. J Neurochem. 2011;117: 1–18. doi: 10.1111/j.1471-4159.2011.07186.x.

[113] Lazenka MF, Selley DE, Sim-Selley LJ. Brain regional differences in CB1 receptor adaptation and regulation of transcription. Life Sci. 2013;92: 446–452. doi: 10.1016/j.lfs.2012.08.023.

[114] Cachope R. Functional diversity on synaptic plasticity mediated by endocannabinoids. Philos Trans R Soc Lond, B, Biol Sci. 2012;367: 3242–3253. doi: 10.1098/rstb.2011.0386.

[115] Glangetas C, Girard D, Groc L, Marsicano G, Chaouloff F, Georges F. Stress switches cannabinoid type-1 (CB1) receptor-dependent plasticity from LTD to LTP in the bed nucleus of the stria terminalis. J Neurosci. 2013;33: 19657–19663. doi: 10.1523/JNEUROSCI.3175-13.2013.

[116] Cui Y, Paillé V, Xu H, Genet S, Delord B, Fino E, et al. Endocannabinoids mediate bidirectional striatal spike-timing-dependent plasticity. J Physiol (Lond). 2015;593: 2833–2849. doi: 10.1113/JP270324.

[117] Crupi R, Marino A, Cuzzocrea S. n-3 fatty acids: role in neurogenesis and neuroplasticity. Curr Med Chem. 2013;20: 2953–2963.

[118] Patten AR, Sickmann HM, Dyer RA, Innis SM, Christie BR. Omega-3 fatty acids can reverse the long-term deficits in hippocampal synaptic plasticity caused by prenatal ethanol exposure. Neurosci Lett. 2013;551: 7–11. doi: 10.1016/j.neulet.2013.05.051.

[119] Arsenault D, Julien C, Chen CT, Bazinet RP, Calon F. Dietary intake of unsaturated fatty acids modulates physiological properties of entorhinal cortex neurons in mice. J Neurochem. 2012;122: 427–443. doi: 10.1111/j.1471-4159.2012.07772.x.

[120] Latour A, Grintal B, Champeil-Potokar G, Hennebelle M, Lavialle M, Dutar P, et al. Omega-3 fatty acids deficiency aggravates glutamatergic synapse and astroglial aging in the rat hippocampal CA1. Aging Cell. 2013;12: 76–84. doi: 10.1111/acel.12026.

[121] McFarland MJ, Barker EL. Lipid rafts: a nexus for endocannabinoid signaling? Life Sci. 2005;77: 1640–1650. doi: 10.1016/j.lfs.2005.05.010.

[122] Barnett-Norris J, Lynch D, Reggio PH. Lipids, lipid rafts and caveolae: their importance for GPCR signaling and their centrality to the endocannabinoid system. Life Sci. 2005;77: 1625–1639. doi: 10.1016/j.lfs.2005.05.040.

[123] Maccarrone M, De Chiara V, Gasperi V, Viscomi MT, Rossi S, Oddi S, et al. Lipid rafts regulate 2-arachidonoylglycerol metabolism and physiological activity in the striatum. J Neurochem. 2009;109: 371–381. doi: 10.1111/j.1471-4159.2009.05948.x.

[124] Lingwood D, Simons K. Lipid rafts as a membrane-organizing principle. Science. 2010;327: 46–50. doi: 10.1126/science.1174621.

[125] Hering H, Lin C-C, Sheng M. Lipid rafts in the maintenance of synapses, dendritic spines, and surface AMPA receptor stability. J Neurosci. 2003;23: 3262–3271.

[126] Wassall SR, Stillwell W. Polyunsaturated fatty acid-cholesterol interactions: domain formation in membranes. Biochim Biophys Acta. 2009;1788: 24–32. doi: 10.1016/j.bbamem.2008.10.011.

[127] Wassall SR, Stillwell W. Docosahexaenoic acid domains: the ultimate non-raft membrane domain. Chem Phys Lipids. 2008;153: 57–63. doi: 10.1016/j.chemphyslip.2008.02.010.

[128] Shaikh SR. Biophysical and biochemical mechanisms by which dietary N-3 polyunsaturated fatty acids from fish oil disrupt membrane lipid rafts. J Nutr Biochem. 2012;23: 101–105. doi: 10.1016/j.jnutbio.2011.07.001.

[129] Appleton KM, Rogers PJ, Ness AR. Updated systematic review and meta-analysis of the effects of n-3 long-chain polyunsaturated fatty acids on depressed mood. Am J Clin Nutr. 2010;91: 757–770. doi: 10.3945/ajcn.2009.28313.

[130] Lin P-Y, Huang S-Y, Su K-P. A meta-analytic review of polyunsaturated fatty acid compositions in patients with depression. Biol Psychiatry. 2010;68: 140–147. doi: 10.1016/j.biopsych.2010.03.018.

[131] McNamara RK, Hahn C-G, Jandacek R, Rider T, Tso P, Stanford KE, et al. Selective deficits in the omega-3 fatty acid docosahexaenoic acid in the postmortem orbitofrontal cortex of patients with major depressive disorder. Biol Psychiatry. 2007;62: 17–24. doi: 10.1016/j.biopsych.2006.08.026.

[132] McNamara RK, Jandacek R, Tso P, Dwivedi Y, Ren X, Pandey GN. Lower docosahexaenoic acid concentrations in the postmortem prefrontal cortex of adult depressed suicide victims compared with controls without cardiovascular disease. J Psychiatr Res. 2013;47: 1187–1191. doi: 10.1016/j.jpsychires.2013.05.007.

[133] Rakofsky JJ, Dunlop BW. Review of nutritional supplements for the treatment of bipolar depression. Depress Anxiety. 2014;31: 379–390. doi: 10.1002/da.22220.

[134] Gertsik L, Poland RE, Bresee C, Rapaport MH. Omega-3 fatty acid augmentation of citalopram treatment for patients with major depressive disorder. J Clin Psychopharmacol. 2012;32: 61–64. doi: 10.1097/JCP.0b013e31823f3b5f.

[135] Carrié I, Clément M, de Javel D, Francès H, Bourre JM. Phospholipid supplementation reverses behavioral and biochemical alterations induced by n-3 polyunsaturated fatty acid deficiency in mice. J Lipid Res. 2000;41: 473–480.

[136] Larrieu T, Hilal ML, Hilal LM, Fourrier C, De Smedt-Peyrusse V, Sans N, et al. Nutritional omega-3 modulates neuronal morphology in the prefrontal cortex along with depression-related behaviour through corticosterone secretion. Transl Psychiatry. 2014;4: e437. doi: 10.1038/tp.2014.77.

[137] Levant B. N-3 (omega-3) polyunsaturated Fatty acids in the pathophysiology and treatment of depression: pre-clinical evidence. CNS Neurol Disord Drug Targets. 2013;12: 450–459.

[138] Venna VR, Deplanque D, Allet C, Belarbi K, Hamdane M, Bordet R. PUFA induce antidepressant-like effects in parallel to structural and molecular changes in the hippocampus. Psychoneuroendocrinology. 2009;34: 199–211. doi: 10.1016/j.psyneuen.2008.08.025.

[139] Ferraz AC, Delattre AM, Almendra RG, Sonagli M, Borges C, Araujo P, et al. Chronic ω-3 fatty acids supplementation promotes beneficial effects on anxiety, cognitive and

depressive-like behaviors in rats subjected to a restraint stress protocol. Behav Brain Res. 2011;219: 116–122. doi: 10.1016/j.bbr.2010.12.028.

[140] Gorzalka BB, Hill MN. Putative role of endocannabinoid signaling in the etiology of depression and actions of antidepressants. Prog Neuropsychopharmacol Biol Psychiatry. 2011;35: 1575–1585. doi: 10.1016/j.pnpbp.2010.11.021.

[141] Valverde O, Torrens M. CB1 receptor-deficient mice as a model for depression. Neuroscience. 2012;204: 193–206. doi: 10.1016/j.neuroscience.2011.09.031.

[142] Bluett RJ, Gamble-George JC, Hermanson DJ, Hartley ND, Marnett LJ, Patel S. Central anandamide deficiency predicts stress-induced anxiety: behavioral reversal through endocannabinoid augmentation. Transl Psychiatry. 2014;4: e408. doi: 10.1038/tp.2014.53.

[143] Qin Z, Zhou X, Pandey NR, Vecchiarelli HA, Stewart CA, Zhang X, et al. Chronic stress induces anxiety via an amygdalar intracellular cascade that impairs endocannabinoid signaling. Neuron. 2015;85: 1319–1331. doi: 10.1016/j.neuron.2015.02.015.

[144] Patel S, Kingsley PJ, Mackie K, Marnett LJ, Winder DG. Repeated homotypic stress elevates 2-arachidonoylglycerol levels and enhances short-term endocannabinoid signaling at inhibitory synapses in basolateral amygdala. Neuropsychopharmacology. 2009;34: 2699–2709. doi: 10.1038/npp.2009.101.

[145] Reich CG, Taylor ME, McCarthy MM. Differential effects of chronic unpredictable stress on hippocampal CB1 receptors in male and female rats. Behav Brain Res. 2009;203: 264–269. doi: 10.1016/j.bbr.2009.05.013.

[146] Wang W, Sun D, Pan B, Roberts CJ, Sun X, Hillard CJ, et al. Deficiency in endocannabinoid signaling in the nucleus accumbens induced by chronic unpredictable stress. Neuropsychopharmacology. 2010;35: 2249–2261. doi: 10.1038/npp.2010.99.

[147] Sumislawski JJ, Ramikie TS, Patel S. Reversible gating of endocannabinoid plasticity in the amygdala by chronic stress: a potential role for monoacylglycerol lipase inhibition in the prevention of stress-induced behavioral adaptation. Neuropsychopharmacology. 2011;36: 2750–2761. doi: 10.1038/npp.2011.166.

[148] Hill MN, Miller GE, Carrier EJ, Gorzalka BB, Hillard CJ. Circulating endocannabinoids and N-acyl ethanolamines are differentially regulated in major depression and following exposure to social stress. Psychoneuroendocrinology. 2009;34: 1257–1262. doi: 10.1016/j.psyneuen.2009.03.013.

[149] Mangieri RA, Piomelli D. Enhancement of endocannabinoid signaling and the pharmacotherapy of depression. Pharmacol Res. 2007;56: 360–366. doi: 10.1016/j.phrs.2007.09.003.

[150] Hill MN, Patel S. Translational evidence for the involvement of the endocannabinoid system in stress-related psychiatric illnesses. Biol Mood Anxiety Disord. 2013;3: 19. doi: 10.1186/2045-5380-3-19.

[151] Larrieu T, Hilal ML, De Smedt-Peyrusse V, Sans N, Layé S. Nutritional Omega-3 deficiency alters glucocorticoid receptor-signaling pathway and neuronal morphology in regionally distinct brain structures associated with emotional deficits, nutritional Omega-3 deficiency alters glucocorticoid receptor-signaling pathway and neuronal morphology in regionally distinct brain structures associated with emotional deficits. Neural Plast. 2015;2016 (2016): e8574830. doi: 10.1155/2016/8574830, 10.1155/2016/8574830.

[152] Malcher-Lopes R, Franco A, Tasker JG. Glucocorticoids shift arachidonic acid metabolism toward endocannabinoid synthesis: a non-genomic anti-inflammatory switch. Eur J Pharmacol. 2008;583: 322–339. doi: 10.1016/j.ejphar.2007.12.033.

[153] Patel S, Roelke CT, Rademacher DJ, Cullinan WE, Hillard CJ. Endocannabinoid signaling negatively modulates stress-induced activation of the hypothalamic-pituitary-adrenal axis. Endocrinology. 2004;145: 5431–5438. doi: 10.1210/en.2004-0638.

[154] Kluger B, Triolo P, Jones W, Jankovic J. The therapeutic potential of cannabinoids for movement disorders. Mov Disord. 2015;30: 313–327. doi: 10.1002/mds.26142.

[155] Hacioglu G, Seval-Celik Y, Tanriover G, Ozsoy O, Saka-Topcuoglu E, Balkan S, et al. Docosahexaenoic acid provides protective mechanism in bilaterally MPTP-lesioned rat model of Parkinson's disease. Folia Histochem Cytobiol. 2012;50: 228–238.

[156] Shchepinov MS, Chou VP, Pollock E, Langston JW, Cantor CR, Molinari RJ, et al. Isotopic reinforcement of essential polyunsaturated fatty acids diminishes nigrostriatal degeneration in a mouse model of Parkinson's disease. Toxicol Lett. 2011;207: 97–103. doi: 10.1016/j.toxlet.2011.07.020.

[157] Tanriover G, Seval-Celik Y, Ozsoy O, Akkoyunlu G, Savcioglu F, Hacioglu G, et al. The effects of docosahexaenoic acid on glial derived neurotrophic factor and neurturin in bilateral rat model of Parkinson's disease. Folia Histochem Cytobiol. 2010;48: 434–441. doi: 10.2478/v10042-010-0047-6.

[158] Bousquet M, Gue K, Emond V, Julien P, Kang JX, Cicchetti F, et al. Transgenic conversion of omega-6 into omega-3 fatty acids in a mouse model of Parkinson's disease. J Lipid Res. 2011;52: 263–271. doi: 10.1194/jlr.M011692.

[159] Bousquet M, Calon F, Cicchetti F. Impact of ω-3 fatty acids in Parkinson's disease. Ageing Res Rev. 2011;10: 453–463. doi: 10.1016/j.arr.2011.03.001.

[160] Dong J, Beard JD, Umbach DM, Park Y, Huang X, Blair A, et al. Dietary fat intake and risk for Parkinson's disease. Mov Disord. 2014;29: 1623–1630. doi: 10.1002/mds.26032.

[161] Calon F, Lim GP, Yang F, Morihara T, Teter B, Ubeda O, et al. Docosahexaenoic acid protects from dendritic pathology in an Alzheimer's disease mouse model. Neuron. 2004;43: 633–645. doi: 10.1016/j.neuron.2004.08.013.

[162] Calon F, Lim GP, Morihara T, Yang F, Ubeda O, Salem N, et al. Dietary n-3 polyunsaturated fatty acid depletion activates caspases and decreases NMDA receptors in the

brain of a transgenic mouse model of Alzheimer's disease. Eur J Neurosci. 2005;22: 617–626. doi: 10.1111/j.1460-9568.2005.04253.x.

[163] Cunnane SC, Chouinard-Watkins R, Castellano CA, Barberger-Gateau P. Docosahexaenoic acid homeostasis, brain aging and Alzheimer's disease: can we reconcile the evidence? Prostaglandins Leukot Essent Fatty Acids. 2013;88: 61–70. doi: 10.1016/j.plefa.2012.04.006.

[164] Piomelli D, Sasso O. Peripheral gating of pain signals by endogenous lipid mediators. Nat Neurosci. 2014;17: 164–174. doi: 10.1038/nn.3612.

[165] Piomelli D, Hohmann AG, Seybold V, Hammock BD. A lipid gate for the peripheral control of pain. J Neurosci. 2014;34: 15184–15191. doi: 10.1523/JNEUROSCI.3475-14.2014.

[166] Rao JS, Lee H-J, Rapoport SI, Bazinet RP. Mode of action of mood stabilizers: is the arachidonic acid cascade a common target? Mol Psychiatry. 2008;13: 585–596. doi: 10.1038/mp.2008.31.

[167] Chauveau F, Cho T-H, Perez M, Guichardant M, Riou A, Aguettaz P, et al. Brain-targeting form of docosahexaenoic acid for experimental stroke treatment: MRI evaluation and anti-oxidant impact. Curr Neurovasc Res. 2011;8: 95–102.

[168] Taha AY, Zahid T, Epps T, Trepanier M-O, Burnham WM, Bazinet RP, et al. Selective reduction of excitatory hippocampal sharp waves by docosahexaenoic acid and its methyl ester analog ex-vivo. Brain Res. 2013;1537: 9–17. doi: 10.1016/j.brainres.2013.09.004.

[169] Trépanier M-O, Taha AY, Mantha RL, Ciobanu FA, Zeng QH, Tchkhartichvili GM, et al. Increases in seizure latencies induced by subcutaneous docosahexaenoic acid are lost at higher doses. Epilepsy Res. 2012;99: 225–232. doi: 10.1016/j.eplepsyres.2011.12.001.

[170] Gaffuri A-L, Ladarre D, Lenkei Z. Type-1 cannabinoid receptor signaling in neuronal development. Pharmacology. 2012;90: 19–39. doi: 10.1159/000339075.

[171] Roland AB, Ricobaraza A, Carrel D, Jordan BM, Rico F, Simon A, et al. Cannabinoid-induced actomyosin contractility shapes neuronal morphology and growth. Elife. 2014;3: e03159. doi: 10.7554/eLife.03159.

Chapter 7

The Endocannabinoid-Like Derivative Oleoylethanolamide at the Gut–Brain Interface: A "Lipid Way" to Control Energy Intake and Body Weight

Maria Beatrice Passani and Roberto Coccurello

Additional information is available at the end of the chapter

http://dx.doi.org/10.5772/63147

Abstract

In the last three decades, we witnessed a concomitant major increase in lifespan and a worldwide increasing incidence of chronic diseases such as obesity and type 2 diabetes. Disruption of energy homeostasis and systemic inflammation appear as common traits of these epidemic human diseases. The conventional endocannabinoid (eCB) system encompasses two G-protein–coupled receptors (GPCRs), their endogenous ligands (anandamide and 2-AG), and the enzymes essential for eCB biosynthesis and hydrolytic inactivation. Nonetheless, the family of eCB-like derivatives is growing constantly including other *N*-acylethanolamines (NAEs) and 2-monoacylglycerols (2-MAGs) that do not bind canonical CB receptors rather other orphan G-protein–coupled receptors or peroxisome proliferator-activated nuclear receptors (PPARs). Here, we focus on the recent knowledge gathered on one such PPAR endocannabinoid ligand, oleoylethanolamide (OEA), from the identification of its synthesis in the small intestine to its anorexiant function with particular emphasis on our discovery of the main brain neurotransmitters system involved in its satiating effects.

Keywords: dietary fatty acids, histamine, PPARα, GPR119, oxytocin

Abbreviations:

2-arachidonoylglycerol (2-AG); 2-linoleoylglycerol (2-LG); 2-monoacylglycerols (2-MAGs); 2-oleoyl glycerol (2-OG); 2-palmitoyl glycerol (2-PG); α/β hydrolase domain 6 (ABHD6) and α/β hydrolase domain 12 (ABHD12); Alzheimer's disease (AD); amyotrophic lateral sclerosis (ALS); anandamide (AEA); calcium-dependent *N*-acyltransferase (Ca-NAT); carnitine palmitoyltransferase-1 (CPT-1); docosahexaenoic acid (DHA); eicosapentaenoic acid (EPA); fatty acids (FAs); fatty acid amide hydrolase (FAAH); free fatty acids (FFAs); frontotemporal dementia (FTD); G-protein–coupled receptors (GPCRs); G-protein–coupled receptor 119 (GPR119); GIP (glucose-dependent insulinotropic peptide);glucagon-like peptide-1 (GLP-1); histidine decarboxylase (HDC); long-chain fatty acids (LCFAs); linoleoylethanolamide (LEA); lipoxygenase (LOX); monoacylglycerol lipase (MAGL); medium-chain fatty acids (MCFAs); monounsaturated fatty acids (MFAs); *N*-acylethanolamines (NAEs); *N*-acylethanolamine hydrolyzing acid amidase (NAAA); *N*-acyltransferase (NAT); *N*-arachidonoylethanolamine (AEA); *N*-acylphosphatidylethanolamine (NAPE); NAPE-hydrolyzing phospholipase D (NAPE-PLD); nucleus of the solitary tract (NST); *N*-oleoylethanolamide (OEA); obese (OB); obesity and type 2 diabetes (OBT2D); palmitoylethanolamide (PEA); paraventricular nucleus (PVN);peptide YY (PYY); peroxisome proliferator-activated receptors (PPARs); polyunsaturated fatty acids (PUFAs); pro-opiomelanocortin (POMC); protein kinase C (PKC); retinoid X receptor (RXR); saturated fatty acids (SFA); stearoylethanolamide (SEA); supraoptic nucleus (SON); transient receptor potential vanilloid type-1 (TRPV1); triacylglycerols (TAGs); type 2 diabetes (T2D); uncoupling protein 1 (Ucp1)

1. Introduction

Here the paradox, "although we are entering in the era of super-ageing population and the expected lifespan is increasing worldwide, overweight and obesity are growing global health threats in children and adult people." Western countries and their inhabitants largely contribute to the scenario. However, although in the United States 35% of the population is obese [1, 2], the rising economies are rapidly filling the gap [3, 4]. In this fatter world, obesity is the major health challenge that is accountable for multiple medical conditions. With a significant impact on morbidity and healthcare costs, obesity increases the risk of associated chronic diseases such as type 2 diabetes (T2D), stroke and heart diseases, hypertension and musculoskeletal disorders, and many types of cancer [5, 6]. In particular, the association between obesity and carcinogenesis as in colorectal, pancreatic, prostate, and breast cancer [7] is supported by the abnormal adipose tissue accumulation and systemic chronic inflammation that characterizes this condition. The concept of adiposopathy or "fat sickness" well translates the idea of adipocyte and adipose tissue dysfunction and chronic inflammation that is at the core of obesity-associated diseases.

Metabolic and neurological disorders have been traditionally viewed independently of one another and considered involving different etiologies and pathogenesis. However, obesity during midlife significantly increases the risk of dementias and Alzheimer's disease (AD) later in life [8, 9]. Thus, the detrimental accretion of "fat sickness" during aging and the problem of the defense of cognitive function are linked to unhealthy eating habits and changes in dietary composition of the current (Westernized) food environment. In the Western diet, not only complex carbohydrate and fibers, but also "good fat" (e.g., monounsaturated and polyunsaturated fats) are replaced in high proportions with easy affordable "bad fats" (e.g., saturated fats and vegetable oils) and refined sugars. The daily intake of saturated fat (SF) and simple

http://dx.doi.org/10.5772/63147

sugars increases the risk of impairment of different cognitive functions and accelerate cognitive decline and AD incidence [10–13].

Unhealthy food can dysregulate the hypothalamic control of energy metabolism and affect hippocampal-dependent cognition, consequently every bit of knowledge about the mechanisms underlying the effects of nutrients on brain function becomes of primary importance.

In this chapter, we consider the role of endocannabinoid (eCB)-like derivatives as a particular class of lipids playing a key function in the control of energy intake, adipose tissue metabolism, management of body weight, and cognitive processing.

2. Obesity culprit of health life in Westernized societies: dietary fatty acids set the scenario for the lipid sensor oleoylethanolamide

Poor dietary habits (i.e., high-fat diet and refined carbohydrates) negatively contribute to excessive energy intake, energy accumulation, and consequent dyslipidemia and metabolic disorders such as obesity and type II diabetes (T2D). Poor dietary habits are considered a pathogenetic factor for the increasing incidence of cognitive dementias and primarily of AD [14, 15]. Deciphering the hidden symmetries underlying energy dysfunction in metabolic syndrome and cognitive decline is one of the main challenges of the next future. Despite the heterogeneity of its nutrients, the so-called Western diet is a dietary monopoly in which saturated fats and simple sugars (simple carbohydrates such as mono and disaccharides) are prevailing.

Indeed, the great convenience and affordability of energy-dense foods that are poor in dietary fiber and sucrose-rich are liable for the growing incidence of obesity. As a matter of fact, while dietary fatty acids (FAs) are essential substrates of oxidation and cell energy sources, the elevated concentration of circulating nonesterified fatty acids (NEFAs) or free fatty acids (FFAs) has been considered for a long time a marker of obesity and a pathogenetic factor in obesity, insulin resistance, and etiology of type 2 diabetes [16, 17]. Paradoxically, insulin-sensitive and highly trained athletes may show ectopic lipid deposition in skeletal muscle [18] proving that lipid accretion is not the only factor liable for deficient insulin signaling.

It is well known that the presence of double bonds determines the group to which FAs belong, from saturated fatty acids (SFA) lacking double bonds to one double-bond-containing monounsaturated fatty acids (MFAs), and polyunsaturated fatty acids (PUFAs) containing at least two double bonds. FFAs are signaling molecules capable to alter membrane fluidity, lipid raft, and therefore signal transduction [19]. Different G-protein–coupled receptors (GPCRs) have been identified to mediate FFA-dependent regulation of several metabolic functions as for instance by means of their anti- or proinflammatory effects [20]. The identification of several FFA receptors (FFARs) on the cell surface has allowed clarifying the existence of different classes of FFARs depending on the length of the carbon chain. Hence, FFA2 (GPR43) and FFA3 (GPR41) receptors are activated by short-chain fatty acids (SCFAs), and FFA1 (GPR40) and FFA4 (GPR120) receptors are activated by medium- and long-chain fatty acids (MCFAs and LCFAs, respectively) [21].

FFAs can also affect metabolism acting as ligands of nuclear hormone receptors such as the family of peroxisome proliferator-activated receptors (PPARs), which are ligand-activated transcription factors regulating key genes involved in lipid and nutrient homeostasis and glucose regulation [22]. PPARs are activated To different degrees by most of FFAs with long chain PUFAs showing great activation potency and *n*-3 PUFA eicosapentaenoic acid (EPA) and docosahexaenoic acid (DHA) as more effective than *n*-6 fatty acids. For this reason, PPARs are regarded as energy sensors, master regulators of energy homeostasis [23]. The PPARs family includes three isoforms, PPARα, PPARβ/δ, and PPARγ(NR1C1, NR1C2, and NR1C3, respectively), differing from one another because of their different tissue distribution, types of ligands, and physiological effects [23, 24]. Nevertheless, PPARs share a common mode of action, i.e., the formation of heterodimers with the nuclear receptor retinoid X receptor (RXR) followed by binding to specific DNA-response elements in target genes [23, 24]. Within this context, the involvement of PPAR-mediated signaling is critical in neural pathways that are essential for metabolic adaptivity to energy depletion, in which LCFAs represent the main energy source [25].

The eCBs are FA derivatives and from this point of view their high affinity for PPARs is not totally unexpected. The eCB signaling is terminated by specific lipases such as fatty acid amide hydrolase (FAAH) and *N*-acylethanolamine hydrolyzing acid amidase (NAAA) for anandamide (AEA) and monoacylglycerol lipase (MAGL), α/β hydrolase domain 6 (ABHD6) and domain 12 (ABHD12) for 2-arachidonyl glycerol (2-AG) [26, 27]. AEA and 2-AG are derivatives of *n*-6 PUFA arachidonic acid (AA) and are hydrolyzed into AA and ethanolamine or AA and glycerol, respectively [28, 29]. eCB also modulate functions that are independent of the stimulation of CB1 and CB2 receptors and transient receptor potential vanilloid type-1 (TRPV1) but are mediated by several "orphan" receptor candidates [30], among which the PPARγ that binds AEA, delta9-tetrahydrocannabinol, ajulemic acid, and 2-AG [31–34].

In this chapter, our focus is on the PPARα isoform that is highly expressed in tissues undergoing oxidative stress and is characterized by an elevated metabolic activity as in cardiac muscle, skeletal muscle, intestine, liver, and brown adipose tissue. PPARα activates the expression of genes involved in fatty acid transport and β-oxidation, thus lowering lipid levels [35]. It is known that PPARα can be activated by synthetic ligands such as the hypolipidemic fibrates (e.g., bezafibrate, clofibrate, and fenofibrate) that are part of the treatment of dyslipidemia and T2D [36]. In fact, the PPARα is considered a key fatty acids sensor that mediates lipid metabolism and the effects of FAs and FAs derivatives on gene expression. PPARα is involved in nutrient metabolism, including the metabolism of lipoproteins, glucose, cholesterol, and amino acids. Besides FAs, among the endogenous ligands of PPARα there are FA-like compounds encompassing acyl-CoAs, eicosanoids, eCBs, and eCB-like derivatives [37, 38].

A pioneeristic evidence of the role of PPARα in the effects of eCB derivatives is represented by the demonstration that fatty acid oxygenases, and in particular the lipoxygenase (LOX) metabolism of 2-AG can increase the transcriptional activity of PPARα [39]. Soon after these discoveries, the structural analog of AEA oleoylethanolamide (OEA) appeared on the scene. OEA belongs to a family of lipid mediators known as fatty acyl ethanolamides or *N*-acylethanolamines (NAEs) that are FA derivatives possessing an amide bond linking an ethanolamine to an acyl group [40–42]. Besides AEA (i.e., *N*-arachidonoylethanolamine) and OEA (*N*-oleoylethanolamide), the NAEs family also includes palmitoylethanolamide (PEA), linoleoylethanolamide (LEA), and stearoylethanolamide (SEA) [43].

Briefly, the complex (and best known) biosynthetic pathways of NAEs initiates from the common precursor N-acylphosphatidylethanolamine (NAPE) and consists in a two-step reaction leading first to NAPE formation by transferring the *sn*-1 fatty acid from a donor phospholipid to phosphatidylethanolamine by a calcium-dependent *N*-acyltransferase (Ca-NAT) [44, 45]. Then, in the second-step, NAPE is hydrolyzed to NAEs via the NAPE-hydrolyzing phospholipase D (NAPE-PLD) [45–47]. Interestingly, each NAE is produced by a corresponding NAPE and those having oleic acid (a monounsatured*n*-9 FA) at the amine position (*N*-oleoyl-PE) generate OEA [45].

Thus, dietary FA intake directly affects and modulates endogenous OEA levels according to nutrient (fat) ingestion or food deprivation-induced restriction of OEA synthesis [48]. Dietary FAs modulate food ingestion in the small intestine (luminal layer) via the increased generation of oleic acid-containing NAPEs, mobilization of NAPE-PLD as well as via the reduction of OEA-degrading FAAH activity [49].

OEA is a well-established anorexiant factor, a lipid-based satiety signal whose increase in the lumen of the small intestine induces a persistent and selective inhibition of food intake without known adverse reactions [42, 48–52]. Anorexiant agents can curb food ingestion via distinct mode of action such as the reduction of meal size ingested. Basically, in nonfood deprived animals, OEA administration increases inter-meal latency (decreasing meal frequency), whereas it decreases also meal size in food deprived animals [42, 52]. Recently, it has also been shown that OEA administration induces a clear leftward shifting (an index of early occurrence) in the temporal development of satiety and the premature onset of satiety [53, 54].

According to the current model of functioning, OEA-mediated satiety signal achieves its anorexiant effects via a multistep process that (upon OEA formation) initiates in the small intestinal lumen via the binding to PPARα, of which OEA is a high affinity agonist [49]. This is further corroborated by the failure of OEA-induced decrease of food intake in mice carrying the deletion of PPARα [49, 52]. OEA is a nanomolar agonist of the PPARα [55], and this nuclear receptor is responsible for most of the actions of OEA described so far. In addition, OEA is also a natural ligand of the G-protein–coupled receptor 119 (GPR119), which is not actually a true FFAs receptor, such as FFA1, FFA2, and FFA3 (see above), rather a novel target for FAs derivatives. The orphan GPR119 has been deorphanized by recognizing in the OEA one of its endogenous high affinity ligands [56]. Besides appetite control, GPR119 is also highly expressed in pancreatic β cells and involved in glucose-dependent insulin secretion as well as secretion of gastrointestinal incretin hormone and peptides (glucagon-like peptide-1 (GLP-1) [57] and GIP (glucose-dependent insulinotropic peptide) from enteroendocrine cells [57] (**Figure 1**). GLP-1 has, among other properties, insulinotropic effects inhibition of gastric emptying, reduction of appetite and promotion of satiety in humans [58] and rodents [59]. Likewise other FAs and FFAs receptors such as GPR120 [60] and FFA1 [61], GPR119 is a lipid sensing receptor [62] that is activated by oleic acid-containing lipids (e.g., *N*-oleoyl-dopamine) and regarded as a potential drug target for the treatment of T2D. In this view, the antidiabetic potential of OEA is still unexplored. The ability of OEA to bind the GPR119 is already demonstrated not to be required for appetite suppression [63]; indeed, deletion of the GPR119 in mice does not prevent the anorexigenic effects of OEA [63, 64]. OEA binding to GPR119 induces secretion of GLP-1 from enteroendocrine L-cells of the ileum [65, 66] and therefore OEA is an *in- vivo* GLP-1 secretagogue. Finally, the TRPV1 must be included [67] especially for its relevance in the "entourage effect" and therefore in the ability to interfere with the eCB system [68].

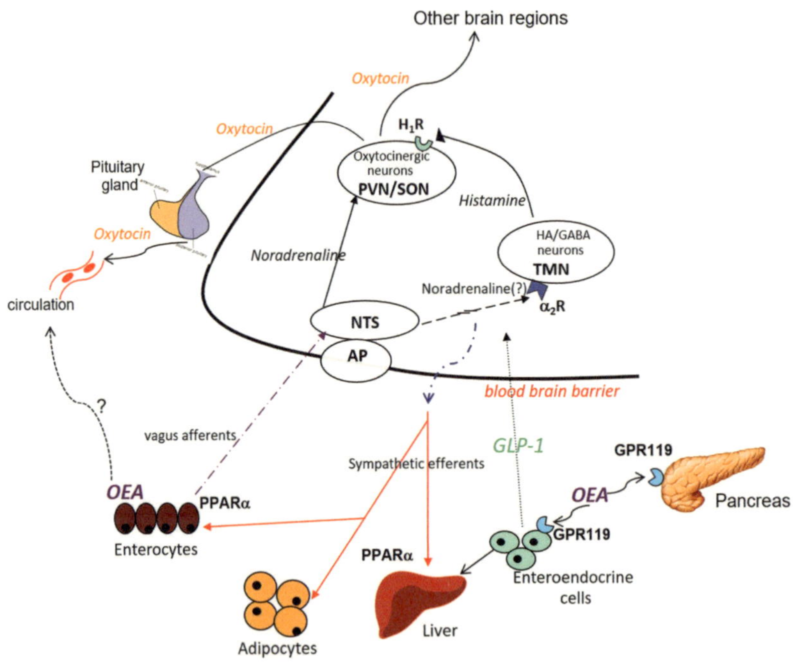

Figure 1. Schematic drawing illustrating the putative interactions between OEA, brain regions, and peripheral organs. OEA activates PPAR-α in the jejunum generating a signal that induces several transcriptional changes leading to increased fatty-acid catabolism, reduced blood lipid levels, and decreased appetite through the activation of brain centers. OEA signaling travels through vagal afferents to the nucleus of the solitary tract (NST). OEA may also reach the area postrema (AP; that lacks a tight blood brain barrier) through the circulation. From the NST noradrenergic afferents regulate oxytocin synthesis in the paraventricular (PVN) and supraoptic nucleus (SON) both directly and via the histaminergic tuberomammillary nucleus (TMN). Efferent neural pathways (for clarity only the sympathetic component is shown here) under the control of brain nuclei may alter energy expenditure and peripheral organs' function. OEA binds also to GPR119 that are expressed on pancreatic β-cells involved in glucose-dependent insulin secretion, as well as on enteroendocrine cells that secrete incretins such as glucagon-like peptide-1 (GLP-1).

3. Placing NAEs and 2-MAGs in the framework of the eCB system and lipid detection: satiety signals and fat sensors

Besides OEA, anorexiant effects have been ascribed also to other NAEs such as PEA and LEA [69]. This study elegantly demonstrates that high-fat feeding reduces intestinal NAEs levels in a dose-dependent fashion also supporting the previous idea that such reduction may also differently affect OEA, PEA and LEA depending on the type of fat (e.g., oleic Vs palmitic oil) ingested [70]. Another key point is the observation that orexigenic AEA and 2-AG levels in the jejunum are upregulated by the arachidonic acid-based diet [70] and that a diet reaching 38% of energy from fat reduces OEA, PEA, and LEA content, irrespective of dietary fat composition [70]. This finding demonstrates the critical importance of long-term exposure to high-fat-like Western diet, rich in saturated (e.g., palmitic acid) and *n*-6 PUFAs dietary fat. Indeed, protracted intake of high-fat diet has been hypothesized to increase the luminal content of FAs and 2-monoacylglycerol thus downregulating the NAT activity lowering the main anorectic NAEs OEA, PEA and LEA [46]. In turn, decreasing the endogenous levels of lipid signals conveying information on meal cessation and satiety removes the control brake on high-fat diet-induced hyperphagia.

The family of eCB-like derivatives includes the additional component of 2-monoacylglycerols (2-MAGs) among which 2-oleoyl glycerol (2-OG), 2-palmitoyl glycerol (2-PG), and 2-linoleoylglycerol (2-LG). Dietary triacylglycerols (TAGs) are the major lipids source for the stimulation of intestinal incretin hormones release. TAG hydrolysis by pancreas lipase produces FAs (two molecules) and 2-MAG (one molecule), with the portion of 2-MAG not degraded contributing to the total levels of 2-MAGs of the intestinal lumen after dietary fat intake [71, 72].

Although we have previously described the high affinity of OEA for GPR119, it is presently not clear the extent to which the low endogenous levels of this lipid-derived signal in the gastrointestinal cells can activate for instance GLP-1 release. Moreover, contrary to the cycles of feeding deprivation and refeeding [49] that produces opposite changes in OEA levels as function of NAPE-PLD activity, prolonged dietary fat intake can reduce intestinal NAEs levels. By contrast, direct effects of dietary fat on incretin secretion (plasma GLP-1 and GIP) have been shown to occur upon 2-OG administration in (fasting) humans volunteers [73]. More recently, it has been demonstrated that the GPR119 activation induced by 2-OG can explain the olive oil-elicited secretion of GLP-1 and peptide YY (PYY) [74]. Similarly, meal rich either in palmitic or linoleic acids will produce TAG deposit in adipose tissue mostly as 2-PG and 2-LG, respectively [75].

This opens a scenario where NAEs, and in particular OEA and 2-MAGs, can play together a concerted (though slightly different) action in fat sensing, lipid detection, and regulation of dietary fat ingestion via satiety signaling. Assuming GPR119 as a fat sensor [62], the high binding potency of full agonists such as OEA [56] is not sufficient to predict higher stimulatory effects on incretin secretion. Although 2-MAGs bind GPR119 less potently than OEA [73] their elevated intestinal levels will increase the probability of GLP-1 activation, especially for 2-OG. Moreover, GLP-1 stimulation is higher upon synthesis of 2-OG than 2-PG, further confirming how much healthier the olive oil-based diet (i.e., Mediterranean diet) can be in comparison with the saturated fat-rich (e.g., palmitic acid) Western diet. An increase of the intestinal levels of 2-MAGs has been described as one key factor underlying the insulin sensitizer effects and antiadipogenic activity of probiotic (*Akkermansia muciniphila*) treatment in high-fat-fed mice [76]. One hypothesis suggests that prolonged high-fat diet intake may downregulate the activity of the NAPE-synthetizing enzyme NAT, thus reducing NAEs levels via a still unknown

2-MAGs-dependent mechanism [46]. In our opinion, this supports the potential *dichotomous role of* 2-MAGs (mainly 2-OG) and NAEs (mainly OEA) that might function as fat sensors and satiety signaling, respectively.

Despite the important knowledge accumulated regarding the hypothalamic mechanisms underlying the control of energy homeostasis and the distinct populations of neurons responsible for appetite regulation [77], very little is known about the central pathways responsible for translating the peripheral information of nutritional status and in orchestrating neural adaptive responses. For instance, we know that different protein kinase C (PKC) isoforms (PKC-δ, PKC-ε, and PKC-θ) are required as dietary fat-associated (e.g., LCFA-CoA) signal transduction pathways and are involved in the development of insulin resistance [78]. In the following sections, we further examine the notion of brain–gut interface, where the OEA signaling originates, the role of OEA in energy homeostasis, and the discovery of the main brain anorexigenic neural pathways engaged by OEA.

4. The notion of brain–gut interface

Fatty acid components are the primary source of calories and constituents of cells and cell membrane-derived modulators such as eCBs and prostanoids. Evolution has endowed our species and other mammals of chemical sensors and neuronal machineries to monitor fat intake and direct foraging behavior to the optimization of fat-rich food collection and consumption. Therefore, a constant updating of the nutritional status and energy expenditure is required for the adequate behavioral responses and homeostatic adjustments. This network links not only peripheral intestinal functions via the production of a number of bioactive molecules with hypothalamic satiety and hunger centers, but also with brain areas devoted to emotional responses and cognitive processes. In modern days, though, fat rich food has lost its survival salience, as it is easily and often inexpensively available to a large part of the population in Western cultures. In fact, a fatty diet has become one of the major causes of obesity, one of today's most blatantly visible – yet most neglected – public health problems. The World Health Organization coined the term "globesity" [3] to pinpoint the escalating global epidemic of overweight and obesity, paradoxically coexisting with undernutrition and malnutrition.

How this "gut–brain axis" network works has only partially been elucidated, however some of the pathways, transmitters, and hormones involved are beginning to be mapped and discovered.

Sensing for dietary fat, begins in the mouth where taste bud cells of the lingual epithelium are activated and transmit an initial set of signals to the nucleus of the solitary tract (NST) in the brain stem [79, 80], and then to brain regions devoted to controlling satiety (e.g., hypothalamic paraventricular, tuberomamillary, arcuate nuclei) as well as to centers that coordinate reward related responses such as the nucleus accumbens [80, 81]. Taken together, all these observations suggest that mammals at least may indeed have a "taste" for fatty food. In the intestine, upon activation by lipids, specialized chemosensory cells release hormones, peptides, lipid-derived mediators that relay signals to the brain via hormonal or neuronal pathways [82, 83]. Among the membrane sensors expressed by these specialized neurons in the oral and intestinal epithelium are the CD36 proteins [79, 84], the G-protein–coupled receptors GPR40 and GPR120 [85]. A decade ago it was discovered that OEA and a subset of structurally similar FAEs are key components of the molecular machinery responsible for monitoring fat intake in the small intestine [48]. Fatty acid ethanolamides provide afferent signals from the digestive tract that travel mostly via vagal afferents [48] to the NST in the brain stem, and activate hypothalamic brain centers that promote satiety, therefore controlling eating behavior (**Figure 1**). It appears then, that the NST serves as a relay station where gustatory information carried by autonomic cephalic nerves, and postingestive information via the vagus nerve converge, filtering out pleasurable sensations (the cephalic phase that assigns rewarding value to food) and metabolic responses (reviewed in [80]).

The concept of brain lipid sensing is not new and is related to the problem of brain detection of body's nutritional status. In addition to fat sensing hypothalamic nuclei, midbrain, and hindbrain circuitry can detect glucose levels (glucose sensing neurons), as in pro-opiomelanocortin (POMC) neurons of high-fat-fed mice that developed insensitivity to glucose load and impaired glucose-elicited ATP production [86]. Glucose and lipid sensing are the two main brain systems for nutrients detection corresponding to insulin and fatty acids signaling acting to preserve energy homeostasis. Moreover, insulin and fat sensing may act either cooperatively or independently of each other to inhibit glucose production and appetite, respectively. The brain lipid sensing system relies on long-chain fatty acids (LCFAs), as lipid signals and oleic acid infusion within the brain inhibits hepatic glucose production, food intake and elicits satiety [87, 88]. In the neurons LCFAs are esterified to LCFA-CoA by acyl-CoA synthetase. In turn, the entry of LCFA-CoA into mitochondria for β-oxidation is regulated by carnitine palmitoyltransferase-1 (CPT-1). The experimental inhibition of hypothalamic CPT-1 increases LCFA-CoA neuronal levels and this event is able to reduce glucose production and to promote premature satiety occurrence [88, 89]. These studies provide evidence that lipid sensing through the gut–brain axis links together different macromolecules involved in nutrients sensing and is critical for glucose homeostasis and appetite control. These reports also indicate that in parallel with the duodenum, LCFA-CoA accumulation is a key event for the inhibition of energy intake and glucose production. Yet again, in case of prolonged intake of high-fat diet, LCFA-CoA fails to accumulate and oleic acid does not reduce hepatic glucose production [90, 91], possibly because of the increase in hypothalamic CPT-1 activity. Remarkably, besides gut nutrient sensing (e.g., intestinal lipid metabolism and cholecystokinin signaling), the brain is able to detect afferent nutrients and peripheral nutritional status to regulate whole-body glucose metabolism and energy homeostasis [86, 92–94].

Efferent neural pathways, i.e., the autonomic nervous system and the hypothalamic-pituitary adrenal axis, under the regulation of the brain may alter energy expenditure and intestinal function [95]. One such pathway originates in the NST toward the digestive tract facilitating fat digestion and absorption (**Figure 1**). Another example of central control of peripheral functions is provided by the influence exerted by the hypothalamic histaminergic neurons, one of the key brain systems regulating eating behavior [96, 97] on peripheral homeostatic responses. Preclinical studies showed that the administration of histamine or of an agonist of the histamine H_1 receptor in the ventricle or the hypothalamic paraventricular nucleus, where activation of these receptors induces satiety, increases mRNA expression levels of uncoupling protein 1 (Ucp1), a marker of energy expenditure, in brown adipose tissue and increases the electrophysiological activity of sympathetic nerves that innervate it [98, 99]. Also, the central administration of histamine augments the lipolytic response in white adipose tissue, whereas pretreatment with a beta adrenergic receptor antagonist blocks the histamine-induced response, suggesting that the effect is mediated by sympathetic nerves that innervate the white adipose tissue [100]. Furthermore, it has been recently proposed [101] that neuronal histamine by activating H_1 receptors downregulates hepatic gluconeogenic gene expression. Interestingly, several of these effects are shared by gut-derived OEA. Another efferent pathway was demonstrated by direct intracerebroventricular infusion of palmitic acid that reduced insulin-mediated suppression of hepatic insulin production. Furthermore, palmitic acid-enriched diet activates PKC-θ in the arcuate nucleus and impairs insulin and leptin signaling [102]. This study elegantly demonstrates the role of PKC-θ activation as one of the pathogenetic mechanisms involved in the genesis of insulin resistance during prolonged high-fat diet intake.

The fascinating aspects of this complex interplay between the intestinal and the central nervous system is that bioactive molecules generated in the digestive tract signal to the brain not only the nutritional status, but may affect also cognitive and emotional responses. As a matter of fact, diet containing balanced PUFAs has become the object of intense research in relation to cognitive aging and neurodegenerative diseases. In this scenario the potential role of gut microbiota in influencing brain function, behavior, in the development of the central nervous system and mental health has recently attracted the attention of neuroscientists and psychiatrists [103–105]. The relevance of the gut–brain axis in health and disease is becoming manifest as preclinical and clinical studies are providing new evidence. In a recent report [106], metabolic changes incorporating fluctuations in weight, insulin resistance, and cholesterol concentrations in several neurodegenerative disorders, such as amyotrophic lateral sclerosis (ALS) and frontotemporal dementia (FTD) have been observed. The authors raise the intriguing possibility of a dysregulated homeostatic balance between peripheral and central signals as partly accountable for the different phenotypes of ALS and FTD patients. In other words, the authors' hypothesis is that neurodegenerative processes affecting brain regions necessary for metabolic regulation concur to the onset of the observed metabolic changes. The gut and the brain, then, use a plethora of signals to communicate, to monitor and integrate gut functions as well as to link emotional and cognitive centers of the brain with peripheral intestinal activity.

It is clear then, that gaining insight into this bidirectional communication network on the one hand poses truly great challenges to the scientific community, on the other it is indispensable to understand the potential for targeting modifiable risk factors in disease development and progression.

5. OEA and the control of energy homeostasis

As previously mentioned, OEA signaling is a biosensor for dietary fat that is generated from oleic acid and conveys a message that translates into a state of satiety characterized by prolonged inter-meal intervals and reduced feeding frequency [48]. OEA is also found in several other organs such as liver, adipose tissue, and brain and its levels can be affected by short-term feeding of nutrients reminiscent of human diets [70]. However, protein and carbohydrates do not stimulate OEA mobilization [52]. OEA biological effects are not limited to moderating food intake, but include stimulation of fat utilization in adipocytes and hepatocytes [107], of fatty acid absorption in the jejunum [108], of incretins secretion from the ileum [65]. The effects of OEA on peripheral organs will be dealt in this paragraph, whereas a separate section will be dedicated to the central actions of OEA.

Digestion of complex dietary lipids in the small-intestinal lumen releases free oleic acid, which is internalized presumably by the transporter CD36 on the luminal membrane of enterocytes in the jejunum [109]. Oleic acid is then directed either toward the formation of chylomicrons or toward the production of OEA through the NAT/NAPE-PLD pathway [109]. Palmitic acid and linoleic acid as well are taken up presumably by the same transporter CD36 into the enterocyte and incorporated into NAPE increasing intestinal levels of PEA and LEA, respectively [46]. Surprisingly, diet-induced obese rats and mice, or rats fed with a diet high in NAEs precursors' content for over 1 week, had decreased intestinal (not hepatic, nor central) levels of the three NAEs [110] independently of the type of dietary fatty acid fed to the rats [70]. This effect is reversible as switching the high-fat diet back to low-fat chow restores the intestinal levels of OEA, LEA, and PEA to normal within 3 days [111]. Therefore, it appears that excessive fat intake may render the mechanism dysfunctional, suggesting that suppressing the satiating effects of gut-derived OEA with a diet rich in fat might contribute to overeating [112].

Food intake and food deprivation also regulate the content of OEA in the jejunum as OEA levels decrease during food deprivation and increase upon refeeding through a concerted regulation of OEA biosynthesis and degradation [49]. However, other visceral organs, such as the liver and pancreas, respond to food deprivation with an increase rather than a decrease in OEA levels, whereas plasma OEA concentrations is modestly affected, implying that nutrients regulate OEA mobilization in a tissue-specific manner [49]. The mechanisms by which nutrients and food deprivation regulate OEA levels in the liver and pancreas is not known, and the biological significance of such a control is not fully explained. Nonetheless, OEA appears to have potential therapeutic effects in liver dysfunctions. A direct comparison of the effect of OEA and fenofibrate (a PPARα agonist used in clinical practice to regulate plasma lipid disorders) on a rat model of nonalcoholic fatty liver disease showed an improved protective effect of OEA and a safer profile with respect to the fibrate [113]. OEA reduces liver triacylglycerol levels and enhances fatty acid oxidation in hepatocytes and these effects are maintained in mice fed a high-fat diet [107]. The authors suggest that changes in lipid metabolism induced by PPARα activation contribute to the weight-reducing action of OEA in obese mice. Furthermore, in rats OEA regulates several hepatic enzymes including liver fatty acid binding protein (responsible for uptake and intracellular trafficking of fatty acids) [113] and the thermogenic uncoupling protein-1 [114]. Also, subchronic administration of a recently synthesized analog of OEA that binds PPARα receptors, elaidyl-sulfamide, was found to lower plasma cholesterol and improve the hepatic function of obese rats [115]. Clearly, these observations warrant further investigation to fully understand the potential therapeutic of OEA and congeners in hepatic function.

The available data on the effects of OEA on the adipose tissue suggest that OEA may work in concert with the sympathetic system to control fat metabolism. The incubation of dissociated rat and mouse adipocytes with OEA increased the release of nonesterified fatty acids and glycerol into the extracellular medium in a dose-dependent manner [107]. Of note, a significant fatty acid mobilization occurred also *in vivo* after systemic administration of OEA to lean rats. Conversely, OEA did not change the plasma levels of glucose, insulin, or glucagon, but markedly increased the transcription of several adipose-tissue genes involved in lipid transport, including CD36 and fatty acid-binding protein [107]. More recently it was reported that administration of OEA caused a significant fat mass reduction and enhanced energy expenditure in rats [114].

One of the first studies in humans showed the potential role of OEA as a regulator of adipose tissue metabolism in obesity and type II diabetes [116]. The study evaluated the levels of endocannabinoids such as AEA, 2-AG, OEA and PEA in the subcutaneous adipose tissue of subjects with both obesity and type II diabetes (OBT2D) and nondiabetic obese (OB) vs normal subjects. All participants in the study showed similar adiposity and whole-body insulin resistance and lower plasma leptin levels when compared with normal controls. However, the levels of OEA, PEA, 2-AG, and AEA were all altered only in OBT2D, but not in OB as compared with normal subjects [116]. The authors suggest that such alterations might contribute to a redistribution of fat accumulation in the subcutaneous adipose tissue relative to visceral adipose tissue and to metabolic dysfunctions that, along with impaired insulin release and sensitivity, are typical of OBT2D patients [116].

6. From gut to the brain: OEA signaling engages the anorexigenic neural pathways

The extensive body of preclinical literature presented so far provides undisputable evidence that OEA functions as a homeostatic signal that regulates metabolic functions, and causes a long-lasting inhibition of food intake in rats, mice, and humans as well [48, 55, 117, 118].

OEA produces its anorexic effects through a mechanism mediated by the vagus nerve, as the hypophagic effect is prevented after vagotomy or reversible blockade of the NST a brain stem area that receives vagal inputs, and it is ineffective when infused directly in the cerebral ventricles [48]. A recent study, though, challenged this suggestion as it reported that in rats that received a subdiaphragmatic vagotomy, OEA maintained its hypophagic effect [119]. Clearly, these inconsistencies require further elucidations. In addition to the vagus nerve, a descending sympathetic pathway originating in the rostral ventrolateral medulla that sends noradrenergic projections to the intestine and other visceral organs, contributes to OEA signaling. Surgical disconnection of this pathway impairs the ability of intraduodenal fat infusions to reduce food intake and inhibits the food-induced OEA synthesis in the jejunum [120].

The central neurotransmitter systems recruited by peripheral OEA to inhibit food intake is beginning to be unraveled. Exogenous administration of OEA increases transcription of the early gene c-Fos, a marker of neuronal activation, in the NST [48], it increases c-Fos mRNA and protein expression in oxytocin-immunoreactive neurons in the paraventricular (PVN) and supraoptic nucleus (SON) [42, 53] in the histaminergic tuberomammillary nucleus [53] and in the area postrema [121], a circumventricular organ that lacks a functional blood brain barrier (**Figure 1**). This latter observation suggests a direct action of OEA in the brain stem by reaching the area postrema from the blood stream [42].

The activation of PVN and SON is paralleled by increased oxytocin mRNA levels, increased peptide neurosecretion, and elevated circulating oxytocin levels [42, 53] (**Figure 1**).In addition, pharmacological blockade of central oxytocin receptors abolishes the hypophagic effects of OEA [42], implying that release of oxytocin in the hypothalamus and/or other brain regions is an obligatory effector of OEA-induced satiety. A noradrenergic pathway from the NST to the hypothalamus seems to mediate OEA effects on feeding behavior and on hypothalamic oxytocin increase, as demonstrated in rats with chemical lesions of hindbrain noradrenergic neurons [122]. Accordingly, in rats, peripheral administration of OEA increases noradrenaline concentrations in the hypothalamus [123]. Recently, we reported that OEA requires the integrity of the central histaminergic system to fully exert its hypophagic effect [53]. Brain histamine has long been known as a mediator of satiety through activation of hypothalamic histamine H_1 receptors [95–97]. In our study [53] we report that mice deficient of the histamine synthesizing enzyme histidine decarboxylase ($HDC^{-/-}$ mice), or pharmacologically deprived of releasable brain histamine did not respond to the hypophagic effect of exogenously administered OEA as normal mice did. We also found that OEA increased c-Fos protein expression in oxytocin neurons of the PVN of wild type, but not $HDC^{-/-}$ mice, suggesting that oxytocin rich nuclei are the likely brain region where histaminergic and OEA indirect signaling converge (**Figure 1**). In this context, it is important to note that OEA does not induce conditioned taste aversion in rats and does not produce behaviors that are indicative of a state of fear or anxiety as it does not change plasma corticosterone levels [124]. Hence, we may exclude that OEA hypophagic actions are attributable to stress or malaise. In fact, the exogenous subchronic oral administration of OEA in rats was shown to have an antidepressant-like action, an effect that is attributed to OEA-induced changes in cerebral noradrenaline and serotonin contents [125].

Despite no data are available indicating that OEA may subserve a neuromodulatory role in the brain, it has been reported that PPARα activity modulates the firing rate of dopaminergic neurons in the rat midbrain through a fast effect on nicotinic receptors [126]. These observations are suggestive of a role of OEA in the modulation of reward and hedonic, nonhomeostatic functions related to the salience of food-related stimuli.

It is well established that stress hormones activated by emotional arousal enhance memories associated with emotional events [127]. Hormonal and neural signaling elicited by feeding as well enhance the consolidation of recent experiences [128]. In this elegant work, the authors used two distinct experimental paradigms in rats to test consolidation of aversive and spatial memories, namely the inhibitory avoidance and the Morris water maze, and found that systemic administration of OEA after training strongly improved the retention of these tasks. The memory-enhancing signal generated by OEA apparently activates the brain **via** the noradrenergic pathway that generates from NST and provides innervation of the basolateral amygdala, being this a pathway crucially implicated in the consolidation of recent emotional memories [129]. It is conceivable, then, that OEA mobilized in the gut after a fat-rich meal initiates an integrated response that prompts enhanced encoding of information about the spatial and emotional context in which the meal was consumed [130]. Synthetic PPARα agonists and inhibitor of FAAHs as well seem to ameliorate memory acquisition in a passive avoidance task in rats [131].

7. Conclusions

The evidence accumulated over the past years strongly support the notion that OEA mediates nutrient- and lipid-specific satiety, fatty acids absorption in enterocytes, lipolysis in adipose tissue, liver and skeletal myocytes, and thermogenic responses [48, 107, 108, 114]. Furthermore, we recently established that the eCB-derivative OEA engages the brain histaminergic [53] and oxytocinergic [42, 53] system to induce satiety and suppression of food intake (**Figure 1**). This study uncovers previously unidentified neural signaling mechanisms involved in the anorectic action of OEA and offers new perspectives for the development of more effective and safer pharmacotherapies to treat obesity and ameliorate the profile of centrally acting drugs [53].

OEA is an ethanolamide of long-chain unsaturated FAs that appears to fulfill most of the criteria used to classify the antiobesity medications, among which safety is of primary importance. Moreover, OEA is an anorexigenic factor that can curb energy intake, stimulate sympathetic activity, and control body weight. Thus, the possibility to investigate the role of OEA in obese patients might not be speculative anymore. A meal rich in oleic acid increases OEA plasma levels in healthy volunteers also reducing the total energy intake 3 hours after oleic acid ingestion [118]. In a recent study [132] on obese patients, it was found that plasma OEA levels positively correlated with body mass index (BMI) whereas an inverse correlation was observed between obesity andbrain areas activity (e.g., insula) associated with reward-signaling. Chronic consumption of "obesogenic" high-fat food can dampen dopamine-mediated signaling of reward and disrupt the relationship between palatable food-associated hedonic eating and neural correlates of reward processing [133–135]. The negative correlation between insular activity and OEA plasma levels in obese subjects raises the possibility that OEA may be involved in the suppression of food-associated liking reaction and that obesity might disturb this function. OEA synthesis is disrupted after prolonged high-fat intake but OEA administration can restore striatal dopamine release and lipid signaling in the gut and increase the hedonic value of less caloric food [136]. Collectively, these data broaden the potential of OEA as dietary fat-derived satiety signal involved in homeostatic feeding as well as in the regulation of hedonic eating.

Acknowledgements

This work was supported by the Italian Ministry of Health – Young Researchers grant GR-2011-02346912. The authors thank Dr. Gustavo Provensi and Dr. Giacomo Giacovazzo for their contributions to unravel the role of the histaminergic system in recruiting OEA-mediated satiety signal. The authors declare no conflict of interest.

Author details

Maria Beatrice Passani[1] and Roberto Coccurello[2*]

*Address all correspondence to: roberto.coccurello@cnr.it

1 Department of Health Sciences Section of Clinical Pharmacology & Oncology, University of Florence, V.le Pieraccini, Firenze, Italy. Position: Maria Beatrice Passani, Associate professor, Department of Health Sciences Section of Clinical Pharmacology & Oncology, University of Florence, Italy

2 National Research Council of Italy (C.N.R.), Institute of Cell Biology and Neurobiology (IBCN), Fondazione S. Lucia (FSL) IRCCS – Via del Fosso di Fiorano, Rome, Italy

References

[1] Flegal KM, Carroll MD, Ogden CL, Curtin LR. Prevalence and trends in obesity among US adults, 1999–2008. JAMA. 2010;303:235–241. DOI: 10.1001/jama.2009.2014

[2] Ogden CL, Carroll MD, Kit BK, Flegal KM. Prevalence of childhood and adult obesity in the United States, 2011–2012. JAMA. 2014;311:806–814. DOI: 10.1001/jama.2014.732

[3] Prentice AM. The emerging epidemic of obesity in developing countries. Int J Epidemiol. 2006;35:93–99. DOI: 10.1093/ije/dyi272

[4] Arnold M, Pandeya N, Byrnes G, Renehan AG, Stevens GA, Ezzati M, et al. Global burden of cancer attributable to high body-mass index in 2012: a population-based study. Lancet Oncol. 2014;16:36–46. DOI: 10.1016/S1470-2045(14)71123-4

[5] Haslam DW, James WPT. Obesity. Lancet. 2005;366:1197–1209. DOI: 10.1016/S0140-6736(05)67483-1

[6] Wiseman M. The second World Cancer Research Fund/American Institute for Cancer Research expert report. Food, nutrition, physical activity, and the prevention of cancer: a global perspective. Proc Nutr Soc. 2008;67:253–256.DOI: 10.1017/S002966510800712X

[7] Renehan AG, Tyson M, Egger M. Body-mass index and incidence of cancer: a systematic review and meta-analysis of prospective observational studies. Lancet.2008;371:569–578. DOI: 10.1016/S0140-6736(08)60269-X

[8] Tolppanen AM, Ngandu T, Kåreholt I, Laatikainen T, Rusanen M, Soininen H, et al. Midlife and late-life body mass index and late-life dementia: results from a prospective population-based cohort. J Alzheimer's Dis. 2014;38:201–209. DOI: 10.3233/JAD-130698

[9] Emmerzaal TL, Kiliaan AJ, Gustafson DR. 2003–2013: A decade of body mass index, Alzheimer's disease, and dementia. J Alzheimer's Dis. 2015; 43:739–755. DOI: 10.3233/JAD-141086

[10] Winocur G, Greenwood CE. Studies of the effects of high fat diets on cognitive function in a rat model. Neurobiol Aging. 2005;26:46–49. DOI: 10.1016/j.neurobiolaging.2005.09.003

[11] Beydoun MA, Beydoun HA, Wang Y. Obesity and central obesity as risk factors for incident dementia and its subtypes: a systematic review and meta-analysis. Obes Rev. 2008;9:204–218. DOI: 10.1111/j.1467-789X.2008.00473.x

[12] De Felice FG, Lourenco M V. Brain metabolic stress and neuroinflammation at the basis of cognitive impairment in Alzheimer's disease. Front Aging Neurosci. 2015;7:94. DOI: 10.3389/fnagi.2015.00094

[13] Prickett C, Brennan L, Stolwyk R. Examining the relationship between obesity and cognitive function: a systematic literature review. Obes Res Clin Pract. 2015;9:93–113. DOI: 10.1016/j.orcp.2014.05.001

[14] Hsu TM, Kanoski SE. Blood-brain barrier disruption: mechanistic links between Western diet consumption and dementia. Front Aging Neurosci. 2014;9:88. DOI: 10.3389/fnagi.2014.00088

[15] Pasinetti GM, Eberstein JA. Metabolic syndrome and the role of dietary lifestyles in Alzheimer's disease. J Neurochem. 2008;106:1503–1514. DOI: 10.1111/j.1471-4159.2008.05454.x

[16] Boden G. Free fatty acids-the link between obesity and insulin resistance. Endocr Pract. 2001;7:44–51. DOI: 10.4158/EP.7.1.44

[17] Karpe F, Dickmann JR, Frayn KN. Fatty acids, obesity, and insulin resistance: Time for a reevaluation. Diabetes. 2011;60:2441–2449. DOI: 10.2337/db11-0425

[18] Goodpaster BH, He J, Watkins S, Kelley DE. Skeletal muscle lipid content and insulin resistance: Evidence for a paradox in endurance-trained athletes. J Clin Endocrinol Metab. 2001;86:5755–5761. http://dx.doi.org/10.1210/jcem.86.12.8075

[19] Ma DWL, Seo J, Switzer KC, Fan YY, McMurray DN, Lupton JR, et al. n-3 PUFA and membrane microdomains: a new frontier in bioactive lipid research. J Nutr Biochem. 2004;15:700–706. DOI: 10.1016/j.jnutbio.2004.08.002

[20] Ichimura A, Hasegawa S, Kasubuchi M, Kimura I. Free fatty acid receptors as therapeutic targets for the treatment of diabetes. Front Pharmacol. 2014;5:236. DOI: 10.3389/fphar.2014.00236

[21] Brown AJ, Goldsworthy SM, Barnes AA, Eilert MM, Tcheang L, Daniels D, et al. The orphan G protein-coupled receptors GPR41 and GPR43 are activated by propionate and other short chain carboxylic acids. J Biol Chem. 2003;278:11312–11319. DOI: 10.1074/jbc.M211609200

[22] Evans RM. PPARs and the complex journey to obesity. Keio J Med.2004;53:53–58. http://doi.org/10.2302/kjm.53.53

[23] Berger J, Moller DE. The mechanisms of action of PPARs. Annu Rev Med. 2002;53:409–435. DOI: 10.1146/annurev.med.53.082901.104018

[24] Schmitz G, Ecker J. The opposing effects of n-3 and n-6 fatty acids. Prog Lipid Res. 2008;47:147–155. DOI: 10.1016/j.plipres.2007.12.004

[25] Nakamura MT, Yudell BE, Loor JJ. Regulation of energy metabolism by long-chain fatty acids. Prog Lipid Res. 2014;53:124–144. DOI: 10.1016/j.plipres.2013.12.001

[26] Sun Y, Alexander SP, Garle MJ, Gibson CL, Hewitt K, Murphy SP, et al. Cannabinoid activation of PPAR alpha; a novel neuroprotective mechanism. Br J Pharmacol. 2007;152:734–743. DOI: 10.1038/sj.bjp.0707478

[27] Blankman JL, Cravatt BF. Chemical probes of endocannabinoid metabolism. Pharmacol Rev. 2013;65:849–871. DOI: 10.1124/pr.112.006387

[28] Freund TF, Katona I, Piomelli D. Role of endogenous cannabinoids in synaptic signaling. Physiol Rev. 2003;83:1017–1066. DOI: 10.1152/physrev.00004.2003

[29] Turcotte C, Chouinard F, Lefebvre JS, Flamand N. Regulation of inflammation by cannabinoids, the endocannabinoids 2-arachidonoyl-glycerol and arachidonoyl-ethanolamide, and their metabolites. J Leukoc Biol. 2015;97:1049–1070. DOI: 10.1189/jlb.3RU0115-021R

[30] Howlett AC, Barth F, Bonner TI, Cabral G, Casellas P, Devane WA, et al. International Union of Pharmacology. XXVII. Classification of cannabinoid receptors. Pharmacol Rev. 2002;54:161–202. DOI: 10.1124/pr.54.2.161

[31] Liu J, Li H, Burstein SH, Zurier RB, Chen JD. Activation and binding of peroxisome proliferator-activated receptor gamma by synthetic cannabinoid ajulemic acid. Mol Pharmacol. 2003;63:983–992. DOI: 10.1124/mol.63.5.983

[32] O'Sullivan SE, Tarling EJ, Bennett AJ, Kendall DA, Randall MD. Novel time-dependent vascular actions of Delta9-tetrahydrocannabinol mediated by peroxisome proliferator-activated receptor gamma. Biochem Biophys Res Commun. 2005;337:824–831. DOI: 10.1016/j.bbrc.2005.09.121

[33] Bouaboula M, Hilairet S, Marchand J, Fajas L, Le Fur G, Casellas P. Anandamide induced PPAR gamma transcriptional activation and 3T3-L1 preadipocyte differentiation. Eur J Pharmacol. 2005;517:174–181. DOI: 10.1016/j.ejphar.2005.05.032

[34] Rockwell CE, Snider NT, Thompson JT, Vanden Heuvel JP, Kaminski NE. Interleukin-2 suppression by 2-arachidonyl glycerol is mediated through peroxisome proliferator-activated receptor gamma independently of cannabinoid receptors 1 and 2. Mol Pharmacol. 2006;70:101–111. DOI: 10.1124/mol.105.019117

[35] Dreyer C, Keller H, Mahfoudi A, Laudet V, Krey G, Wahli W. Positive regulation of the peroxisomal beta-oxidation pathway by fatty acids through activation of peroxisome proliferator-activated receptors (PPAR). Biol Cell. 1993;77:67–76. DOI: 10.1016/S0248-4900(05)80176-5

[36] Rakhshandehroo M, Knoch B, Müller M, Kersten S. Peroxisome proliferator-activated receptor alpha target genes. PPAR Res. vol. 2010, Article ID 612089, 20 pages, 2010. DOI: 10.1155/2010/612089

[37] Kliewer SA, Sundseth SS, Jones SA, Brown PJ, Wisely GB, Koble CS, et al. Fatty acids and eicosanoids regulate gene expression through direct interactions with peroxisome proliferator-activated receptors alpha and gamma. Proc Natl Acad Sci U S A. 1997;94:4318–4323

[38] Blankman JL, Simon GM, Cravatt BF. A comprehensive profile of brain enzymes that hydrolyze the endocannabinoid 2-arachidonoylglycerol. Chem Biol. 2007;14:1347–1356. DOI: 10.1016/j.chembiol.2007.11.006

[39] Kozak KR, Gupta RA, Moody JS, Ji C, Boeglin WE, Dubois RN, et al. 15-Lipoxygenase metabolism of 2-arachidonylglycerol: generation of a peroxisome proliferator-activated receptor α agonist. J Biol Chem. 2002;277:23278–23286. DOI: 10.1074/jbc.M201084200

[40] Schmid HHO, Berdyshev EV. Cannabinoid receptor-inactive N-acylethanolamines and other fatty acid amides: metabolism and function. Prostaglandins Leukot Essent Fat Acids. 2002;66:363–376. DOI: 10.1054/plef.2001.0348

[41] Romano A, Karimian Azari E, Tempesta B, Mansouri A, Micioni Di Bonaventura M V., Ramachandran D, et al. High dietary fat intake influences the activation of specific hindbrain and hypothalamic nuclei by the satiety factor oleoylethanolamide. Physiol Behav. 2014;136:55–62. DOI: 10.1016/j.physbeh.2014.04.039

[42] Gaetani S, Fu J, Cassano T, Dipasquale P, Romano A, Righetti L, et al. The fat-induced satiety factor oleoylethanolamide suppresses feeding through central release of oxytocin. J Neurosci. 2010;30:8096–8101. DOI: 10.1523/JNEUROSCI.0036-10.2010

[43] Hansen HS. Palmitoylethanolamide and other anandamide congeners. Proposed role in the diseased brain. Exp Neurol. 2010;224:48–55. DOI: 10.1016/j.expneurol.2010.03.022

[44] Hansen HS, Moesgaard B, Hansen HH, Petersen G. N-acylethanolamines and precursor phospholipids -- relation to cell injury. Chem Phys Lipids. 2000;108:135–150. DOI: 10.1016/S0009-3084(00)00192-4

[45] Ueda N, Tsuboi K, Uyama T. Enzymological studies on the biosynthesis of N-acylethanolamines. Biochim Biophys Acta. 2010;1801:1274–1285. DOI: 10.1016/j.bbalip.2010.08.010

[46] Hansen HS. Role of anorectic N-acylethanolamines in intestinal physiology and satiety control with respect to dietary fat. Pharmacol Res. 2014;86:18–25. DOI: 10.1016/j.phrs.2014.03.006

[47] Okamoto Y, Morishita J, Tsuboi K, Tonai T, Ueda N. Molecular Characterization of a phospholipase D generating anandamide and its congeners. J Biol Chem. 2004;279:5298–5305. DOI: 10.1074/jbc.M306642200

[48] Rodríguez de Fonseca F, Navarro M, Gómez R, Escuredo L, Nava F, Fu J, et al. An anorexic lipid mediator regulated by feeding. Nature. 2001;414:209–212. DOI: 10.1038/35102582

[49] Fu J, Astarita G, Gaetani S, Kim J, Cravatt BF, Mackie K, et al. Food intake regulates oleoylethanolamide formation and degradation in the proximal small intestine. J Biol Chem. 2007;282:1518–1528. DOI: 10.1074/jbc.M607809200

[50] Oveisi F, Gaetani S, Eng KTP, Piomelli D. Oleoylethanolamide inhibits food intake in free-feeding rats after oral administration. Pharmacol Res. 2004;49:461–466. DOI: 10.1016/j.phrs.2003.12.006

[51] Nielsen MJ, Petersen G, Astrup A, Hansen HS. Food intake is inhibited by oral oleoylethanolamide. J Lipid Res. 2004;45:1027–1029. DOI: 10.1194/jlr.C300008-JLR200

[52] Schwartz GJ, Fu J, Astarita G, Li X, Gaetani S, Campolongo P, et al. The lipid messenger OEA links dietary fat intake to satiety. Cell Metab. 2008;8:281–288. DOI: 10.1016/j.cmet.2008.08.005

[53] Provensi G, Coccurello R, Umehara H, Munari L, Giacovazzo G, Galeotti N, et al. Satiety factor oleoylethanolamide recruits the brain histaminergic system to inhibit food intake. Proc Natl Acad Sci U S A. 2014;111:11527–11532. DOI: 10.1073/pnas.1322016111

[54] Romano A, Coccurello R, Giacovazzo G, Bedse G, Moles A, Gaetani S. Oleoylethanolamide: a novel potential pharmacological alternative to cannabinoid antagonists for the control of appetite. Biomed Res Int. 2014;2014:203425. DOI: 10.1155/2014/203425

[55] Fu J, Gaetani S, Oveisi F, Lo Verme J, Serrano A, Rodriguez De Fonseca F, et al. Oleoylethanolamide regulates feeding and body weight through activation of the nuclear receptor PPAR-alpha. Nature. 2003;425:90–93. DOI: 10.1038/nature01921

[56] Overton HA, Babbs AJ, Doel SM, Fyfe MCT, Gardner LS, Griffin G, et al. Deorphanization of a G protein-coupled receptor for oleoylethanolamide and its use in the

discovery of small-molecule hypophagic agents. Cell Metab. 2006;3:167–175. DOI: 10.1016/j.cmet.2006.02.004

[57] Flock G, Holland D, Seino Y, Drucker DJ. GPR119 regulates murine glucose homeostasis through incretin receptor-dependent and independent mechanisms. Endocrinology. 2011;152:374–383. DOI: 10.1210/en.2010-1047

[58] Verdich C, Flint A, Gutzwiller JP, Näslund E, Beglinger C, Hellström PM, et al. A meta-analysis of the effect of glucagon-like peptide-1 (7–36) amide on Ad Libitum energy intake in humans. J Clin Endocrinol Metab. 2001;86:4382–4389. DOI: http://dx.doi.org/10.1210/jcem.86.9.7877

[59] Tang-Christensen M, Larsen PJ, Göke R, Fink-Jensen A, Jessop DS, Møller M, et al. Central administration of GLP-1-(7–36) amide inhibits food and water intake in rats. Am J Physiol. 1996;271:R848–R856

[60] Hirasawa A, Tsumaya K, Awaji T, Katsuma S, Adachi T, Yamada M, et al. Free fatty acids regulate gut incretin glucagon-like peptide-1 secretion through GPR120. Nat Med. 2005;11:90–94. DOI: 10.1038/nm1168

[61] Edfalk S, Steneberg P, Edlund H. Gpr40 is expressed in enteroendocrine cells and mediates free fatty acid stimulation of incretin secretion. Diabetes. 2008;57:2280–2287. DOI: 10.2337/db08-0307

[62] Hansen HS, Rosenkilde MM, Holst JJ, Schwartz TW. GPR119 as a fat sensor. Trends Pharmacol Sci. 2012;33:374–381. DOI: 10.1016/j.tips.2012.03.014

[63] Lan H, Vassileva G, Corona A, Liu L, Baker H, Golovko A, et al. GPR119 is required for physiological regulation of glucagon-like peptide-1 secretion but not for metabolic homeostasis. J Endocrinol. 2009;201:219–230. DOI: 10.1677/JOE-08-0453

[64] Lo Verme J, Gaetani S, Fu J, Oveisi F, Burton K, Piomelli D. Regulation of food intake by oleoylethanolamide. Cell Mol Life Sci. 2005;62:708–716. DOI: 10.1007/s00018-004-4494-0

[65] Lauffer LM, Iakoubov R, Brubaker PL. GPR119 is essential for oleoylethanolamide-induced glucagon-like peptide-1 secretion from the intestinal enteroendocrine L-cell. Diabetes. 2009;58:1058–1066. DOI: 10.2337/db08-1237

[66] Chu Z-L, Carroll C, Chen R, Alfonso J, Gutierrez V, He H, et al. N-Oleoyldopamine enhances glucose homeostasis through the activation of GPR119. Mol Endocrinol. 2010;24:161–170. DOI: 10.1210/me.2009-0239

[67] Ahern GP. Activation of TRPV1 by the satiety factor oleoylethanolamide. J Biol Chem. 2003;278:30429–30434. DOI: 10.1074/jbc.M305051200

[68] Ho W-S V, Barrett DA, Randall MD. "Entourage" effects of N-palmitoylethanolamide and N-oleoylethanolamide on vasorelaxation to anandamide occur through TRPV1 receptors. Br J Pharmacol. 2008;155:837–846. DOI: 10.1038/bjp.2008.324

[69] Diep TA, Madsen AN, Holst B, Kristiansen MM, Wellner N, Hansen SH, et al. Dietary fat decreases intestinal levels of the anorectic lipids through a fat sensor. FASEB J. 2011;25:765–774. DOI: 10.1096/fj.10-166595

[70] Artmann A, Petersen G, Hellgren LI, Boberg J, Skonberg C, Nellemann C, et al. Influence of dietary fatty acids on endocannabinoid and N-acylethanolamine levels in rat brain, liver and small intestine. Biochim Biophys Acta. 2008;1781:200–212. DOI: 10.1016/j.bbalip.2008.01.006

[71] Mu H, Høy CE. The digestion of dietary triacylglycerols. Prog Lipid Res. 2004; 43:105–133. DOI: 10.1016/S0163-7827(03)00050-X

[72] Mu H, Porsgaard T. The metabolism of structured triacylglycerols. Prog Lipid Res. 2005;44:430–448. DOI: 10.1016/j.plipres.2005.09.002

[73] Hansen KB, Rosenkilde MM, Knop FK, Wellner N, Diep TA, Rehfeld JF, et al. 2-Oleoyl glycerol is a GPR119 agonist and signals GLP-1 release in humans. J Clin Endocrinol Metab. 2011;96:e1409–1417. DOI: 10.1210/jc.2011-0647

[74] Mandøe MJ, Hansen KB, Hartmann B, Rehfeld JF, Holst JJ, Hansen HS. The 2-monoacylglycerol moiety of dietary fat appears to be responsible for the fat-induced release of GLP-1 in humans1. Am J Clin Nutr. 2015;102:548–55. DOI: 10.3945/ajcn.115.106799

[75] Perona JS, Portillo MP, Teresa Macarulla M, Tueros AI, Ruiz-Gutiérrez V. Influence of different dietary fats on triacylglycerol deposition in rat adipose tissue. Br J Nutr. 2000;84:765–74. DOI: 10.1017/S0007114500002130

[76] Everard A, Belzer C, Geurts L, Ouwerkerk JP, Druart C, Bindels LB, et al. Cross-talk between *Akkermansiamuciniph*ila and intestinal epithelium controls diet-induced obesity. Proc Natl Acad Sci U S A. 2013;110:9066–9071. DOI: 10.1073/pnas.1219451110/-/DCSupplemental

[77] Coll AP, Yeo GSH. The hypothalamus and metabolism: integrating signals to control energy and glucose homeostasis. Curr Opin Pharmacol. 2013;13:970–976. DOI: 10.1016/j.coph.2013.09.010

[78] Turban S, Hajduch E. Protein kinase C isoforms: mediators of reactive lipid metabolites in the development of insulin resistance. FEBS Lett. 2011;585:269–274. DOI: 10.1016/j.febslet.2010.12.022

[79] Gaillard D, Laugerette F, Darcel N, El-Yassimi A, Passilly-Degrace P, Hichami A, et al. The gustatory pathway is involved in CD36-mediated orosensory perception of long-chain fatty acids in the mouse. FASEB J. 2008;22:1458–1468. DOI: 10.1096/fj.07-8415com

[80] Gaillard D, Passilly-Degrace P, Besnard P. Molecular mechanisms of fat preference and overeating. Ann NY Acad Sci. 2008;1141:163–175. DOI: 10.1196/annals

[81] Liang N-C, Hajnal A, Norgren R. Sham feeding corn oil increases accumbens dopamine in the rat. Am J Physiol Regul Integr Comp Physiol. 2006;291:R1236–R1239. DOI: 10.1196/annals.1441.028

[82] DiPatrizio N V., Piomelli D. Intestinal lipid-derived signals that sense dietary fat. J Clin Invest. 2015;125:891–898. DOI: 10.1172/JCI76302

[83] Côté CD, Zadeh-Tahmasebi M, Rasmussen BA, Duca FA, Lam TKT. Hormonal signaling in the gut. J Biol Chem. 2014;289:11642–11649. DOI: 10.1074/jbc.O114.556068

[84] Laugerette F, Passilly-Degrace P, Patris B, Niot I, Febbraio M, Montmayeur JP, et al. CD36 involvement in orosensory detection of dietary lipids, spontaneous fat preference, and digestive secretions. J Clin Invest. 2005;115:3177–3184. DOI: 10.1172/JCI25299

[85] Cartoni C, Yasumatsu K, Ohkuri T, Shigemura N, Yoshida R, Godinot N, et al. Taste preference for fatty acids is mediated by GPR40 and GPR120. J Neurosci. 2010;30:8376–8382. DOI: 10.1523/JNEUROSCI.0496-10.2010

[86] Parton LE, Ye CP, Coppari R, Enriori PJ, Choi B, Zhang C-Y, et al. Glucose sensing by POMC neurons regulates glucose homeostasis and is impaired in obesity. Nature. 2007;449:228–232. DOI: 10.1038/nature06098

[87] Obici S, Feng Z, Morgan K, Stein D, Karkanias G, Rossetti L. Central administration of oleic acid inhibits glucose production and food intake. Diabetes. 2002;51:271–275. DOI: 10.2337/diabetes.51.2.271

[88] Coccurello R, Caprioli A, Bellantuono S, D'Amato FR, Conti R, Giannessi F, et al. Effects of the increase in neuronal fatty acids availability on food intake and satiety in mice. Psychopharmacology. 2010;210:85–95. DOI: 10.1007/s00213-010-1820-0

[89] Obici S, Feng Z, Arduini A, Conti R, Rossetti L. Inhibition of hypothalamic carnitine palmitoyltransferase-1 decreases food intake and glucose production. Nat Med. 2003;9:756–761. DOI: 10.1038/nm873

[90] Morgan K, Obici S, Rossetti L. Hypothalamic responses to long-chain fatty acids are nutritionally regulated. J Biol Chem. 2004;279:31139–31148. DOI: 10.1074/jbc.M400458200

[91] Pocai A, Lam TKT, Obici S, Gutierrez-Juarez R, Muse ED, Arduini A, et al. Restoration of hypothalamic lipid sensing normalizes energy and glucose homeostasis in overfed rats. J Clin Invest. 2006;116:1081–1091. DOI: 10.1172/JCI26640

[92] Lam TKT, Gutierrez-Juarez R, Pocai A, Rossetti L. Regulation of blood glucose by hypothalamic pyruvate metabolism. Science. 2005;309:943–947. DOI: 10.1126/science.1112085

[93] Plum L, Belgardt BF, Brüning JC. Central insulin action in energy and glucose homeostasis. J Clin Invest. 2006;116:1761–1766. DOI: 10.1172/JCI29063

[94] Chari M, Lam CKL, Wang PYT, Lam TKT. Activation of central lactate metabolism lowers glucose production in uncontrolled diabetes and diet-induced insulin resistance. Diabetes. 2008;57:836–840. DOI: 10.2337/db07-1464

[95] Carabotti M, Scirocco A, Maselli MA, Severi C. The gut-brain axis: interactions between enteric microbiota, central and enteric nervous systems. Ann Gastroenterol. 2015;28:203–209. DOI: 10.1172/JCI76304

[96] Passani MB, Blandina P, Torrealba F. The histamine H3 receptor and eating behavior. J Pharmacol Exp Ther. 2011;336:24–29. DOI: 10.1124/jpet.110.171306

[97] Provensi G, Blandina P, Passani MB. The histaminergic system as a target for the prevention of obesity and metabolic syndrome. Neuropharmacology. 2015; http://dx.doi.org/10.1016/j.neuropharm.2015.07.002

[98] Masaki T, Chiba S, Yasuda T, Noguchi H, Kakuma T, Watanabe T, et al. Involvement of hypothalamic histamine H1 receptor in the regulation of feeding rhythm and obesity. Diabetes. 2004;53:2250–2260. DOI: 10.2337/diabetes.53.9.2250

[99] Yasuda T, Masaki T, Sakata T, Yoshimatsu H. Hypothalamic neuronal histamine regulates sympathetic nerve activity and expression of uncoupling protein 1 mRNA in brown adipose tissue in rats. Neuroscience. 2004;125:535–540. DOI: 10.2337/diabetes.53.9.2250

[100] Masaki T, Yoshimatsu H, Chiba S, Watanabe T, Sakata T. Central infusion of histamine reduces fat accumulation and upregulates UCP family in leptin-resistant obese mice. Diabetes. 2001;50:376–384. DOI: 10.2337/diabetes.50.2.376

[101] Kimura K, Nakamura Y, Inaba Y, Matsumoto M, Kido Y, Asahara SI, et al. Histidine augments the suppression of hepatic glucose production by central insulin action. Diabetes. 2013;62:2266–2277. DOI: 10.2337/db12-1701

[102] Benoit SC, Kemp CJ, Elias CF, Abplanalp W, Herman JP, Migrenne S, et al. Palmitic acid mediates hypothalamic insulin resistance by altering PKC-theta subcellular localization in rodents. J Clin Invest. 2009;119:2577–2589. DOI: 10.1172/JCI36714

[103] Foster JA, Lyte M, Meyer E, Cryan JF. Gut microbiota and brain function: an evolving field in neuroscience. Int J Neuropsychopharmacol. 2015;pyv114. DOI: 10.1093/ijnp/pyv114

[104] Dinan TG, Cryan JF. Regulation of the stress response by the gut microbiota: implications for psychoneuroendocrinology. Psychoneuroendocrinology. 2012;37:1369–1378. DOI: 10.1016/j.psyneuen.2012.03.007

[105] Erny D, Hrabě de Angelis AL, Jaitin D, Wieghofer P, Staszewski O, David E, et al. Host microbiota constantly control maturation and function of microglia in the CNS. Nat Neurosci. 2015;18:965–977. DOI: 10.1038/nn.4030

[106] Ahmed RM, Irish M, Piguet O, Halliday GM, Ittner LM, Farooqi S, et al. Amyotrophic lateral sclerosis and frontotemporal dementia: distinct and overlapping changes in

eating behaviour and metabolism. Lancet Neurol. 2016;15:332–342. DOI: 10.1016/S1474-4422(15)00380-4

[107] Guzmán M, Lo Verme J, Fu J, Oveisi F, Blázquez C, Piomelli D. Oleoylethanolamide stimulates lipolysis by activating the nuclear receptor peroxisome proliferator-activated receptor◎alpha (PPAR-alpha). J Biol Chem. 2004;279:27849–27854. DOI: 10.1074/jbc.M404087200

[108] Yang Y, Chen M, Georgeson KE, Harmon CM. Mechanism of oleoylethanolamide on fatty acid uptake in small intestine after food intake and body weight reduction. Am J Physiol Regul Integr Comp Physiol. 2007;292:R235–R241. DOI: 10.1152/ajpregu.00270.2006

[109] Piomelli D.A fatty gut feeling. Trends Endocrinol Metab.2013;24:332–341. DOI: 10.1016/j.tem.2013.03.001

[110] Igarashi M, DiPatrizio N V, Narayanaswami V, Piomelli D. Feeding-induced oleoylethanolamide mobilization is disrupted in the gut of diet-induced obese rodents. Biochim Biophys Acta. 2015;1851:1218–1226. DOI: 10.1016/j.bbalip.2015.05.006

[111] Diep TA, Madsen AN, Krogh-Hansen S, Al-Shahwani M, Al-Sabagh L, Holst B, et al. Dietary non-esterified oleic acid decreases the jejunal levels of anorectic N-acylethanolamines. PLoS One. 2014;9: e100365DOI: 10.1371/journal.pone.0100365

[112] Hansen HS, Diep TA. N-acylethanolamines, anandamide and food intake. Biochem Pharmacol. 2009;78:553–560. DOI: 10.1016/j.bcp.2009.04.024

[113] Li L, Li L, Chen L, Lin X, Xu Y, Ren J, et al. Effect of oleoylethanolamide on diet-induced nonalcoholic fatty liver in rats. J Pharmacol Sci. 2015;127:244–250. DOI: 10.1016/j.jphs.2014.12.001

[114] Suárez J, Rivera P, Arrabal S, Crespillo A, Serrano A, Baixeras E, et al. Oleoylethanolamide enhances β-adrenergic-mediated thermogenesis and white-to-brown adipocyte phenotype in epididymal white adipose tissue in rat. Dis Model Mech. 2014;7:129–141. DOI: 10.1242/dmm.013110

[115] Decara JM, Romero-Cuevas M, Rivera P, Macias-González M, Vida M, Pavón FJ, et al. Elaidyl-sulfamide, an oleoylethanolamide-modelled PPARα agonist, reduces body weight gain and plasma cholesterol in rats. Dis Model Mech. 2012;5:660–670. DOI: 10.1242/dmm.009233

[116] Annuzzi G, Piscitelli F, Di Marino L, Patti L, Giacco R, Costabile G, et al. Differential alterations of the concentrations of endocannabinoids and related lipids in the subcutaneous adipose tissue of obese diabetic patients. Lipids Heal Dis. 2010;9:43. DOI: 10.1186/1476-511X-9-43

[117] Gaetani S, Oveisi F, Piomelli D. Modulation of meal pattern in the rat by the anorexic lipid mediator oleoylethanolamide. Neuropsychopharmacology. 2003;28:1311–1316. DOI: 10.1038/sj.npp.1300166

[118] Mennella I, Savarese M, Ferracane R, Sacchi R, Vitaglione P. Oleic acid content of a meal promotes oleoylethanolamide response and reduces subsequent energy intake in humans. Food Funct. 2015;6:204–210. DOI: 10.1039/c4fo00697f

[119] Azari EK, Ramachandran D, Weibel S, Arnold M, Romano A, Gaetani S, et al. Vagal afferents are not necessary for the satiety effect of the gut lipid messenger oleoylethanolamide (OEA). Am J Physiol Regul Integr Comp Physiol. 2014;307:R167–R178. DOI: 10.1152/ajpregu.00067.2014

[120] Sclafani A, Ackroff K, Schwartz GJ. Selective effects of vagal deafferentation and celiac-superior mesenteric ganglionectomy on the reinforcing and satiating action of intestinal nutrients. Physiol Behav. 2003;78:285–294. DOI: 10.1016/S0031-9384(02)00968-X

[121] Romano a., Karimian Azari E, Tempesta B, Mansouri a., Micioni Di Bonaventura M V., Ramachandran D, et al. High dietary fat intake influences the activation of specific hindbrain and hypothalamic nuclei by the satiety factor oleoylethanolamide. Physiol Behav. 2014;136:55–62. DOI: 10.1016/j.physbeh.2014.04.039

[122] Romano A, Cassano T, Tempesta B, Cianci S, Dipasquale P, Coccurello R, et al. The satiety signal oleoylethanolamide stimulates oxytocin neurosecretion from rat hypothalamic neurons. Peptides. 2013;49:21–26. DOI: 10.1016/j.peptides.2013.08.006

[123] Serrano A, Pavón FJ, Tovar S, Casanueva F, Señarís R, Diéguez C, et al. Oleoylethanolamide: Effects on hypothalamic transmitters and gut peptides regulating food intake. Neuropharmacology. 2011;60:593–601. DOI: 10.1016/j.neuropharm.2010.12.007

[124] Proulx K, Cota D, Castaneda TR, Tschop MH, D'Alessio DA, Tso P, et al. Mechanisms of oleoylethanolamide-induced changes in feeding behavior and motor activity. Am J Physiol Regul Integr Comp Physiol. 2005;289:R729–R737. DOI: 10.1152/ajpregu.00029.2005

[125] Yu H-L, Sun L-P, Li M-M, Quan Z-S. Involvement of norepinephrine and serotonin system in antidepressant-like effects of oleoylethanolamide in the mice models of behavior despair. Neurosci Lett. 2015;593:24–28. DOI: 10.1016/j.neulet.2015.03.019

[126] Melis M, Carta S, Fattore L, Tolu S, Yasar S, Goldberg SR, et al. Peroxisome proliferator-activated receptors-alpha modulate dopamine cell activity through nicotinic receptors. Biol Psychiatry. 2010;68:256–264. DOI: 10.1016/j.biopsych.2010.04.016

[127] McGaugh JL, Roozendaal B. Role of adrenal stress hormones in forming lasting memories in the brain. Curr Opin Neurobiol. 2002;12:205–210. DOI: 10.1016/S0959-4388(02)00306-9

[128] Campolongo P, Roozendaal B, Trezza V, Hauer D, Schelling G, McGaugh JL, et al. Endocannabinoids in the rat basolateral amygdala enhance memory consolidation and enable glucocorticoid modulation of memory. Proc Natl Acad Sci U S A. 2009;106:4888–4893. DOI: 10.1073/pnas.0900835106

[129] McGaugh JL. Memory—a century of consolidation. Science. 2000;287:248–251. DOI: 10.1126/science.287.5451.248

[130] Campolongo P, Roozendaal B, Trezza V, Cuomo V, Astarita G, Fu J, et al. Fat-induced satiety factor oleoylethanolamide enhances memory consolidation. Proc Natl Acad Sci U S A. 2009;106:8027–8031. DOI: 10.1073/pnas.0903038106

[131] Mazzola C, Medalie J, Scherma M, Panlilio L V, Solinas M, Tanda G, et al. Fatty acid amide hydrolase (FAAH) inhibition enhances memory acquisition through activation of PPAR-alpha nuclear receptors. Learn Mem. 2009;16:332–337. DOI: 10.1101/lm.1145209

[132] Grosshans M, Schwarz E, Bumb JM, Schaefer C, Rohleder C, Vollmert C, et al. Oleoylethanolamide and human neural responses to food stimuli in obesity. JAMA Psychiatry. 2014;71:1254–1261. DOI: 10.1001/jamapsychiatry.2014.1215

[133] Kenny PJ. Common cellular and molecular mechanisms in obesity and drug addiction. Nat Rev Neurosci. 2011;12:638–651. DOI: 10.1038/nrn3105

[134] Volkow ND, Wang GJ, Baler RD. Reward, dopamine and the control of food intake: implications for obesity. Trends Cogn Sci. 2011;15:37–46. DOI: 10.1016/j.tics.2010.11.001

[135] Berthoud H-R. The neurobiology of food intake in an obesogenic environment. Proc Nutr Soc. 2012;71:478–487. DOI: 10.1017/S0029665112000602

[136] Tellez LA, Medina S, Han W, Ferreira JG, Licona-Limón P, Ren X, et al. A gut lipid messenger links excess dietary fat to dopamine deficiency. Science. 2013;341:800–802. DOI: 10.1126/science.1239275

Chapter 8

Cannabinoid CB1/CB2 Receptors in the Heart: Expression, Regulation, and Function

Elena Kaschina

Additional information is available at the end of the chapter

http://dx.doi.org/10.5772/

Abstract

Endocannabinoids exert their actions in the heart and vessels, at least in part, by stimulating the cannabinoid CB1 and the CB2 receptor subtypes which belong to a group of seven transmembrane-spanning receptors and are coupled to Gi/o-proteins. Activation of cardiovascular CB1 receptors leads to depressed cardiac contractility and hypotension. Conversely, in most studies, the CB1 receptor antagonists are cardioprotective against ischemia–reperfusion injury, myocardial ischemia, heart failure, and cardiomyopathies. Evidence to date indicates that CB2 receptor activation is cardioprotective. CB2 receptor-mediated effects such as anti-inflammation and anti-fibrosis may be in part opposite to the actions of the CB1 receptor. The aim of this review is to up-date on recent experimental findings and controversies on the role of endocannabinoid system in the myocardial injury with emphasis on pathophysiological processes such as left ventricular remodeling, cardiac fibrosis, hypertrophy, and endothelial dysfunction. Recent experimental studies employing genetic deficiency of CB1 and CB2 receptors and endocannabinoid anandamide metabolizing enzymes are reviewed. Moreover, the protective mechanisms which are mediated by cannabinoid receptors during ischemic preconditioning as well as in the early and late phase after myocardial infarction are discussed in the context of possible therapeutic implications.

Keywords: cannabinoid receptors, CB1, CB2, heart, myocardial infarction, heart remodeling

1. Introduction

Endocannabinoids, its degrading enzymes and the cannabinoid CB1 and CB2 receptors are present in rodent and human cardiovascular tissues. In addition to its role in the control of the central nervous system, the endocannabinoid system (ECS) may play a pivotal part in cardiovascular regulation by heart diseases (reviewed in [1-3]).

In normal physiological conditions, ECS is not highly regulated. However, by cardiovascular pathologies, this system is activated and may reflect a protective response which limits cardiac injury. Activated ECS has been implicated in acute cardiovascular conditions such as hemorrhagic, septic, and cardiogenic shock as well as in chronic diseases such as coronary heart disease, heart failure, and cardiomyopathy.

Endocannabinoids exert their actions in the heart and vessels, at least in part, by stimulating the cannabinoid CB1 and the CB2 receptor subtypes which belong to a group of seven transmembrane-spanning receptors and are coupled to Gi/o-proteins [4, 5]. Signaling through the CB1 receptor elicits hypotension, bradycardia, and negative inotropy [6]. Moreover, this receptor subtype is implicated in inflammation, apoptosis, oxidative stress [7], and metabolic dysregulation [8], thereby contributing to tissue injury. The CB2 receptors, on the contrary, may play a compensatory anti-inflammatory, anti-oxidative, and anti-atherogenic role [9, 10] contributing to cardiovascular protection.

Nevertheless, the role of cannabinoid receptors in the heart under several pathological conditions remains controversial. Recent studies on hemodynamic, antiarrhythmic, and cardiometabolic effects of cannabinoids have been highlighted in several excellent reviews [2, 3, 11-14]. Hence, these topics are not in the scope of this chapter.

The aim of this review was to up-date on recent findings and controversies on the role of ECS in the myocardial injury with emphasis on pathophysiological processes such as left ventricular remodeling, cardiac fibrosis, hypertrophy, and endothelial dysfunction. Starting with the localization of the cannabinoid system components in the heart under normal and pathological conditions, the role of both CB1/CB2 receptors in the regulation of the cardiac function will be analyzed. Experimental studies in mice deficient in cannabinoid receptors and endocannabinoid anandamide metabolizing enzymes greatly expanded our knowledge on the role of ECS. Hence, lessons from these studies will also be discussed. Moreover, the protective mechanisms which are mediated by cannabinoid receptors during ischemic preconditioning as well as in the early and late phase after myocardial infarction will be described in the context of possible therapeutic implications.

2. Endocannabinoids and cannabinoid receptors in the heart

The major endocannabinoids, anandamide, and 2-arachidonoylglycerol (2-AG) have been detected in the rat heart by Schmid et al. [15]. These findings were later confirmed by Wagner et al. [16] who also revealed the presence of CB1 receptors via immunohistochemistry in isolated rat hearts. Finally, the presence of both CB1 and CB2 receptors has been confirmed in myocardium of rat [17, 18], mice [19], and guinea pigs [20]. Messenger RNA and immunoreactivity for CB1 receptors have also been reported from murine cardiomyocytes [21], and only one receptor subtype, CB1, was present on neonatal cardiomyocytes [22].

In human heart, CB1 mRNA expression has been first found by Galiegue et al. [23] and later confirmed in isolated human atrial muscle on the protein level by Bonz et al. [24]. Moreover, human primary cardiomyocytes [9] and coronary vascular smooth muscle [25] also expressed CB1 receptors. Finally, it has been recently demonstrated that mRNA transcripts of CB1 and CB2 receptors are expressed in an almost equal proportion on healthy human left ventricular myocardium [26].

Hence, the main components of the ECS are present in rodent and human healthy heart. Their regulation under pathophysiological conditions has been intensively investigated during the last decade in different models of cardiac injury and in human diseases.

To begin with, circulating levels of endocannabinoids were elevated after cardiac injury, such as **myocardial infarction** in the rat [27] and **ischemia/reperfusion** in mice [28]. The CB2 receptors were upregulated in ischemic cardiomyocytes [28] and in cardiomyocytes following cultivation under hypoxia [29]. Our group found general induction of CB1 and CB2 receptor gene expression due to experimental myocardial infarction in the rat 6 weeks after operation [30].

Interestingly, in **heart failure** induced by doxorubicin, tissue anandamide content was elevated, whereas the expression of CB1/CB2 receptors in the heart was not changed [21]. Also **diabetic cardiomyopathy** in mice was characterized by increased myocardial endocannabinoid anandamide levels, although in this model, the CB1 receptors were upregulated parallel to increased oxidative/nitrative stress and activation of *p38* [31].

In humans, the endocannabinoid 2-AG level elevated in the infarct-side coronary artery of **acute myocardial infarction** patients along with increased reactive oxygen species and *tumor necrosis factor-α* levels [19]. Furthermore, elevated endocannabinoid plasma levels have been associated with coronary circulatory dysfunction in human obesity [32].

Aortic stenosis patients, who are known to develop heart hypertrophy, have significantly higher concentration of anandamide, its degrading enzyme fatty acid amide hydrolase (*FAAH*) and expression of CB2 receptors, which are predominantly located on cardiomyocytes [33]. Similarly, in patients suffering from **heart failure**, peripheral blood levels of endocannabinoids were elevated, whereas the expression of CB1 receptors was downregulated 0.7-fold and CB2 receptors was upregulated more than 11-fold indicating a shift toward CB2 expression [26].

Recently, in **human epicardial adipose tissue**, expression of the CB1/CB2 receptors and *FAAH* content was compared between patients with and without ischemic heart disease [34]. In ischemic hearts, the CB1-to-CB2 expression ratio shifted toward CB1 and was accompanied by higher *PKA* activation. In contrast, in nonischemics, CB2, *FAAH, PLC,* and *PKC* as well as *ERK1/2* were increased.

Concerning intracellular localization of the cannabinoid receptors, evidence is now provided for CB1 receptors. They were found in specific restricted regions within cardiac myocytes as demonstrated by array tomography in mice heart tissues [35]. Moreover, Currie et al. [36] suggested the existence of cardiac nuclear CB receptors.

Altogether, endocannabinoids and both CB1/CB2 receptors are present in human and murine hearts. The receptors co-localize with cardiac myocytes, coronary vascular smooth muscle, and endothelial cells as well as with epicardial adipose tissues.

Increased circulating and myocardial endocannabinoids levels as well as regulation of CB1 and CB2 receptors in heart diseases may reflect a protective response of the local ECS to limit cardiac injury. Whereas the CB1 receptors expression levels are controversially regulated depending on the heart disease model and cardiac function, the CB2 receptors are mostly upregulated. Thus, the endocannabinoid—CB2 receptor protective axis may play a major role in limiting injury.

3. Cardiac function

In healthy individuals, activation of ECS does not significantly regulate cardiac functions. In the intact heart of rodents, endogenous CB1/CB2 receptor agonists are also not involved in the electrophysiological processes and cardiac rhythm regulation [37]. Conversely, CB1 receptor antagonists do not affect cardiac hemodynamic in normotensive rodents [6, 30].

As previously described, in cardiac disorders and after myocardial infarction, circulating levels of endocannabinoids are elevated and the majority of studies suggest that this elevation improves cardiac performance [3, 27].

However, administration of anandamide, D9-tetrahydrocannabinol (*Δ*-9-THC), or synthetic cannabinoids causes complex hemodynamic changes and changes in heart rate and contractility [6]. Moreover, there are reports of adverse cardiovascular effects following cannabis or synthetic cannabinoid use, including myocardial infarction, arrhythmias, and sudden death [38, 39]. These negative effects may be related to increased sympathetic activity and inhibition of parasympathetic activity, leading to tachycardia, increased oxygen demand, and arrhythmias [40].

Regulation of cardiac contractility by the cannabinoid system is complex and includes actions on the nervous system and local cardiac mechanisms.

It has been previously assumed that cardiovascular effects of cannabinoids were centrally mediated through activation of receptors in the brain. However, evidence from studies mentioned below suggests that most effects are mediated locally through cardiac cannabinoid receptors. The activation of presynaptic CB1 receptors might decrease the release of noradrenalin contributing to negative inotropy [41]. Albeit, in some studies, effects on cardiac contractility were independent of the endogenous noradrenalin release [42]. Other possible mechanisms of negative inotropic effects include inhibition of voltage-dependent Na^+ and L-type Ca^{2+} channels in myocytes [43] and suppression of Na^+/Ca^{2+} exchanger current [44, 45].

It is now becoming clear that negative inotropy is mediated through the CB1 receptor. This has been shown in papillary muscles, isolated hearts, and in rodent *in vivo* models [6]. Conversely, our group observed that an inhibition of CB1 receptors with rimonabant increased heart inotropy in rats after myocardial infarction but not in healthy rats. This implies chronic activation of the endocannabinoid system after cardiac ischemia [30]. In this study, where hemodynamic parameters were measured 6 weeks after myocardial infarction using heart catheter, the CB1 receptor antagonist rimonabant significantly increased maximal and minimal peak rate of left ventricular pressure increase (dP/dt_{max} and dP/dt_{min}), preventing a decrease in contractility post myocardial infarction. Moreover, in the rat model of metabolic syndrome, the CB1 receptor blockade also improved systolic cardiac function raising fractional shortening and ejection fraction [30]. The positive inotropic effect of CB1 antagonism in these studies was associated with increased cardiac protein expression of *sarcoplasmic reticulum* Ca^{2+}*ATPase* (*SERCA2a*) which is known to raise intracellular calcium concentration.

In contrast to CB1 receptor activation, CB2 receptor activation does not modulate the ion channel function (reviewed in [46]). Hence, it is not pronounced that the CB2 receptor mediates contractility effects. However, in one study, CB2 receptors developed positive contractile response in rat isolated atria associated with increased *cAMP* production [42].

Given that endocannabinoids are cleaved by hydrolysis as well as cycloxygenase-2, lipoxygenases, and cytochrom P450-mediated oxidative metabolism, the generated autacoids may exert additional cardiovascular effects [6]. This fact requires further investigations.

4. Lessons from knockout mice

4.1. CB1 receptor knockout mice ($CB1^{-/-}$)

The generation of mice deficient in CB1 or CB2 receptors has greatly expanded our knowledge on the role of these receptor subtypes in heart disease.

In $CB1^{-/-}$ mice, basal blood pressure and heart rate are normal [47]. Compared with wild type, CB1 knockouts showed a marked increase of mortality due to acute [48] and chronic heart failure [49] after pressure overload due to transverse aortic constriction. Moreover, in the late period after aortic constriction, compared to wild-type mice, $CB1^{-/-}$ mice had significantly worse cardiac functional parameters associated with the activation of the *epidermal growth factor* receptor and *mitogen-activated protein kinases P38* and *ERK*. These findings suggest a protective role of the CB1 receptor stimulation in the heart [49].

On the other hand, genetic deletion of the CB1 receptor attenuated the diabetes-induced cardiac dysfunction [31]. Moreover, this study suggests that over-activation of this receptor subtype may play an important role in the pathogenesis of diabetic cardiomyopathy by facilitating angiotensin AT1 receptor signaling, *MAPK* activation, oxidative/nitrative stress, inflammation, cell death, fibrosis, and contractile dysfunction. Conversely, CB1 receptor inhibition may be of significant benefit in the treatment of diabetic cardiovascular complications.

In summary, there are controversies concerning the role of the CB1 receptor activation in cardiac pathology: It may be both deleterious and beneficial depending on the disease model. By over-activation of this receptor, the pathological reactions may be provoked.

4.2. CB2 receptor knockout mice ($CB2^{-/-}$)

In the $CB2^{-/-}$ mice, initially, an absence of immunomodulatory effects of endocannabinoids was observed [50, 51]. Later, Defer et al. [52] showed the importance of the CB2 receptor in cardioprotection. In the infarction/reperfusion model in $CB2^{-/-}$ mice, increased infarct size was associated with enhanced apoptosis and remodeling. Moreover, in the late remodeling phase after myocardial infarction, $CB2^{-/-}$ mice developed left ventricular dysfunction, exacerbated fibrosis, and dilative cardiomyopathy [52].

The role of the CB2 receptor during the initial phase of **ischemic cardiomyopathy** development prior to the onset of ventricular dysfunction or infarction has been studied in the $CB2^{-/-}$ mice by repetitive periods of ischemia/reperfusion [53]. $CB2^{-/-}$ mice showed an increased rate of apoptosis, irreversible loss of cardiomyocytes, persistent left ventricular dysfunction, increased inflammatory response, and decreased anti-oxidative capacity 60 days after the injury.

Further studies of remodeling processes in reperfused infarction in the $CB2^{-/-}$ mice again confirmed the cardioprotective role of this receptor subtype [54]. In contrast to a rapid formation of granulation tissue and a compacted non-transmural scar in wild-type mice after 7 days of reperfusion, $CB2^{-/-}$ mice showed a non-compacted transmural scar and a significantly worse cardiac function. Adverse myocardial remodeling in $CB2^{-/-}$ mice has been associated with macrophage infiltration and low induction of tenascin C, collagen-Iα, or lysil oxidase [54].

Hence, it seems that the CB2 receptor is implicated in multiple pathophysiological processes after heart injury: It modulates inflammatory response, collagen deposition, and organization of stable scar during remodeling.

4.3. Fatty acid amide hydrolase knockout mice ($FAAH^{-/-}$)

Inhibition of the endocannabinoid anandamide metabolizing enzyme, the fatty acid amide hydrolase (*FAAH*), is another strategy to study the impact of endocannabinoid system in health and disease. $FAAH^{-/-}$ mice had a normal hemodynamic profile, despite of 2.5-fold increase in the myocardial anandamide levels [55]. Albeit by aging, these mice exhibit less cardiac dysfunction, decreased levels of oxidative stress, and inflammation compared to the wild type [56]. Thus, an increased endocannabinoid activity by aging could be beneficial in the context of anti-inflammatory and anti-atherosclerotic effects.

However, in the doxorubicin model of heart failure, $FAAH^{-/-}$ mice compared to their wild type were characterized by increased mortality due to cardiac dysfunction and myocardial oxidative–nitrative stress [57]. This study suggests that in heart failure model associated with mitochondrial dysfunction and ROS generation, *FAAH* plays a key role in controlling the anandamide-induced myocardial cell death. Moreover, this cardiac injury was, at least in part, mediated by the activation of CB1 receptors by endocannabinoids, since these effects could be attenuated by selective CB1 antagonists [57].

5. Ischemia–reperfusion injury

Short ischemia/reperfusion episodes—known as ischemic preconditioning—protect the myocardium against infarction [58]. This endogenous cardioprotective mechanism could be experimentally activated at two time points: The early preconditioning when the treatment is applied 1–4 h before ischemia and the delayed preconditioning when the treatment is applied 24–72 h before induction of myocardial infarction. Importantly, endogenous cannabinoid 2-AG is increased by preconditioning in the heart [59].

Initial studies on the role of cannabinoids in cardiac ischemia were predominantly performed *ex vivo* in papillary muscles or isolated heart. In these models, endocannabinoids ameliorated ischemia/reperfusion injury and reduced the early phase of heart remodeling (reviewed in [13, 60, 61]). It also has been pointed at the role of CB2 receptor activation in remote ischemic preconditioning [62-65]. Albeit, Underdown et al. [66] suggested that anandamide reduced infarct size in rat isolated hearts by interaction with a new cannabinoid receptor subtype, distinct from CB1 or CB2 receptors.

Further studies, which aimed to elucidate the role of CB1/2 receptors in the heart, were performed in the animal model of myocardial infarction via ligation of the left coronary artery. Most investigations used an indirect approach by blocking the beneficial effects of endocannabinoids activation either by CB1 or CB2 receptor antagonists.

In the rat model of coronary occlusion/reperfusion, both anandamide and non-selective CB1/CB2 receptors agonist HU-210 decreased the incidence of ventricular arrhythmias and reduced infarct size through the activation of the CB2 but not the CB1 receptors [67]. Also in mouse myocardial ischemia/reperfusion model, the protective effect of a CB1/CB2 receptors agonist WIN55212-2 was abolished by the selective CB2 antagonist AM630 and not affected by the selective CB1 antagonist AM251 [68]. In this study, cardioprotection was associated with a decreased *myeloperoxidase* activity and downregulation of *interleukin-1beta* and *CXC chemokine ligand 8* in the heart [68]. Likewise, pretreatment with the CB2 antagonist AM630 abolished the protective effects of remote preconditioning on infarct size and arrhythmias, whereas pretreatment with the CB1 antagonist AM251 had no significant effect on ischemia-induced arrhythmias or the infarct size [69].

Direct CB2 receptor activation by selective agonist JWH-133 during heart ischemia also reduced the infarct size [70] and prevented apoptosis through inhibition of the intrinsic mitochondria-mediated apoptotic pathway and involvement of the *PI3K/Akt* signal pathway [71].

Recently, Waldman et al. [72] observed a specific effect of non-selective activation of CB1/CB2 receptors by *Δ*-9-THC on ischemia/reperfusion in mice. Administrated in a very low dose (0.002 mg/kg), which is 3–4 orders of magnitude lower than the conventional doses, *Δ*-9-THC reduced infarct size and accumulation of neutrophils in the heart. This study also provided evidence for a wide therapeutic time window (2–48 h before ischemia) using extremely low dose of the cannabinoid drug.

Summarizing, during early and delayed ischemic preconditioning, cannabinoids activate long-lasting protective mechanisms in the heart predominantly via the CB2 receptors. The cellular mechanisms, by which endocannabinoids have a protective function by ischemia/reperfusion, include anti-apoptosis [71], prevention of inflammation [68, 72], induction of the heat shock protein 72 as well as prevention of calcium overload, and oxidative stress (reviewed in [13]).

6. Myocardial infarction and left ventricular remodeling

Acute phase post-myocardial infarction is characterized by cell death and inflammatory response, whereas in the late phase post infarction, collagen deposition, interstitial fibrosis, and extracellular matrix degradation contribute to cardiac remodeling processes [73]. Pathological left ventricular remodeling leads to progressive left ventricular dilatation and dysfunction, cardiac fibrosis, and the development of heart failure. Recent data provide evidence that cannabinoids might modulate many of these pathological processes, although the direct role of receptor subtype and interaction mechanisms is not clearly defined.

Administration of CB1 selective antagonist AM251 for 12 weeks promoted **left ventricular remodeling** indicated by left ventricular volume in rats with large myocardial infarction, whereas the nonselective cannabinoid agonist HU-210 enhanced left ventricular performance [16]. Hence, in this study, the CB1 blockade had negative effects on cardiac function post myocardial infarction, although this observation was significant only in rats with large myocardial infarction.

On the other hand, recent studies suggest that the blockade of the CB1 receptor may be protective. For example, chronic treatment with the CB1 receptor antagonist rimonabant reduced infarct size in wild-type mice but not in $CB1^{-/-}$ mice in acute ischemia/reperfusion injury. Importantly, the protective effects were independent from weight reduction and adiponectin levels [74].

Our group described the protective effects of the CB1 receptor antagonist rimonabant on cardiac remodeling in a rat model of myocardial infarction and in metabolic syndrome [30]. Pretreatment with rimonabant prevented left ventricular dilatation and cardiac dysfunction in the early and late phase after myocardial infarction. This was evidenced by an improvement of functional cardiac parameters such as left ventricular internal diameter, ejection fraction, fractional shortening and dP/dt_{max}, dP/dt_{min} [30]. Moreover, rimonabant prevented electrocardiographic abnormalities and elevation of serum *brain natriuretic peptide* (*BNP*) levels, increased the cardiac protein expression of *SERCA2a* and improved pulse wave reflection. Importantly, preventive treatment was even more effective compared to post-ischaemic treatment regime. This finding is in agreement with the study performed by Lim et al. [74] where rimonabant administration 7 days—but not shortly—before ischemia reduced infarct size via a CB1-related mechanism. This fact confirms the importance of ECS in ischemic preconditioning.

Left ventricular remodeling post-myocardial infarction is also associated with **hypertrophy** in noninfarcted myocytes due to wall stress and activation of the local hormones. Antigrowth effect of anandamide was recently demonstrated in neonatal rat ventricular myocytes [75]. In this study, the ability of R-methanandamide to suppress myocyte enlargement and fetal gene activation was mediated by CB2 and CB1 receptors, respectively.

The late phase post-myocardial infarction is characterized by **cardiac fibrosis** associated with altered cardiac performance and arrhythmogenesis. Endocannabinoids may modulate either pro- or anti-fibrosis, depending on their interaction with CB1 or CB2 receptors, respectively [76, 77]. In the heart and aorta, CB1 antagonist rimonabant decreased collagen accumulation and prevented the upregulation of pro-fibrotic protein *TGF-β1* in the remote myocardium after ischemia [30]. On the other hand, genetic deletion of CB2 receptors increased *TGF-β1* and collagen production in the chronic heart failure model [52], indicating again that CB1 and CB2 receptors have opposing effects on fibrotic processes.

Furthermore, **extracellular matrix degradation** contributes to left ventricular wall-thinning in the remote region after myocardial infarction [78]. Since CB1 antagonist rimonabant dose-dependently reduced the activity of matrix metalloprotease MMP-9 in cardiac fibroblasts [30], CB1 receptors might be involved in proteolytic mechanisms. In addition, CB1/CB2 receptors are present in immune cells [23] through which they could modulate cytokine secretion and influence matrix remodeling.

Endothelial dysfunction and collagen accumulation contribute to increased pulse wave reflection and increase after load in patients with heart failure. It was initially suggested that inhibition of CB1 receptor deteriorates endothelial function after experimental myocardial infarction [16]. However, recent investigations showed that the inhibition of CB1 receptor is beneficial by endothelial dysfunction. It improved endothelium-dependent relaxation of aortic rings via a mechanism that involves downregulation of AT1 receptor expression [79] and ameliorated pulse wave reflection after experimental myocardial infarction in the rat [30].

As mentioned above in **heart failure,** ECS may become over-activated and contribute to depressed cardiac function, which can be attenuated by CB1 antagonists (reviewed in [14]). In doxorubicin-induced heart failure mouse model, pretreatment with CB1 antagonists improved doxorubicin-induced cardiac dysfunction by anti-inflammatory, antioxidative, and cytoprotective mechanisms [21]. Importantly, this and other studies suggested that beneficial effects of CB1 antagonists on contractile functions may extend beyond inhibition of CB1-mediated negative inotropic effect. Moreover, the protective role of CB1 inhibition may be partly explained by the activation of unopposed CB2 receptors because tissue endocannabinoids levels are elevated by cardiac diseases. The cellular CB2 receptor-mediated mechanisms, in turn, include increased *nitric oxide* (*NO*) production by induction of *NO synthase* (*iNOS*) [16], prevention of calcium overload through inhibition of I_{NCX} [45], prevention of *TNF-alpha* induced chemotaxis [70], and activation of anti-apoptotic [71], anti-inflammatory, and anti-atherogenic pathways (reviewed in [11]).

7. Conclusion

Endocannabinoids exert their actions in the heart mostly via the stimulation of the CB1 and the CB2 receptors. These receptors modulate pathophysiological processes following myocardial injury such as left ventricular remodeling, cardiac fibrosis, hypertrophy, and endothelial dysfunction.

Activation of cardiovascular CB1 receptors leads to depressed cardiac contractility and hypotension. Conversely, in most studies, the CB1 receptor antagonists are cardioprotective against ischemia–reperfusion injury, myocardial ischemia, heart failure, arrhythmias, and cardiomyopathies. The CB1 receptor antagonists also exert beneficial anti-apoptotic, anti-inflammatory, and anti-oxidative actions which are beyond inhibition of CB1-mediated negative inotropic effect.

Evidence to date indicates that CB2 receptor activation is cardioprotective. CB2 receptor-mediated effects such as anti-inflammation and anti-fibrosis may be in part opposite to the actions of the CB1 receptor. Given that tissue endocannabinoids levels are increased by cardiac injury, the protective role of CB1 inhibition may be partly explained by the activation of unopposed CB2 receptors. This fact requires further investigations. Moreover, little is known about the interaction of the CB1/CB2 receptors with other receptors like angiotensin-II receptors or PPARs as well as the role of new discovered putative endothelial cannabinoid receptor CBe and endocannabinoid metabolic products in cardiac diseases.

The endocannabinoid system indeed could represent a novel pharmacological target in treatment of cardiac disease. However, therapeutic use of cannabinoids, their synthetic analogs and cannabinoid receptor agonists/antagonists remain limited due to their psychotropic adverse effects. Therefore, it is necessary to develop newer compounds without actions on central nervous system.

Author details

Elena Kaschina

Address all correspondence to: elena.kaschina@charite.de

Center for Cardiovascular Research (CCR), Institute of Pharmacology, Charité-University Medicine Berlin, Berlin, Germany

References

[1] Pertwee RG. Pharmacological actions of cannabinoids. Handb Exp Pharmacol. 2005;168:1–51

[2] Pacher P, Bátkai S, Kunos G. Cardiovascular pharmacology of cannabinoids. In: Pertwee R, editor. Cannabinoids. Springer, New York: 2005b. pp. 599–627

[3] O'Sullivan SE. Endocannabinoids and the cardiovascular system in health and disease. Handb Exp Pharmacol. 2015;231:393–422. doi:10.1007/978-3-319-20825-1_14. Review. [PMID: 26408169]

[4] Matsuda LA, Lolait SJ, Brownstein MJ, Young CA, Bonner TI. Structure of a cannabinoid receptor and functional expression of the cloned cDNA. Nature (Lond). 1990;346:561–564. [PubMed: 2165569]

[5] Munro S, Thomas KL, Abu-Shaar M. Molecular characterization of a peripheral receptor for cannabinoids. Nature (Lond). 1993;365:61–65. [PubMed: 7689702]

[6] Bátkai S, Pacher P. Endocannabinoids and cardiac contractile function: pathophysiological implications. Pharmacol Res. 2009;60(2):99–106. Review. [PMID: 19569260]

[7] Mukhopadhyay P, Rajesh M, Batkai S, Patel V, Kashiwaya Y, Liaudet L, et al. CB1 cannabinoid receptors promote oxidative stress and cell death in murine models of doxorubicin-induced cardiomyopathy and in human cardiomyocytes. Cardiovasc Res. 2010a;85:773–784

[8] Matias I, Di Marzo V. Endocannabinoids and the control of energy balance. Trends Endocrinol Metab. 2007;18(1):27–37

[9] Mukhopadhyay P, Rajesh M, Pan H, Patel V, Mukhopadhyay B, Batkai S, et al. Cannabinoid-2 receptor limits inflammation, oxidative/nitrosative stress, and cell death in nephropathy. Free Radic Biol Med. 2010b;48:457–467

[10] Steffens S, Veillard NR, Arnaud C, Pelli G, Burger F, Staub C, Karsak M, Zimmer A, Frossard JL, Mach F. Low dose oral cannabinoid therapy reduces progression of atherosclerosis in mice. Nature (Lond). 2005;434:782–786. [PubMed: 15815632]

[11] Steffens S, Pacher P. Targeting cannabinoid receptor CB (2) in cardiovascular disorders: promises and controversies. Br J Pharmacol. 2012;167(2):313–323. doi:10.1111/j.1476-5381.2012.02042.x. [PMID: 22612332]

[12] Li Q, Ma HJ, Zhang H, Qi Z, Guan Y, Zhang Y. Electrophysiological effects of anandamide on rat myocardium. Br J Pharmacol. 2009;158(8):2022–2029. [PMID: 20050190]

[13] Maslov LN, Khaliulin I, Zhang Y, Krylatov AV, Naryzhnaya NV, Mechoulam R, Petrocellis L, Downey JM. Prospects for creation of cardioprotective drugs based on cannabinoid receptor agonists. J Cardiovasc Pharmacol Ther. 2015. pii: 1074248415612593

[14] Mukhopadhyay P, Mohanraj R, Bátkai S, Pacher P. CB1 cannabinoid receptor inhibition: promising approach for heart failure? Congest Heart Fail. 2008;14(6):330–334. doi:10.1111/j.1751-7133.2008.00016.x. Review. [PMID: 19076859]

[15] Schmid PC, Schwartz KD, Smith CN, Krebsbach RJ, Berdyshev EV, Schmid HH. A sensitive endocannabinoid assay. The simultaneous analysis of N-acylethanolamines and 2-monoacylglycerols. Chem Phys Lipids. 2000;104(2):185–191

[16] Wagner JA, Hu K, Karcher J, Bauersachs J, Schafer A, Laser M, Han H, Ertl G. CB1 cannabinoid receptor antagonism promotes remodeling and cannabinoid treatment prevents endothelial dysfunction and hypotension in rats with myocardial infarction. Br J Pharmacol. 2003;138:1251–1258. [PubMed: 12711625]

[17] Bouchard JF, Lepicier P, Lamontagne D. Contribution of endocannabinoids in the endothelial protection afforded by ischemic preconditioning in the isolated rat heart. Life Sci. 2003;72:1859–1870. [PubMed: 12586223]

[18] Lepicier P, Bouchard JF, Lagneux C, Lamontagne D. Endocannabinoids protect the rat isolated heart against ischaemia. Br J Pharmacol. 2003;139:805–815. [PubMed: 12813004]

[19] Wang PF, Jiang LS, Bu J, Huang XJ, Song W, Du YP, He B. Cannabinoid-2 receptor activation protects against infarct and ischemia-reperfusion heart injury. J Cardiovasc Pharmacol. 2012;59(4):301–307. doi:10.1097/FJC.0b013e3182418997

[20] Currie S, Rainbow RD, Ewart MA, Kitson S, Pliego EH, Kane KA, McCarron JG. IP(3)R-mediated Ca(2+) release is modulated by anandamide in isolated cardiac nuclei. J Mol Cell Cardiol. 2008;45(6):804–811. doi:10.1016/j.yjmcc.2008.07.005. Epub: 2008 Jul 22

[21] Mukhopadhyay P, Bátkai S, Rajesh M, Czifra N, Harvey-White J, Haskó G, Zsengeller Z, Gerard NP, Liaudet L, Kunos G, et al. Pharmacological inhibition of CB1 cannabinoid receptor protects against doxorubicin-induced cardiotoxicity. J Am Coll Cardiol. 2007;50(6):528–536

[22] Shmist YA, Goncharov I, Eichler M, Shneyvays V, Isaac A, Vogel Z, Shainberg A. Delta-9-tetrahydrocannabinol protects cardiac cells from hypoxia via CB2 receptor activation and nitric oxide production. Mol Cell Biochem. 2006;283(1–2):75–83

[23] Galiegue S, Mary S, Marchand J, Dussossoy D, Carriere D, Carayon P, et al. Expression of central and peripheralcannabinoid receptors in human immune tissues and leukocyte subpopulations. Eur J Biochem. 1995;232:54–61

[24] Bonz A, Laser M, Kullmer S, Kniesch S, Babin-Ebell J, Popp V, Ertl G, Wagner JA. Cannabinoids acting on CB1 receptors decrease contractile performance in human atrial muscle. J Cardiovasc Pharmacol. 2003;41:657–664. [PubMed: 12658069]

[25] Rajesh M, Mukhopadhyay P, Haskó G, Pacher P. Cannabinoid CB1 receptor inhibition decreases vascular smooth muscle migration and proliferation. Biochem Biophys Res Commun. 2008;377:1248–1252

[26] Weis F, Beiras-Fernandez A, Sodian R, Kaczmarek I, Reichart B, Beiras A, Schelling G, Kreth S. Substantially altered expression pattern of cannabinoid receptor 2 and activated endocannabinoid system in patients with severe heart failure. J Mol Cell Cardiol. 2010;48(6):1187–1193

[27] Wagner JA, Hu K, Bauersachs J, Karcher J, Wiesler M, Goparaju SK, Kunos G, Ertl G. Endogenous cannabinoids mediate hypotension after experimental myocardial infarction. J Am Coll Cardiol. 2001a;38:2048–2054. [PubMed: 11738314]

[28] Duerr GD, Heinemann JC, Gestrich C, Heuft T, Klaas T, Keppel K, Roell W, Klein A, Zimmer A, Velten M, Kilic A, Bindila L, Lutz B, Dewald O. Impaired border zone formation and adverse remodeling after reperfused myocardial infarction in cannabinoid CB2 receptor deficient mice. Life Sci. 2015;138:8–17. doi:10.1016/j.lfs.2014.11.005. Epub: 2014 Nov 14. [PMID: 25447445]

[29] Heinemann JC, Duerr GD, Keppel K, Breitbach M, Fleischmann BK, Zimmer A, Wehner S, Welz A, Dewald O. CB2 receptor-mediated effects of pro-inflammatory macrophages influence survival of cardiomyocytes. Life Sci. 2015;138:18–28. doi:10.1016/j.lfs.2014.11.027. Epub 2014 Dec 9. [PMID: 25497711]

[30] Slavic S, Lauer D, Sommerfeld M, Kemnitz UR, Grzesiak A, Trappiel M, Thöne-Reineke C, Baulmann J, Paulis L, Kappert K, Kintscher U, Unger T, Kaschina E. Cannabinoid receptor 1 inhibition improves cardiac function and remodelling after myocardial infarction and in experimental metabolic syndrome. J Mol Med (Berl). 2013;91(7):811–23. doi:10.1007/s00109-013-1034-0. Epub: 2013 May 1. [PMID: 23636507]

[31] Rajesh M, Bátkai S, Kechrid M, Mukhopadhyay P, Lee WS, Horváth B, Holovac E, Cinar R, Liaudet L, Mackie K, Haskó G, Pacher P. Cannabinoid 1 receptor promotes cardiac dysfunction, oxidative stress, inflammation, and fibrosis in diabetic cardiomyopathy. Diabetes. 2012;61(3):716–727. doi:10.2337/db11-0477. Epub: 2012 Feb 7. [PMID: 22315315]

[32] Quercioli A, Pataky Z, Vincenti G, Makoundou V, Di Marzo V, Montecucco F, Carballo S, Thomas A, Staub C, Steffens S, Seimbille Y, Golay A, Ratib O, Harsch E, Mach F, Schindler TH. Elevated endocannabinoid plasma levels are associated with coronary circulatory dysfunction in obesity. Eur Heart J. 2011;32(11):1369–1378. doi:10.1093/eurheartj/ehr029. Epub: 2011 Feb 8

[33] Duerr GD, Heinemann JC, Dunkel S, Zimmer A, Lutz B, Lerner R, Roell W, Mellert F, Probst C, Esmailzadeh B, Welz A, Dewald O. Myocardial hypertrophy is associated with inflammation and activation of endocannabinoid system in patients with aortic valve stenosis. Life Sci. 2013;92(20–21):976–983. doi:10.1016/j.lfs.2013.03.014. Epub: 2013 Apr 6. [PMID: 23567807]

[34] Cappellano G, Uberti F, Caimmi PP, Pietronave S, Mary DA, Dianzani C, Micalizzi E, Melensi M, Boldorini R, Nicosia G, Crosio E, Chiocchetti A, Aina F, Prat M, Dianzani U, Vacca G, Ariatti C, Grossini E. Different expression and function of the endocannabinoid system in human epicardial adipose tissue in relation to heart disease. Can J Cardiol. 2013;29(4):499–509. doi:10.1016/j.cjca.2012.06.003. Epub: 2012 Aug 24

[35] Saatch S, Smith SJ, Micheva KD. Array tomography for cardiovascular imaging: description of technique and potential application. In: Shenasa M, editor. Cardiac mapping, 4th Edition, Wiley-Blackwell, 2012, 966 p.

[36] Currie S, Rainbow RD, Ewart MA, Kitson S, Pliego EH, Kane KA, McCarron JG. IP(3)R-mediated Ca(2+) release is modulated by anandamide in isolated cardiac nuclei. J Mol Cell Cardiol. 2008;45(6):804–11. doi:10.1016/j.yjmcc.2008.07.005. Epub: 2008 Jul 22

[37] Krylatov AV, Maslov LN, Ermakov SY, Lasukova OV, Barzakh EI, Crawford D, Pertwee RG. Significance of cardiac cannabinoid receptors in regulation of cardiac rhythm, myocardial contractility, and electrophysiologic processes in heart. Izv Akad Nauk Ser Biol. 2007;(1):35–44

[38] Fisher BA, Ghuran A, Vadamalai V, Antonios TF. Cardiovascular complications induced by cannabis smoking: a case report and review of the literature. Emerg Med J. 2005;22:679–680

[39] Clark BC, Georgekutty J, Berul CI. Myocardial ischemia secondary to synthetic cannabinoid (K2) use in pediatric patients. J Pediatr. 2015;167(3):757–761.e1. doi: 10.1016/j.jpeds.2015.06.001. Epub: 2015 Jul 9. [PMID: 26165442]

[40] Ghuran A, Nolan J. Recreational drug misuse: issues for the cardiologist. Heart. 2000;83:627–633

[41] Molderings GJ, Likungu J, Göthert M. Presynaptic cannabinoid and imidazoline receptors in the human heart and their potential relationship. Naunyn Schmiedebergs Arch Pharmacol. 1999;360(2):157–164. [PMID: 10494885]

[42] Sterin-Borda L, Del Zar CF, Borda E. Differential CB1 and CB2 cannabinoid receptor-inotropic response of rat isolated atria: endogenous signal transduction pathways. Biochem Pharmacol. 2005;69:1705–1713. [PubMed: 15885656]

[43] Al Kury LT, Voitychuk OI, Yang KH, Thayyullathil FT, Doroshenko P, Ramez AM, Shuba YM, Galadari S, Howarth FC, Oz M. Effects of the endogenous cannabinoid anandamide on voltage-dependent sodium and calcium channels in rat ventricular myocytes. Br J Pharmacol. 2014;171(14):3485–3498. doi:10.1111/bph.12734. [PMID: 24758718]

[44] Al Kury LT, Yang KH, Thayyullathil FT, Rajesh M, Ali RM, Shuba YM, Howarth FC, Galadari S, Oz M. Effects of endogenous cannabinoid anandamide on cardiac Na^+/Ca^{2+} exchanger. Cell Calcium. 2014;55(5):231–237. doi:10.1016/j.ceca.2014.02.017. Epub: 2014 Mar 11

[45] Li Q, Cui N, Du Y, Ma H, Zhang Y. Anandamide reduces intracellular Ca^{2+} concentration through suppression of Na^+/Ca^{2+} exchanger current in rat cardiac myocytes. Plos One. 2013. doi:10.1371/journal.pone.0063386

[46] Bosier B, Muccioli GG, Hermans E, Lambert DM. Functionally selective cannabinoid receptor signalling: therapeutic implications and opportunities. Biochem Pharmacol.

2010;80(1):1–12. doi:10.1016/j.bcp.2010.02.013. Epub: 2010 Mar 3. Review. [PMID: 20206137]

[47] Ledent C, Valverde O, Cossu G, Petitet F, Aubert JF, Beslot F, Bohme GA, Imperato A, Pedrazzini T, Roques BP, et al. Unresponsiveness to cannabinoids and reduced addictive effects of opiates in CB1 receptor knockout mice. Science (Wash DC). 1999;283:401–404

[48] Liao Y, Bin J, Asakura M, Xuan W, Chen B, Huang Q, Xu D, Ledent C, Takashima S, Kitakaze M. Deficiency of type 1 cannabinoid receptors worsens acute heart failure induced by pressure overload in mice. Eur Heart J. 2012;33(24):3124–3133. doi:10.1093/eurheartj/ehr246. Epub: 2011 Jul 23. [PMID: 21785110]

[49] Liao Y, Bin J, Luo T, Zhao H, Ledent C, Asakura M, Xu D, Takashima S, Kitakaze M. CB1 cannabinoid receptor deficiency promotes cardiac remodeling induced by pressure overload in mice. Int J Cardiol. 2013;167(5):1936–1944. doi:10.1016/j.ijcard.2012.05.033. Epub: 2012 May 31. [PMID: 22656047]

[50] Buckley NE, McCoy KL, Mezey E, Bonner T, Zimmer A, Felder CC, et al. Immunomodulation by cannabinoids is absent in mice deficient for the cannabinoid CB_2 receptor. Eur J Pharmacol. 2000;396:141–149

[51] Buckley NE. The peripheral cannabinoid receptor knockout mice: an update. Br J Pharmacol. 2008;153(2):309–318. Epub: 2007 Oct 29. Review. [PMID: 1796574]

[52] Defer N, Wan J, Souktani R, Escoubet B, Perier M, Caramelle P, et al. The cannabinoid receptor type 2 promotes cardiac myocyte and fibroblast survival and protects against ischemia/reperfusion-induced cardiomyopathy. FASEB J. 2009;23:2120–2130

[53] Duerr GD, Heinemann JC, Suchan G, Kolobara E, Wenzel D, Geisen C, Matthey M, Passe-Tietjen K, Mahmud W, Ghanem A, Tiemann K, Alferink J, Burgdorf S, Buchalla R, Zimmer A, Lutz B, Welz A, Fleischmann BK, Dewald O. The endocannabinoid-CB2 receptor axis protects the ischemic heart at the early stage of cardiomyopathy. Basic Res Cardiol. 2014;109(4):425. doi:10.1007/s00395-014-0425-x. Epub: 2014 Jul 1. [PMID: 24980781]

[54] Duerr GD, Heinemann JC, Gestrich C, Heuft T, Klaas T, Keppel K, Roell W, Klein A, Zimmer A, Velten M, Kilic A, Bindila L, Lutz B, Dewald O. Impaired border zone formation and adverse remodeling after reperfused myocardial infarction in cannabinoid CB2 receptor deficient mice. Life Sci. 2015;138:8–17. doi:10.1016/j.lfs.2014.11.005. Epub: 2014 Nov 14

[55] Pacher P, Bátkai S, Osei-Hyiaman D, Offertáler L, Liu J, Harvey-White J, Brassai A, Járai Z, Cravatt BF, Kunos G. Hemodynamic profile, responsiveness to anandamide, and baroreflex sensitivity of mice lacking fatty acid amide hydrolase. Am J Physiol Heart Circ Physiol. 2005;289(2):H533–H541. Epub: 2005 Apr 8. [PMID: 15821037]

[56] Batkai, S, Rajesh M, Mukhopadhyay P, Hasko G, Liaudet L, Cravat B F, Csiszar A, Ungvari Z, Pacher P. Decreased age-related cardiac dysfunction, myocardial nitrative

stress, inflammatory gene expression, and apoptosis in mice lacking fatty acid amide hydrolase. Am J Physiol Heart Circ Physiol. 2007;293:H909–H918

[57] Mukhopadhyay P, Horváth B, Rajesh M, Matsumoto S, Saito K, Bátkai S, Patel V, Tanchian G, Gao RY, Cravatt BF, Haskó G, Pacher P. Fatty acid amide hydrolase is a key regulator of endocannabinoid-induced myocardial tissue injury. Free Radic Biol Med. 2011;50(1):179–195. doi:10.1016/j.freeradbiomed.2010.11.002. Epub: 2010 Nov 9

[58] Murry CE, Jennings RB, Reimer KA. Preconditioning with ischemia: a delay of lethal cell injury in ischemic myocardium. Circulation. 1986;74(5):1124–1136

[59] Wagner JA, Abesser M, Harvey-White J, Ertl G. 2-Arachidonylglycerol acting on CB1 cannabinoid receptors mediates delayed cardioprotection induced by nitric oxide in rat isolated hearts. J Cardiovasc Pharmacol. 2006;47(5):650–655. [PMID: 16775503]

[60] Hiley CR, Ford WR. Endocannabinoids as mediators in the heart: a potential target for therapy of remodelling after myocardial infarction? Br J Pharmacol. 2003;138:1183–1184

[61] Pacher P, Haskó G. Endocannabinoids and cannabinoid receptors in ischaemia-reperfusion injury and preconditioning. Br J Pharmacol. 2008;153(2):252–262. Epub: 2007 Nov 19. Review. [PMID: 18026124]

[62] Lagneux C, Lamontagne D. Involvement of cannabinoids in the cardioprotection induced by lipopolysaccharide. Br J Pharmacol. 2001;132(4):793–796

[63] Joyeux M, Arnaud C, Godin-Ribuot D, Demenge P, Lamontagne D, Ribuot C. Endocannabinoids are implicated in the infarct size-reducing effect conferred by heat stress preconditioning in isolated rat hearts. Cardiovasc Res. 2002;55(3):619–625

[64] Bouchard JF, Lepicier P, Lamontagne D. Contribution of endocannabinoids in the endothelial protection afforded by ischemic preconditioning in the isolated rat heart. Life Sci. 2003;72:1859–1870. [PubMed: 12586223]

[65] Lepicier P, Bouchard JF, Lagneux C, Lamontagne D. Endocannabinoids protect the rat isolated heart against ischaemia. Br J Pharmacol. 2003;139:805–815. [PubMed: 12813004]

[66] Underdown NJ, Hiley CR, Ford WR. Anandamide reduces infarct size in rat isolated hearts subjected to ischaemia-reperfusion by a novel cannabinoid mechanism. Br J Pharmacol. 2005;146:809–816. [PubMed: 16158067]

[67] Krylatov AV, Ugdyzhekova DS, Bernatskaya NA, Maslov LN, Mekhoulam R, Pertwee RG, Stephano GB. Activation of type II cannabinoid receptors improves myocardial tolerance to arrhythmogenic effects of coronary occlusion and reperfusion. Bull Exp Biol Med. 2001;131:523–525. [PubMed: 11586395]

[68] Di Filippo C, Rossi F, Rossi S, D'Amico M. Cannabinoid CB2 receptor activation reduces mouse myocardial ischemia-reperfusion injury: involvement of cytokine/chemokines and PMN. J Leukoc Biol. 2004;75:453–459. [PubMed: 14657208]

[69] Hajrasouliha AR, Tavakoli S, Ghasemi M, Jabehdar-Maralani P, Sadeghipour H, Ebrahimi F, et al. Endogenous cannabinoids contribute to remote ischemic precondi-

tioning via cannabinoid CB2 receptors in the rat heart. Eur J Pharmacol. 2008;579:246–252

[70] Montecucco F, Lenglet S, Braunersreuther V, Burger F, Pelli G, Bertolotto M, et al. CB (2) cannabinoid receptor activation is cardioprotective in a mouse model of ischemia/reperfusion. J Mol Cell Cardiol. 2009;46:612–620

[71] Li Q, Wang F, Zhang YM, Zhou JJ, Zhang Y. Activation of cannabinoid type 2 receptor by JWH133 protects heart against ischemia/reperfusion-induced apoptosis. Cell Physiol Biochem. 2013;31(4–5):693–702. doi:10.1159/000350088. Epub: 2013 May 17

[72] Waldman M, Hochhauser E, Fishbein M, Aravot D, Shainberg A, Sarne Y. An ultra-low dose of tetrahydrocannabinol provides cardioprotection. Biochem Pharmacol. 2013;85(11):1626–33. doi:10.1016/j.bcp.2013.03.014

[73] Gajarsa JJ, Kloner RA. Left ventricular remodeling in the post-infarction heart: a review of cellular, molecular mechanisms, and therapeutic modalities. Heart Fail Rev. 2011;16(1):13–21. doi:10.1007/s10741-010-9181-7

[74] Lim SY, Davidson SM, Yellon DM, Smith CCT. The cannabinoid CB1 receptor antagonist, rimonabant, protects against acute myocardial infarction. Basic Res Cardiol. 2009;104(6):781–792

[75] Lu Y, Akinwumi BC, Shao Z, Anderson HD. Ligand activation of cannabinoid receptors attenuates hypertrophy of neonatal rat cardiomyocytes. J Cardiovasc Pharmacol. 2014;64(5):420–430. doi:10.1097/FJC.0000000000000134. [PMID: 24979612]

[76] Julien B, Grenard P, Teixeira-Clerc F, Van Nhieu JT, Li L, Karsak M, Zimmer A, Mallat A, Lotersztajn S. Antifibrogenic role of the cannabinoid receptor CB2 in the liver. Gastroenterology. 2005;128:742–755. [PubMed: 15765409]

[77] Siegmund SV, Uchinami H, Osawa Y, Brenner DA, Schwabe RF. Anandamide induces necrosis in primary hepatic stellate cells. Hepatology. 2005;41:1085–1095. [PubMed: 15841466]

[78] Spinale FG. Myocardial matrix remodeling and the matrix metalloproteinases: influence on cardiac form and function. Physiol Rev. 2007;87(4):1285–1342. Review. [PMID: 17928585]

[79] Tiyerili V, Zimmer S, Jung S, Wassmann K, Naehle CP, LütjohannD, Zimmer A, Nickenig G, Wassmann S. CB1 receptor inhibition leads to decreased vascular AT1 receptor expression, inhibition of oxidative stress and improved endothelial function. Basic Res Cardiol. 2010;105(4):465–477

The Role for the Endocannabinoid System in Cardioprotection and Myocardial Adaptation

Oliver Dewald and Georg D. Duerr

Additional information is available at the end of the chapter

http://dx.doi.org/10.5772/62485

Abstract

Results from different studies showing CB2 receptor-associated cardioprotective action are still fairly controversial and no single specific mechanism could be identified. Several groups investigated the involvement of the endocannabinoid system in cellular systems and function of cardiomyocytes, fibroblasts, macrophages and endothelial cells. While some studies are limited in their translational relevance, a few recent studies describe a myocardial ischemia and reperfusion scenario in a fashion comparable to the clinical situation. Recent studies provided evidence for involvement of the CB2 receptor–endocannabinoid axis in prevention of cardiomyocyte apoptosis including modulation of antioxidative enzymes and contractile elements expression. CB2 receptor has further been shown to specifically modulate the inflammatory response and macrophage function after myocardial ischemia. These effects have an impact on the subsequent myocardial remodeling, where the CB2 receptor modulates function of myofibroblasts, collagen production and limitation of myocardial infarction size. Recent experimental and clinical data showed the association of the endocannabinoid system in myocardial hypertrophy. In conclusion, increasing amount of evidence supports a crucial role of the endocannabinoid system in cardioprotection and myocardial remodeling, while some of them even suggest model-independent systemic effects in adaptation of cardiomyocytes or components of the extracellular matrix.

Keywords: endocannabinoids, myocardial ischemia, reperfusion, cardioprotection, remodeling

1. Introduction

Cannabinoids have been described as potent regulators of a variety of neurological functions influencing pain control, behaviour and memory. The discovery of the cannabinoid receptors

CB1 and CB2 led to initial description of CB1 receptor to be restricted to neurons while CB2 receptor was found on immunological cells. Later studies reported these receptors being also localized on vascular cells [1] and in the heart [2]. Furthermore, production of ligands to the cannabinoid receptors—endogenous cannabinoids—was reported in endothelial cells [3]. Experiments performed *in vitro* and *in vivo* showed that the effects of endocannabinoids on the cardiovascular system are pleiotropic and only partially understood to date. Due to the socioeconomic impact of cardiovascular diseases, a better understanding of the pathology and associated mechanisms is needed for development of novel therapeutic strategies. Since modern therapies are aiming to disease prevention with early treatment, the mechanisms of cardioprotection gained a significant attention and have been investigated more deeply. The cardioprotective mechanisms provide limitation of the myocardial damage after injury and are very complex. Growing evidence supporting the role of inflammation in cardioprotection [4] and modulation of inflammatory response by endocannabinoids led to investigations of the endocannabinoids in myocardial injury and protection.

2. Mechanisms of cardioprotection

Myocardial protection is a very complex system involving not only intracellular mechanisms in cardiomyocytes, but also bearing a large contribution of cells within the local microenvironment in the heart. The contradictions in the experimental evidence for specific mechanisms in the cardiomyocytes are not only related to differences in experimental setup, but also most probably associated to variations in mediators and cells within the local microenvironment. These factors make it difficult to draw clear conclusions from experimental data which will lead to new targets for therapy. Therefore, significant efforts have been made to enlighten the complexity of cardioprotection.

A number of signalling cascades and systems are involved in cardioprotection. Based on strong experimental and clinical evidence, the first line of intervention is aiming at the earliest possible restoration of the blood flow, i.e., reperfusion. The very early observation of timely onset of reperfusion leading to preservation of myocardial function [5, 6] provided ground for the clinical introduction of early percutaneous coronary intervention. Subsequently, Murry introduced the concept of ischemic preconditioning based upon four episodes of five minutes ischemia interrupted by each five minutes of reperfusion before a myocardial infarction was induced (40 minutes ischemia) and thereby resulting in decreased infarct size [7]. Interestingly, this effect was not found after a three-hour ischemia period underlining the ultimate goal of early reperfusion. This concept of myocardial conditioning was first applied in temporal relation to the myocardial injury, thereby defining preconditioning and postconditioning [8]. Studies extended this concept by introduction of spatial component in remote preconditioning, where short, repetitive limb occlusions provide protection to the following longer episode of myocardial ischemia [9, 10]. The latter concept was clinically implemented and proved to be beneficial to the patients [11]. Numerous studies described a wide range of molecules and signalling cascades involved utilizing different models, species, and pharmacological or genetic manipulation. So far there are only scattered reports investigating the role of endocannabinoids in ischemic preconditioning. One of the studies applied heat stress preconditioning 24 hours before isolation of the hearts, which then underwent 30 min ischemia and 120 minutes reperfusion *ex vivo* using Langendorff system [12]. The application of selective CB2 receptor antagonist SR144528 reduced the protective effects of heart preconditioning on infarct size. The authors therefore suggested a potential protective role of CB2 receptor in ischemia and reperfusion (I/R).

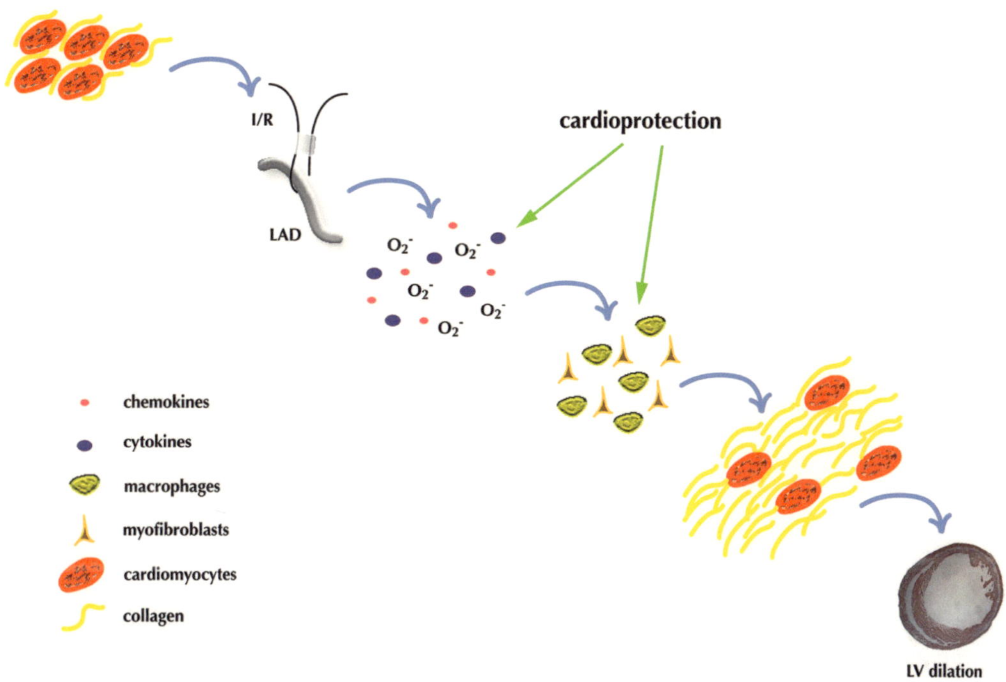

Figure 1. Cascade of events after reperfusion of ischemic myocardium. I/R, ischemia and reperfusion; LAD, left anterior descending artery; LV, left ventricular.

Another important area of cardioprotection originated in studies describing effects of modulation of inflammatory response during reperfusion injury. The very early studies reported detrimental outcome in patients treated with methylprednisolone after reperfusion of myocardial infarction [13]. Despite this drawback, it was the experimental work in subsequent years which provided solid evidence for beneficial effects of reperfusion [14]. The effects of inflammation in reperfusion must also be differentiated in a temporal and spatial context, because reperfusion initially induces a strong inflammatory response. In short-term (few days), this leads to a stronger functional impairment of the heart than without reperfusion, but the long-term effects of reperfusion have been proven to preserve the myocardial function and could even prevent development of dysfunction. The ischemia of myocardial tissue leads to accumulation of free radicals and toxic metabolic products while the adenosine triphosphate storages are depleted and cellular homeostasis is increasingly impaired. The reperfusion of ischemic myocardium is associated with activation of the complement system and a strong increase in reactive oxygen species (ROS). The subsequent response includes activation of tumour necrosis factor α (*TNF-α*) and initiation of a cytokine response [15] leading to a cascade of events (**Figure 1**). Activation of *TNF-α* leads to induction of interleukin (*IL-*)*8* and CC chemokine ligand (*CCL*)*2*, which – in combination with complement factor C5a activation —attracts neutrophil granulocytes to the ischemic myocardium [16]. The extravasation of neutrophils and the expression of intercellular adhesion molecule (*ICAM-*)*1* lead to direct adhesion of neutrophils on cardiomyocytes with damaging effects involving ROS [17]. The ROS cause an oxidative burst leading to irreversible cellular damage [18] and is counteracted by different scavenger enzymes, e.g., peroxidases, superoxide dismutases (SODs) or catalase. The damaged cardiomyocytes release chemokine *CCL2* and cytokine transforming growth factor (*TGF-*)*β* and thereby promote invasion of mononuclear cells [19].

Differentiation of monocytes to macrophages in myocardium leads to even further increased production of inflammatory cytokines, while macrophages initiate their production of growth factors, e.g., basic fibroblast growth factor or vascular endothelial growth factor. As a result, proliferation of fibroblasts, differentiation of myofibroblasts and neoangiogenesis are initiated and all aiming at granulation tissue formation and tissue remodeling. These events involve different macrophage subpopulations, which are differentiated upon polarization of the lymphocytes response from *Th1* to *Th2* type [20]. While previous studies described classical proinflammatory M1 and alternative anti-inflammatory M2 subtype of macrophages, novel studies provide evidence of even more subtypes of these crucial cells in tissue repair. The application of so called cardiosphere-derived cells led to differentiation of a unique cardioprotective subtype of macrophages in infarcted rat hearts not bearing M1 or M2 markers and resulting in reduction of infarct size [21]. The inflammatory response has to be deactivated at the certain point of granulation tissue formation in order to provide rapid tissue remodeling and formation of a stable scar. This resolution of inflammatory response is mediated by anti-inflammatory cytokines, e.g., *IL-10*, which also inhibit matrix metalloproteinases (MMP) and stimulate their counter actors, tissue inhibitors of MMP (TIMP) [22]. Therefore, the regulation of macrophage function during myocardial remodeling gained a strong attention in recent years.

Among other factors, specific chemokines have been associated with modulation of macrophage function. Chemokines are a subgroup of cytokines having distinct effects on mononuclear cells and macrophages, but also on neutrophils and endothelial cells. One of the most potent monocyte chemoattractants is the chemokine *CCL2*, which is associated with transendothelial migration and differentiation of monocytes into macrophages [23–25]. *CCL2* is induced by proinflammatory cytokines *TNF-α* and *IL-1β* [24] and mediates mononuclear cell migration into reperfused myocardial infarction [26]. It has also been associated with differentiation of myofibroblasts and collagen production. Reperfusion of myocardial infarction in *CCL*-deficient ($CCL2^{-/-}$) mice was associated with prolonged inflammatory response and delayed formation of granulation tissue resulting in attenuated myocardial remodeling [27]. This was accompanied by decreased differentiation of myofibroblasts and significantly larger left ventricular diameter when compared with wild-type (WT) mice. Another study provided additional evidence for a crucial role of chemokine *CCL2* in the ischemic heart. In a model

http://dx.doi.org/10.5772/62485

of repetitive brief I/R there was a significant reduction in collagen deposition and fibrosis associated with no ventricular dysfunction in *CCL2*$^{-/-}$ mice when compared to interstitial fibrosis and moderate dysfunction in WT animals [28]. Therefore, modulation of macrophage function *via* pharmacological manipulation of chemokine expression profile could be a promising target in development of novel clinical strategies.

3. Experimental evidence for involvement of endocannabinoids in cardioprotection

One of the first publications reported a CB1 receptor-mediated decrease in contractility of human atrial muscle [2]. Cannabinoids also led to a reduction of left ventricular systolic pressure [29]. There is a certain variability in results between *in vivo* and *ex vivo* effects of cannabinoids reported in the myocardium [30], the vasculature [31], the peripheral [32] and the central nervous system. The alterations in vascular tone were accompanied by changes in myocardial contractility and chronotropy and were associated to both CB1 receptor as well as vanilloid receptor [33]. In regard to pathophysiology, beneficial effects were reported for the experimental treatment of atherosclerosis using Δ-9-tetrahydrocannabinol (THC) [34]. In contrast, the results of endocannabinoid effects in the heart were heterogenous. One group reported triggering of heart attacks after use of marijuana [35], while other groups described protective effects in ischemic heart disease upon a decrease in mortality after experimental myocardial infarction [36], or anandamide-induced reduction of infarction size [37]. Still, the underlying mechanisms are not well understood and many investigations aim to shed more light into this clinically important filed. Myocardial I/R is always associated with inflammatory response and it is therefore likely that the endocannabinoid system may act in this process *via* the CB2 receptor as it modulates the function of macrophages [38]. A cardioprotective role has been postulated upon induction of *extracellular signal-regulated kinases (ERK)1/2* after 30 minutes of myocardial ischemia and 10 minutes reperfusion in mice [39]. Another study provided *in vitro* evidence of CB2 receptor-related cardioprotection *in vitro* using hydrogen peroxide treatment leading to increased apoptosis of cardiomyocytes and higher differentiation potential of myofibroblasts [40]. The same report described CB2 receptor-dependent down regulation of *caspase 3* after one hour ischemia and three days reperfusion, but provided surprising results in WT mice with normal left ventricular function after four weeks of reperfusion accompanied by infarct size of only 4% of left ventricular area. Other studies aimed to provide more insights into CB2 receptor mediated mechanisms in cardioprotection.

Application of a non-specific (acting on CB1 and CB2 receptor) agonist WIN55212-2 was shown to reduce infarct size in a mouse model of coronary occlusion without reperfusion, while it decreased myeloperoxidase activity of neutrophils [41]. CB2 receptor can influence the *Th1*/*Th2*-polarization of lymphocytes *in vitro*, which is an important step in differentiation of macrophage subpopulations. This is relevant for cardiac repair since macrophage subpopulations are involved in granulation tissue formation [20], remodeling and scar formation *via* modulation of fibroblasts and differentiation of myofibroblasts. The myofibroblasts are the major source of extracelullar matrix components and thereby play a crucial role in tissue remodeling. In this context, CB2 receptor has been associated with regulation of myofibroblast differentiation in a murine liver fibrosis model [42].

Recent work from our group investigated the role of endocannabinoids and CB2 receptor in a mouse model of non-infarcted ischemic cardiomyopathy induced by brief repetitive I/R. Repetitive daily episode of 15 minute ischemia followed by reperfusion until the next day lead to a transient inflammatory reaction, development of interstitial fibrosis and left ventricular dysfunction [43]. We could show that fibrosis and dysfunction are reversible after 60 days of recovery after the last episode of I/R, where normal left ventricular myocardium is found. This is of clinical interest since: (a) repetitive episodes of ischemia are the hallmark of angina pectoris in patients and (b) these functional and morphological characteristics are also found in human hibernating myocardium with restoration of normal function after revascularization [8]. Mice with overexpression of SOD showed significantly less inflammation and fibrotic depositions associated with almost normal left ventricular function in this model and thereby revealed the importance of ROS in development of fibrosis and left ventricular dysfunction [43]. Another study in the same mouse model revealed a crucial role for the chemokine *CCL2* in development of interstitial fibrosis and left ventricular dysfunction [28]. It was therefore a logical next step to utilize CB2-deficient ($Cnr2^{-/-}$) mice in model of repetitive, brief I/R [44]. In an initial set of experiments, we found persistent induction of CB2 receptor in WT hearts upon repetitive I/R. Since there is no reliable CB2 antibody for histological detection in mice available we isolated cardiomyocytes using Langendorff apparatus and after their purification we could demonstrate induction of *Cnr2* mRNA selectively in cardiomyocytes. $Cnr2^{-/-}$ mice underwent the repetitive I/R protocol and presented with small infarcted areas—microinfarctions—indicating irreversible loss of cardiomyocytes already after three days I/R. The discontinuation of the I/R protocol led to no restoration of the left ventricular function in $Cnr2^{-/-}$ mice after 60 days, in contrast to full recovery in WT mice. WT hearts showed a transient increase in production of anandamide in parallel to the inflammatory reaction, whereas 2-arachidonoylglycerol (2-AG) level was elevated only after 7 days I/R. These data clearly showed not only the involvement of CB2 receptor and endocannabinoids in ischemic myocardium, but also provided a time course of their expression. The study revealed increased apoptosis and ROS production in $Cnr2^{-/-}$ hearts when compared to the WT mice. The investigation of mechanisms associated to the increased apoptosis in $Cnr2^{-/-}$ hearts revealed a CB2 receptor-associated regulation in expression of contractile elements and antioxidative enzymes (**Figure 2**). Analysis of inflammatory response revealed a CB2 receptor dependent induction of the cytokine *IL-1β* and the chemokines *CCL2, CCL3* and *CCL4* in this model. Interestingly, $Cnr2^{-/-}$ mice were able to induce the inflammatory response by a stronger induction of monocyte-colony stimulating factor *(M-CSF)* and *TNF-α* than the WT mice. This led to persistent macrophage infiltration of the ischemic myocardium in $Cnr2^{-/-}$ mice, while they were also unable to induce the anti-inflammatory cytokine *IL-10* and thereby resolve the inflammatory response. Magnetic sorting of macrophages using flow cytometry and their mRNA expression profile provided evidence for a delayed initiation of the anti-inflammatory M2a subpopulation of macrophages in $Cnr2^{-/-}$ mice. Additional experiments using reconstituted chimeric mice provided additional evidence for the pivotal role of macrophages in the irreversible loss of cardiomyocytes in $Cnr2^{-/-}$ mice.

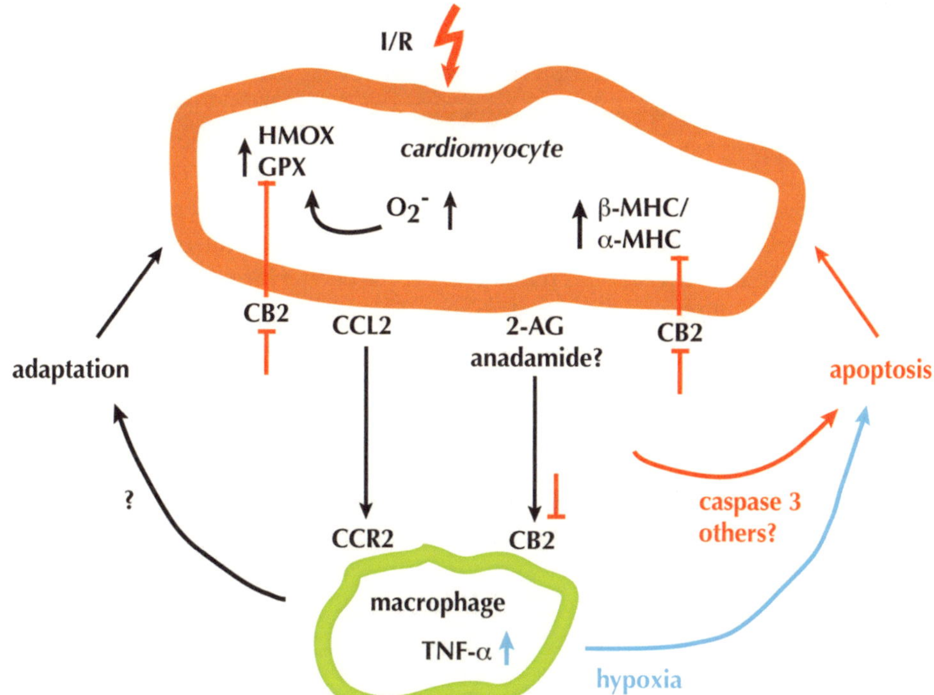

Figure 2. CB2 receptor-dependent mechanisms of cardioprotection in ischemic non-infarcted murine myocardium. I/R, ischemia and reperfusion; HMOX, heme oxygenase; GPX, glutathione peroxidase; MHC, myosin heavy chain; 2-AG, 2-arachidonoylglycerol; TNF-α, tumour necrosis factor α.

The consequences of prolonged inflammatory response were not limited to cardiomyocyte loss, but also involved adverse remodeling process in $Cnr2^{-/-}$ hearts. A morphological differentiation of collagen deposition revealed a comparable collagen area between the two genotypes, but significantly less interstitial fibrosis and concentration of collagen in microinfarctions in $Cnr2^{-/-}$ hearts [44]. At the molecular level this was associated with significantly less mRNA expression of *collagen III*, which is the reversible form of the deposited collagen isoforms. The significantly lower differentiation of myofibroblasts was associated with a low expression or early remodeling marker *tenascin C in vivo* and *in vitro*. Taken together, the survival of non-infarcted ischemic myocardium is dependent on a complex involvement of endocannabinoids and CB2 receptor in molecular and cellular mechanisms of cardioprotection.

Based on these findings we utilized $Cnr2^{-/-}$ mice in a model of reperfused myocardial infarction. One hour of ischemia was followed by reperfusion for different time periods up to seven days and led to a significantly worse left ventricular function in $Cnr2^{-/-}$ mice when compared to the WT mice [45]. Histological analysis showed expansion of the infarcted area as a transmural lesion in $Cnr2^{-/-}$ when compared to the non-transmural scar formation in WT mice. Myocardial infarction was associated with increased production of anandamide and 2-AG, but also of their associated lipids oleoyl ethanolamine and palmitoyl ethanolamide in both genotypes. The molecular analysis showed a similar pattern as in non-infarcted repetitive I/R, with an impaired induction of antioxidative enzymes and unfavourable expression of contractile elements in *Cnr2*$^{-/-}$ mice. Molecular analysis revealed an *IL-1β*- and *TNF-α*-associated induction of inflammatory response with only low-level chemokine response after six hours of reperfusion in *Cnr2*$^{-/-}$ mice. In contrast WT mice showed a regular pattern with a significant increase in expression of *TNF-α* and chemokines *CCL2, CCL3* and *CCL4*. The significantly higher density of macrophages was associated with their prolonged action in infarction until seven days reperfusion and their completely transmural involvement in *Cnr2*$^{-/-}$ mice [45]. The analysis of myocardial remodeling revealed significantly less myofibroblasts and a lower induction of *tenascin C* in *Cnr2*$^{-/-}$ hearts. The most important finding was the lack of *thrombospondin 1* induction in *Cnr2*$^{-/-}$ hearts, which was responsible for the impaired formation of the infarction border zone and thereby failed limitation of the myocardial injury.

In summary, our *in vivo* studies showed substantial involvement of endocannabinoids and CB2 receptor in cardioprotective mechanisms and subsequent myocardial remodeling in the murine heart. While their clinical relevance still remains to be investigated, it is even more important to better understand the molecular mechanisms and the impact of cellular interactions mediated by this system.

4. Endocannabinoids in cellular mechanisms of myocardial adaptation

Several studies investigated the effects of cannabinoid receptors in regulation of cellular homeostasis and pathology, but their methodological differences and model-related problems do not allow to drawn clear and direct conclusions. A number of pharmacological studies investigated the impact of cannabinoid receptors on blood pressure *in vivo* and *ex vivo* [46] and some of these studies showed associated negative inotropic effects mediated by CB1 receptor. This was further supported by the evidence for CB1 receptor-mediated contractile dysfunction in experimental models of hepatic cirrhosis [47]. Still, none of these studies provided insights into specific cell actions of CB1 receptor. A study using 30 min left anterior descending artery (LAD) occlusion and 2.5 hours of reperfusion thereafter showed CB2 receptor effects by using non-specific agonist WIN55212-2 and reversal of its action with CB2 receptor antagonist AM630 [41]. Thereby, the authors described CB2 receptor-mediated effects on inflammatory response and myeloperoxidase activity indicating general leukocyte involvement. Another study utilized selective CB2 receptor agonist JWH-133 and showed cardioprotective effects based on activation of *ERK1/2* and the signal transducer and activator of transcription *(STAT)3*-mediated pathway [39]. The same study described also attenuated neutrophil recruitment towards inflammatory cytokine *TNF-α in vitro*.

Potential cardioprotective effects were described for cannabidiol based on the lower incidence of arrhythmia in rat hearts after ischemia and reperfusion, but the authors only speculated about involvement of cardiac current and channels [48]. The already above mentioned study suggested CB2 receptor-related cardioprotection after hydrogen peroxide treatment leading to increased apoptosis of cardiomyocytes and higher differentiation

http://dx.doi.org/10.5772/62485

potential of myofibroblasts *in vitro* [40]. Our own work provided evidence for increased mRNA expression of *Cnr2* in purified cardiomyocytes after three days of brief repetitive I/R [44]. Cardiomyocytes were isolated using enzyme digestion in Langendorff apparatus and subsequent separation of them from fibroblasts was achieved using a short stay in cell culture where fibroblasts attach rapidly to the dish. We also used embryonic cardiomyocyte cell culture (having a large proportion of concomitant fibroblasts needed for survival) and were able to show a lower induction of antioxidative enzyme *heme oxygenase 1* and chemokine *CCL2* in *Cnr2*$^{-/-}$ cells under hypoxic conditions (2% O_2). In order to eliminate the confounding effects of fibroblasts, we utilized puromycin-purified embryonic stem cell-derived cardiomyocytes (97%-pure cardiomyocyte cell culture) [49]. This pure cardiomyocyte culture confirmed our findings on *heme oxygenase 1* and *CCL2*, and in addition provided evidence for hypoxia-dependent up regulation of CB2 receptor [44]. These data clearly showed specific CB2 receptor-related effects in cardiomyocytes.

Based on our data from cardiomyocytes *in vitro* and macrophage modulation *in vivo* we further investigated cellular interactions between cardiomyocytes and macrophages [50]. Initially we demonstrated the topical expression of CB2 receptor on WT cardiomyocytes and both WT macrophage subtypes M1 and M2 in cell culture, which increased under hypoxic conditions (2% O_2) and even more when proinflammatory cytokine interferon *(IFN)-γ* was added into the culture medium [50]. In order to exclude methodological problems of cell culture we quantified the number of vital WT cardiomyocytes in the culture after 12 and 24 hours cultivation under normoxia and hypoxia and found comparable cell numbers in both conditions, while the number was slightly lower after 24 hours indicating only minor loss due to apoptosis. Next, we compared apoptosis in WT vs. *Cnr2*$^{-/-}$ cardiomyocytes and found significantly higher amount of apoptotic cells among the *Cnr2*$^{-/-}$ cardiomyocytes. This raised the question whether the increased apoptosis alone is solely responsible for the loss of cardiomyocytes observed in our *in vivo* model, and we therefore investigated the function of macrophages in the next step. We stimulated the macrophages with *IFN-γ* in order to stimulate the differentiation into M1 subtype [50]. In order to measure the migration potential of this subtype we used either supernatant from the cardiomyocytes cell culture after 24 hours hypoxia or potent chemoattractants *CCL2* and *M-CSF* in a Boyden chamber, which are both strongly induced after myocardial infarction in mice [51]. We found a significantly stronger migration potential of *Cnr2*$^{-/-}$ M1 macrophages towards the supernatant of hypoxic cardiomyocytes than in WT M1 macrophages. This finding indicated a more aggressive nature of *Cnr2*$^{-/-}$ M1 macrophages and we subsequently utilized them in co-culture with cardiomyocytes. The co-culture experiments revealed significantly higher loss of embryonic cardiomyocytes and their apoptosis when combined with *Cnr2*$^{-/-}$ than with WT M1 macrophages. In addition, we found that production of *TNF-α* in M1 macrophages was dependent on stimulation of CB2 receptor by anandamide [50]. In summary, we were able to identify at least some of the mechanisms behind the aggressive nature of macrophages in *Cnr2*$^{-/-}$ mice and their interaction with cardiomyocytes under conditions, which are comparable to the *in vivo* situation. Still, it remains to be elucidated in future studies which molecular pathways are involved in this cellular interaction and expand it towards other cells in the heart.

5. Clinical perspective for endocannabinoids in myocardial adaptation

A number of clinical studies described the involvement of endocannabinoids in human cardiac conditions. One study described an increased level of endocannabinoids in the blood stream and higher expression of CB2 receptor in the heart of patients with terminal heart failure [52]. Another study from the same group described significant reduction of plasma anandamide concentration after induction of general anaesthesia using isoflurane [53]. In the same patient population they reported a significant increase in 2-AG after onset of cardiopulmonary bypass during heart surgery, but remained only speculative on the clinical relevance of these findings by suggesting association with inflammatory response. A recent study from our group showed activation of the endocannabinoid system and up regulation of its receptors in myocardial hypertrophy in patients with aortic valve stenosis [54]. We were able to identify expression of CB2 receptor predominantly on cardiomyocytes, but also on myofibroblasts and mononuclear cells in hypertrophic myocardium. The same study revealed a persistent low-grade inflammation and active remodeling in hypertrophied hearts and this shows parallels to our experimental findings discussed above.

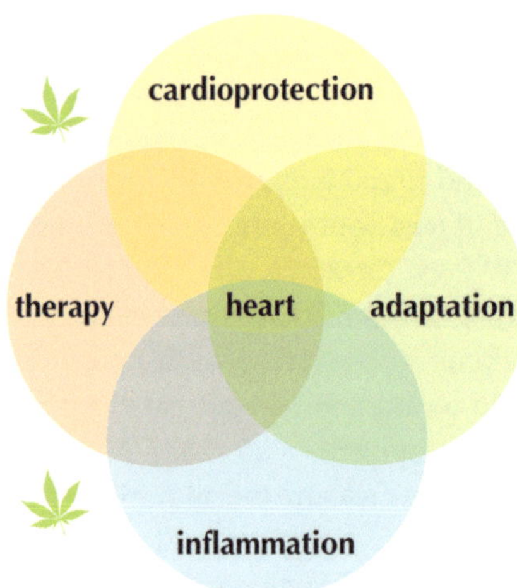

Figure 3. Complex relations in a clinical scenario targeting endocannabinoid system.

The endocannabinoid system gained clinical relevance in the last few years because of a CB1-receptor antagonist based therapy (rimonabant) being approved for clinical use in severely obese patients, but then disappeared rather early due to unwanted and detrimental side effects [55]. Still, one study investigated the effect of rimonabant on progression of atherosclerosis in patients with abdominal obesity and coronary artery disease (STRADIVARIUS randomized controlled trial). The results were disappointing for the primary endpoint, since no effect could be identified on the disease progression [56]. Still, the secondary endpoint of normalized total atheroma volume was met and this could be the basis for future studies. In the light of our results on the role of the chemokine *CCL2* and the CB2 receptor in myocardial remodeling and adaptation to injury [27, 43–45], it has to be emphasised, that we need to expand our knowledge of cellular interactions and mechanisms in other disease models. The complexity of this system and its interaction are shown in **Figure 3**. The next step will be the investigation of highly specific compounds acting on cannabinoid receptors. Nevertheless, the modulation of inflammatory response remains to be a potential therapeutical target in cardioprotection.

6. Conclusions

Growing amount of evidence supports the role of the endocannabinoid system and cannabinoid receptors in cardioprotection and myocardial adaptation. Several mechanisms have been described in specific cells *in vitro* and some of these show parallels with the *in vivo* data. The data on CB2 receptor-mediated adaptation of injured myocardium show a spatiotemporal resolution of its actions on different cells in the heart and shed more light into the finely balanced system of cardioprotection. Therefore, an even better mechanistic understanding of the cannabinoid system and its action on the cardiovascular system in the healthy and the diseased state are needed than the present one we have. This will eventually allow the identification of promising new pathways and/or targets for the treatment of cardiovascular diseases.

Acknowledgements

OD was supported by DFG FOR926 grants DE802/2-1 and 2-2. GDD was supported by a BONFOR grant from the Medical School, University of Bonn, Germany.

Author details

Oliver Dewald* and Georg D. Duerr

*Address all correspondence to: o.dewald@uni-bonn.de

Department of Cardiac Surgery, University Clinical Centre Bonn, Germany

References

[1] Zoratti C, Kipmen-Korgun D, Osibow K, Malli R, Graier WF: Anandamide initiates Ca(2+) signaling via CB2 receptor linked to phospholipase C in calf pulmonary endothelial cells. British Journal of Pharmacology. 2003; 140:1351-1362. DOI:10.1038/sj.bjp.0705529

[2] Bonz A, Laser M, Kullmer S, Kniesch S, Babin-Ebell J, Popp V, Ertl G, Wagner JA: Cannabinoids acting on CB1 receptors decrease contractile performance in human atrial muscle. Journal of Cardiovascular Pharmacology. 2003; 41:657-664.

[3] Deutsch DG, Goligorsky MS, Schmid PC, Krebsbach RJ, Schmid HH, Das SK, Dey SK, Arreaza G, Thorup C, Stefano G, Moore LC: Production and physiological actions of anandamide in the vasculature of the rat kidney. The Journal of Clinical Investigation. 1997; 100:1538-1546. DOI:10.1172/JCI119677

[4] Frangogiannis NG: The inflammatory response in myocardial injury, repair, and remodelling. Nature reviews. Cardiology. 2014; 11:255-265. DOI:10.1038/nrcardio.2014.28

[5] Ginks WR, Sybers HD, Maroko PR, Covell JW, Sobel BE, Ross J, Jr.: Coronary artery reperfusion. II. Reduction of myocardial infarct size at 1 week after the coronary occlusion. The Journal of Clinical Investigation. 1972; 51:2717-2723. DOI:10.1172/JCI107091

[6] Maroko PR, Libby P, Ginks WR, Bloor CM, Shell WE, Sobel BE, Ross J, Jr.: Coronary artery reperfusion. I. Early effects on local myocardial function and the extent of myocardial necrosis. The Journal of Clinical Investigation. 1972; 51:2710-2716. DOI:10.1172/JCI107090

[7] Murry CE, Jennings RB, Reimer KA: Preconditioning with ischemia: a delay of lethal cell injury in ischemic myocardium. Circulation. 1986; 74:1124-1136.

[8] Heusch G: Molecular basis of cardioprotection: signal transduction in ischemic pre-, post-, and remote conditioning. Circulation Research. 2015; 116:674-699. DOI:10.1161/CIRCRESAHA.116.305348

[9] Przyklenk K, Bauer B, Ovize M, Kloner RA, Whittaker P: Regional ischemic 'preconditioning' protects remote virgin myocardium from subsequent sustained coronary occlusion. Circulation. 1993; 87:893-899.

[10] Whittaker P, Przyklenk K: Reduction of infarct size in vivo with ischemic preconditioning: mathematical evidence for protection via non-ischemic tissue. Basic Research in Cardiology. 1994; 89:6-15.

[11] Thielmann M, Kottenberg E, Kleinbongard P, Wendt D, Gedik N, Pasa S, Price V, Tsagakis K, Neuhauser M, Peters J, Jakob H, Heusch G: Cardioprotective and prognostic effects of remote ischaemic preconditioning in patients undergoing coronary artery bypass surgery: a single-centre randomised, double-blind, controlled trial. Lancet. 2013; 382:597-604. DOI:10.1016/S0140-6736(13)61450-6

[12] Joyeux M, Arnaud C, Godin-Ribuot D, Demenge P, Lamontagne D, Ribuot C: Endocannabinoids are implicated in the infarct size-reducing effect conferred by heat stress preconditioning in isolated rat hearts. Cardiovascular Research. 2002; 55:619-625.

[13] Roberts R, DeMello V, Sobel BE: Deleterious effects of methylprednisolone in patients with myocardial infarction. Circulation. 1976; 53:I204-206.

[14] Frangogiannis NG, Smith CW, Entman ML: The inflammatory response in myocardial infarction. Cardiovascular Research. 2002; 53:31-47.

[15] Frangogiannis NG, Shimoni S, Chang SM, Ren G, Dewald O, Gersch C, Shan K, Aggeli C, Reardon M, Letsou GV, Espada R, Ramchandani M, Entman ML, Zoghbi WA: Active interstitial remodeling: an important process in the hibernating human myocardium. Journal of the American College of Cardiology. 2002; 39:1468-1474.

[16] Kukielka GL, Smith CW, LaRosa GJ, Manning AM, Mendoza LH, Daly TJ, Hughes BJ, Youker KA, Hawkins HK, Michael LH, et al.: Interleukin-8 gene induction in the myocardium after ischemia and reperfusion in vivo. The Journal of Clinical Investigation. 1995; 95:89-103. DOI:10.1172/JCI117680

[17] Entman ML, Youker K, Shoji T, Kukielka G, Shappell SB, Taylor AA, Smith CW: Neutrophil induced oxidative injury of cardiac myocytes. A compartmented system requiring CD11b/CD18-ICAM-1 adherence. The Journal of Clinical Investigation. 1992; 90:1335-1345. DOI:10.1172/JCI115999

[18] Kloner RA, Bolli R, Marban E, Reinlib L, Braunwald E: Medical and cellular implications of stunning, hibernation, and preconditioning: an NHLBI workshop. Circulation. 1998; 97:1848-1867.

[19] Kumar AG, Ballantyne CM, Michael LH, Kukielka GL, Youker KA, Lindsey ML, Hawkins HK, Birdsall HH, MacKay CR, LaRosa GJ, Rossen RD, Smith CW, Entman ML: Induction of monocyte chemoattractant protein-1 in the small veins of the ischemic and reperfused canine myocardium. Circulation. 1997; 95:693-700.

[20] Nahrendorf M, Swirski FK, Aikawa E, Stangenberg L, Wurdinger T, Figueiredo JL, Libby P, Weissleder R, Pittet MJ: The healing myocardium sequentially mobilizes two monocyte subsets with divergent and complementary functions. The Journal of Experimental Medicine. 2007; 204:3037-3047. DOI:10.1084/jem.20070885

[21] de Couto G, Liu W, Tseliou E, Sun B, Makkar N, Kanazawa H, Arditi M, Marban E: Macrophages mediate cardioprotective cellular postconditioning in acute myocardial infarction. The Journal of Clinical Investigation. 2015; 125:3147-3162. DOI:10.1172/JCI81321

[22] Lacraz S, Nicod LP, Chicheportiche R, Welgus HG, Dayer JM: IL-10 inhibits metalloproteinase and stimulates TIMP-1 production in human mononuclear phagocytes. The Journal of Clinical Investigation. 1995; 96:2304-2310. DOI:10.1172/JCI118286

[23] Gerszten RE, Garcia-Zepeda EA, Lim YC, Yoshida M, Ding HA, Gimbrone MA, Jr., Luster AD, Luscinskas FW, Rosenzweig A: MCP-1 and IL-8 trigger firm adhesion of monocytes to vascular endothelium under flow conditions. Nature. 1999; 398:718-723. DOI:10.1038/19546

[24] Weber C, Draude G, Weber KS, Wubert J, Lorenz RL, Weber PC: Downregulation by tumor necrosis factor-alpha of monocyte CCR2 expression and monocyte chemotactic protein-1-induced transendothelial migration is antagonized by oxidized low-density lipoprotein: a potential mechanism of monocyte retention in atherosclerotic lesions. Atherosclerosis. 1999; 145:115-123.

[25] Weber C, Erl W, Weber KS, Weber PC: Effects of oxidized low density lipoprotein, lipid mediators and statins on vascular cell interactions. Clinical Chemistry and Laboratory Medicine. 1999; 37:243-251. DOI:10.1515/CCLM.1999.043

[26] Frangogiannis NG, Youker KA, Rossen RD, Gwechenberger M, Lindsey MH, Mendoza LH, Michael LH, Ballantyne CM, Smith CW, Entman ML: Cytokines and the microcirculation in ischemia and reperfusion. Journal of Molecular and Cellular Cardiology. 1998; 30:2567-2576. DOI:10.1006/jmcc.1998.0829

[27] Dewald O, Zymek P, Winkelmann K, Koerting A, Ren G, Abou-Khamis T, Michael LH, Rollins BJ, Entman ML, Frangogiannis NG: CCL2/Monocyte Chemoattractant Protein-1 regulates inflammatory responses critical to healing myocardial infarcts. Circulation Research. 2005; 96:881-889. DOI:10.1161/01.RES.0000163017.13772.3a

[28] Frangogiannis NG, Dewald O, Xia Y, Ren G, Haudek S, Leucker T, Kraemer D, Taffet G, Rollins BJ, Entman ML: Critical role of monocyte chemoattractant protein-1/CC chemokine ligand 2 in the pathogenesis of ischemic cardiomyopathy. Circulation. 2007; 115:584-592. DOI:10.1161/CIRCULATIONAHA.106.646091

[29] Ford WR, Honan SA, White R, Hiley CR: Evidence of a novel site mediating anandamide-induced negative inotropic and coronary vasodilatator responses in rat isolated hearts. British Journal of Pharmacology. 2002; 135:1191-1198. DOI:10.1038/sj.bjp.0704565

[30] Lake KD, Compton DR, Varga K, Martin BR, Kunos G: Cannabinoid-induced hypotension and bradycardia in rats mediated by CB1-like cannabinoid receptors. The Journal of Pharmacology and Experimental Therapeutics. 1997; 281:1030-1037.

[31] Jarai Z, Wagner JA, Varga K, Lake KD, Compton DR, Martin BR, Zimmer AM, Bonner TI, Buckley NE, Mezey E, Razdan RK, Zimmer A, Kunos G: Cannabinoid-induced mesenteric vasodilation through an endothelial site distinct from CB1 or CB2 receptors. Proceedings of the National Academy of Sciences of the United States of America. 1999; 96:14136-14141.

[32] Ishac EJ, Jiang L, Lake KD, Varga K, Abood ME, Kunos G: Inhibition of exocytotic noradrenaline release by presynaptic cannabinoid CB1 receptors on peripheral sympathetic nerves. British Journal of Pharmacology. 1996; 118:2023-2028.

[33] Pacher P, Batkai S, Kunos G: Haemodynamic profile and responsiveness to anandamide of TRPV1 receptor knock-out mice. The Journal of Physiology. 2004; 558:647-657. DOI:10.1113/jphysiol.2004.064824

[34] Steffens S, Veillard NR, Arnaud C, Pelli G, Burger F, Staub C, Karsak M, Zimmer A, Frossard JL, Mach F: Low dose oral cannabinoid therapy reduces progression of atherosclerosis in mice. Nature. 2005; 434:782-786. DOI:10.1038/nature03389

[35] Mittleman MA, Lewis RA, Maclure M, Sherwood JB, Muller JE: Triggering myocardial infarction by marijuana. Circulation. 2001; 103:2805-2809.

[36] Wagner JA, Hu K, Bauersachs J, Karcher J, Wiesler M, Goparaju SK, Kunos G, Ertl G: Endogenous cannabinoids mediate hypotension after experimental myocardial infarction. Journal of the American College of Cardiology. 2001; 38:2048-2054.

[37] Underdown NJ, Hiley CR, Ford WR: Anandamide reduces infarct size in rat isolated hearts subjected to ischaemia-reperfusion by a novel cannabinoid mechanism. British Journal of Pharmacology. 2005; 146:809-816. DOI:10.1038/sj.bjp.0706391

[38] Munro S, Thomas KL, Abu-Shaar M: Molecular characterization of a peripheral receptor for cannabinoids. Nature. 1993; 365:61-65. DOI:10.1038/365061a0

[39] Montecucco F, Lenglet S, Braunersreuther V, Burger F, Pelli G, Bertolotto M, Mach F, Steffens S: CB(2) cannabinoid receptor activation is cardioprotective in a mouse model of ischemia/reperfusion. Journal of Molecular and Cellular Cardiology. 2009; 46:612-620. DOI:10.1016/j.yjmcc.2008.12.014

[40] Defer N, Wan J, Souktani R, Escoubet B, Perier M, Caramelle P, Manin S, Deveaux V, Bourin MC, Zimmer A, Lotersztajn S, Pecker F, Pavoine C: The cannabinoid receptor type 2 promotes cardiac myocyte and fibroblast survival and protects against ischemia/reperfusion-induced cardiomyopathy. FASEB Journal: Official Publication of the Federation of American Societies for Experimental Biology. 2009; 23:2120-2130. DOI: 10.1096/fj.09-129478

[41] Di Filippo C, Rossi F, Rossi S, D'Amico M: Cannabinoid CB2 receptor activation reduces mouse myocardial ischemia-reperfusion injury: involvement of cytokine/chemokines and PMN. Journal of Leukocyte Biology. 2004; 75:453-459. DOI:10.1189/jlb.0703303

[42] Julien B, Grenard P, Teixeira-Clerc F, Van Nhieu JT, Li L, Karsak M, Zimmer A, Mallat A, Lotersztajn S: Antifibrogenic role of the cannabinoid receptor CB2 in the liver. Gastroenterology. 2005; 128:742-755.

[43] Dewald O, Frangogiannis NG, Zoerlein M, Duerr GD, Klemm C, Knuefermann P, Taffet G, Michael LH, Crapo JD, Welz A, Entman ML: Development of murine ischemic cardiomyopathy is associated with a transient inflammatory reaction and depends on reactive oxygen species. Proceedings of the National Academy of Sciences of the United States of America. 2003; 100:2700-2705. DOI:10.1073/pnas.0438035100

[44] Duerr GD, Heinemann JC, Suchan G, Kolobara E, Wenzel D, Geisen C, Matthey M, Passe-Tietjen K, Mahmud W, Ghanem A, Tiemann K, Alferink J, Burgdorf S, Buchalla R, Zimmer A, Lutz B, Welz A, Fleischmann BK, Dewald O: The endocannabinoid-

CB2 receptor axis protects the ischemic heart at the early stage of cardiomyopathy. Basic Research in Cardiology. 2014; 109:425. DOI:10.1007/s00395-014-0425-x

[45] Duerr GD, Heinemann JC, Gestrich C, Heuft T, Klaas T, Keppel K, Roell W, Klein A, Zimmer A, Velten M, Kilic A, Bindila L, Lutz B, Dewald O: Impaired border zone formation and adverse remodeling after reperfused myocardial infarction in cannabinoid CB2 receptor deficient mice. Life Sciences. 2015; 138:8-17. DOI:10.1016/j.lfs.2014.11.005

[46] Batkai S, Pacher P: Endocannabinoids and cardiac contractile function: pathophysiological implications. Pharmacological Research. 2009; 60:99-106.

[47] Batkai S, Mukhopadhyay P, Harvey-White J, Kechrid R, Pacher P, Kunos G: Endocannabinoids acting at CB1 receptors mediate the cardiac contractile dysfunction in vivo in cirrhotic rats. American journal of physiology. Heart and Circulatory Physiology. 2007; 293:H1689-1695. DOI:10.1152/ajpheart.00538.2007

[48] Walsh SK, Hepburn CY, Kane KA, Wainwright CL: Acute administration of cannabidiol in vivo suppresses ischaemia-induced cardiac arrhythmias and reduces infarct size when given at reperfusion. British Journal of Pharmacology. 2010; 160:1234-1242. DOI:10.1111/j.1476-5381.2010.00755.x

[49] Kolossov E, Bostani T, Roell W, Breitbach M, Pillekamp F, Nygren JM, Sasse P, Rubenchik O, Fries JW, Wenzel D, Geisen C, Xia Y, Lu Z, Duan Y, Kettenhofen R, Jovinge S, Bloch W, Bohlen H, Welz A, Hescheler J, Jacobsen SE, Fleischmann BK: Engraftment of engineered ES cell-derived cardiomyocytes but not BM cells restores contractile function to the infarcted myocardium. The Journal of Experimental Medicine. 2006; 203:2315-2327. DOI:10.1084/jem.20061469

[50] Heinemann JC, Duerr GD, Keppel K, Breitbach M, Fleischmann BK, Zimmer A, Wehner S, Welz A, Dewald O: CB2 receptor-mediated effects of pro-inflammatory macrophages influence survival of cardiomyocytes. Life Sciences. 2015; 138:18-28. DOI:10.1016/j.lfs.2014.11.027

[51] Dewald O, Ren G, Duerr GD, Zoerlein M, Klemm C, Gersch C, Tincey S, Michael LH, Entman ML, Frangogiannis NG: Of mice and dogs: species-specific differences in the inflammatory response following myocardial infarction. The American Journal of Pathology. 2004; 164:665-677. DOI:10.1016/S0002-9440(10)63154-9

[52] Weis F, Beiras-Fernandez A, Sodian R, Kaczmarek I, Reichart B, Beiras A, Schelling G, Kreth S: Substantially altered expression pattern of cannabinoid receptor 2 and activated endocannabinoid system in patients with severe heart failure. Journal of Molecular and Cellular Cardiology. 2010; 48:1187-1193. DOI:10.1016/j.yjmcc.2009.10.025

[53] Weis F, Beiras-Fernandez A, Hauer D, Hornuss C, Sodian R, Kreth S, Briegel J, Schelling G: Effect of anaesthesia and cardiopulmonary bypass on blood endocannabinoid

concentrations during cardiac surgery. British Journal of Anaesthesia. 2010; 105:139-144. DOI:10.1093/bja/aeq117

[54] Duerr GD, Heinemann JC, Dunkel S, Zimmer A, Lutz B, Lerner R, Roell W, Mellert F, Probst C, Esmailzadeh B, Welz A, Dewald O: Myocardial hypertrophy is associated with inflammation and activation of endocannabinoid system in patients with aortic valve stenosis. Life Sciences. 2013; 92:976-983. DOI:10.1016/j.lfs.2013.03.014

[55] Topol EJ, Bousser MG, Fox KA, Creager MA, Despres JP, Easton JD, Hamm CW, Montalescot G, Steg PG, Pearson TA, Cohen E, Gaudin C, Job B, Murphy JH, Bhatt DL, Investigators C: Rimonabant for prevention of cardiovascular events (CRESCENDO): a randomised, multicentre, placebo-controlled trial. Lancet. 2010; 376:517-523. DOI: 10.1016/S0140-6736(10)60935-X

[56] Nissen SE, Nicholls SJ, Wolski K, Rodes-Cabau J, Cannon CP, Deanfield JE, Despres JP, Kastelein JJ, Steinhubl SR, Kapadia S, Yasin M, Ruzyllo W, Gaudin C, Job B, Hu B, Bhatt DL, Lincoff AM, Tuzcu EM, Investigators S: Effect of rimonabant on progression of atherosclerosis in patients with abdominal obesity and coronary artery disease: the STRADIVARIUS randomized controlled trial. JAMA. 2008; 299:1547-1560. DOI: 10.1001/jama.299.13.1547

Chapter 10

Cannabinoids: Drug or Medication?

Léa Giron and Katia Befort

Additional information is available at the end of the chapter

http://dx.doi.org/10.5772/63172

Abstract

This chapter aims at exploring the use and misuse of cannabinoids as it has become a major societal issue. In the first section, we describe the historical use of cannabis as a natural cure in ancient civilizations. We then explore the current use of cannabinoids in medicine, which includes innovative strategies for treating various diseases such as multiple sclerosis or cancer-induced pain. In the second section, we consider how the discovery and characterization of the endocannabinoid system have increased knowledge of this system's mode of action. Consumption of cannabis for recreational use however is a significant public health issue today. Scientific advances are confronted with the adverse health effects that are demonstrated in preclinical and clinical studies based on the psychotic and addictive properties of this compound. In the third section, we therefore provide an overview of the recent findings on the endocannabinoid system using animal models with proposed molecular mechanisms and potential interactions with other neuromodulatory systems like the opioid system. Finally, through alternative strategies to current treatments with both phyto- and synthetic cannabinoids, we try to reconcile the beneficial aspects of the use of cannabinoids for medication and the aspects associated with addictive properties.

Keywords: animal models, cannabis, dependence, endocannabinoid, pharmacology, therapies

Abbreviations

2-AG, 2-arachidonoylglycerol; AEA, anandamide, *N*-arachidonoyl-ethanolamide; AIDS, acquired immune deficiency syndrome; ALS, amyotrophic lateral sclerosis; CBD, cannabidiol; CBN, cannabinol; CB1, type 1 cannabinoid receptor; CB2, type 2 cannabinoid receptor; CNS, central nervous system; CPA, conditioned place aversion; CPP, conditioned place preference; DA, dopamine; DAGL, diacylglycerol lipase; FAAH, fatty acid amide hydrolase;

G protein, guanine nucleotide binding protein; GABA, c-aminobutyric acid; GPCR, G-protein-coupled receptor; iv, intravenous; MGL, monoacylglycerol lipase; MS, multiple sclerosis; NAPE-PLD, *N*-acyl phosphatidylethanolamine phospholipase D; Δ^9-THC, delta-9-tetrahydrocannabinol

1. Cannabis as medication

1.1. Historical uses of cannabis

Cannabis is a botanical genus belonging to annual plants from the *Cannabaceae* family. According to botanical classification, this genus only contains one species *Cannabis sativa* L. subdivided into three subtypes: *sativa*, *indica*, and *ruderalis*. *Cannabis sativa* was one of the first plants cultivated by humans. In the 4th millenary BC in China, cannabis was mainly produced for its stalk fibers, which were used to manufacture strings, ropes, textiles, and paper. It was also consumed for its fruits [1]. Cannabis has been used as a natural medication for thousands of years. It can be traced back to 2700 BC, but at that time it was only transmitted by oral traditions [1]. The first written evidence of its therapeutic use was reported during the first century of the Christian era, with the world's oldest pharmacopoeia, the Chinese Pharmacopoeia *Shen Nong Ben Cao Jing* [2]. The main uses of cannabis were for treatment of rheumatic pain, constipation, disorders of the female reproductive system, and also malaria. In India, its use was mostly for analgesic, anticonvulsivant, tranquilizer, antispasmodic, digestive, appetite stimulant, or antitussive properties. Cannabis also spread throughout Asia for use in religious rituals as it was described as a magic and medicinal plant in the *Atharva Veda* (4th Veda) sacred text of Hindu and Vedic traditions [1].

As cannabis has been prohibited by law, it has been difficult to follow its use for its recreational properties. It has probably been used for recreational purpose since the beginning of the Christian era. Additionally, its consumption for its psychoactive effects became quite popular in the 1950s in the United States of America with the rise of jazz. It then spread among young people within Western countries with, for example, the explosion of its popularity in the 1960s–1970s with the hippie movement. Nowadays, cannabis and related compounds are the most abused illicit substances in Europe, the United States, and Australia [3–5]. Consumption of cannabis is still often underestimated in our modern societies, but the current prevalence has been estimated by the World Health Organization as about 3.9% among the global population (15–64 years old) [6].

1.2. Phytocannabinoids

Today in the common language, the terms "cannabis" or "marijuana" stand for mixtures of dried herbs (also named Bhang). In particular, the dried flowering tops, leaves, and stalks of the mature female plant (Ganja) are commonly used as cannabis herbs [2]. Resinous extracts of compressed flowering tops called "hashish" or "hash" are also consumed and are stronger than marijuana [7]. Interestingly, the plant *Cannabis sativa* contains more than 400 different chemical compounds including over 60 cannabinoids which are specific to the plants of the genus *Cannabis*. These molecules are called phytocannabinoids. The most potent one is the (−)-Δ^9-tetrahydrocannabinol (Δ^9-THC) and has been purified and isolated in 1964 by Raphael Mechoulam's team [8]. This molecule is the main psychoactive component of *Cannabis sativa* and is therefore responsible for most of the psychoactive and physical effects of cannabis consumption [9]. It has been described as a partial agonist for both cannabinoid receptors, CB1 and CB2 (see below) [10]. The other main active constituents of cannabis are the (−)-Δ^8-tetrahydrocannabinol (Δ^8-THC), the cannabinol (CBN), and the cannabidiol (CBD) [11]. The Δ^8-THC is slightly less potent than Δ^9-THC, as CBN, and is present in very small quantities in the plant. CBD is devoid of psychoactive effects and of most of the other Δ^9-THC-like effects, but has other interesting features such as antiepileptic, antianxiety, antinausea, and antischizophrenic properties [12]. Phytocannabinoids other than Δ^9-THC can show additive, synergistic, or antagonist effects with Δ^9-THC and these interactions may modulate its actions when cannabis is consumed as an herbal mixture [13]. Noteworthy, Δ^9-THC content may strongly vary upon the origin of the plants and the type of cannabis preparations. Since Δ^9-THC is the main active compound of cannabis, refined farming methods and plant genetic crossbreeding technologies have been developed in order to increase Δ^9-THC content and therefore to increase the potency of cannabis [13]. Depending on their relative content of Δ^9-THC and CBD, cannabis plants are classified in three different types: "drug-type" plants (Δ^9-THC/CBD > 1), "intermediate-type" plants (Δ^9-THC/CBD = 1), and "fiber-type" plants (Δ^9-THC/CBD < 1) [14]. In addition to the relative content in various phytocannabinoids, consumption patterns also impact the effects of cannabis.

1.3. Modes of cannabis consumption

Although cannabis is often mixed with tobacco, then rolled and smoked as "joints," it can also be consumed in other forms [13]. It can be smoked from pipe or even from "buckets" by inhaling from a mass of plant or resin ignited in a plastic bottle. Moreover, it is ingested in the form of candies or baked into cakes (cookies, muffins). In the latter case, cannabis is mixed with butter to form "marijuana butter," also called "cannabutter" or "Marrakech butter," and then mixed with other baking ingredients ("space cake"). Finally, more rarely, macerated extracts of cannabis can be taken. Contrary to other drugs of abuse that can also be injected, cannabis is unsuitable for intravenous use due to its relative insolubility in water. When cannabis is taken as joints, the association of the phytocannabinoids with nicotine will produce the hedonic effects sought by the smokers. It is therefore more difficult to study these effects and the specific properties coming from cannabis alone. There are many factors influencing the global effect of cannabis in humans resulting from combination of the relative content in different phytocannabinoids (e.g., Δ^9-THC, CBD), the route of administration, the mode of consumption (concomitant intake of nicotine, polyconsumption), the previous experiences of the consumer with drugs, and the intake conditions [15]. Unlike other drugs of abuse such as heroin, cocaine, or benzodiazepines, the risk of overdose of cannabis is rather low and no sudden deaths directly linked to cannabis herbs have been reported so far [13].

1.4. Psychological and systemic effects of cannabis

People primarily use cannabis for its positive effect on mood. Indeed, it results in an euphoria or "high," characterized by a sensation of relaxation, decreased anxiety, awareness, depression, and increased sociability depending on the intake conditions [16]. Nevertheless, paradoxical reactions with dysphoria, anxiety, severe panic, and psychosis can be observed when high doses of Δ^9-THC are taken. In some cases, similar effects can also occur at the first consumption or for more psychologically vulnerable people [16]. Therefore, psychotropic effects of cannabis are dose-dependent and variable depending on the quantity of cannabis consumed and on its Δ^9-THC content.

Cannabis use induces some adverse effects. It impairs cognitive and psychomotor functioning [17]. Its consumption induces slowed reaction time, motor incoordination, short-term memory loss, as well as attention disorders, and so it thus disturbs driving capacities, explaining the observed link between cannabis consumption and road accidents [13]. Furthermore, chronic use of cannabis may lead to long-term effects on attention and memory and these disturbances may last weeks or even several months after stopping cannabis consumption [18]. Moreover, cannabis can increase the risk of psychotic symptoms. It has been shown to induce the emergence of chronic psychosis such as schizophrenia in young consumers [19–21]. Finally, high and frequent cannabis consumption can lead to dependence and therefore to development of tolerance and withdrawal syndromes (see below).

At the systemic level, cannabis has mainly cardiorespiratory effects [18]. Its impact on the cardiovascular system can be reflected by induction of dose-dependent tachycardia, vasodilatation, and reddening of the ocular conjunctiva, the latter being a typical sign of cannabis consumption. Postural hypotension and fainting can also be observed. Moreover, relationships between cannabis consumption and cardiac arrhythmias, cardiovascular ischemias, coronary insufficiency, and other cases of fatal cardiac accidents have been reported [2, 22, 23]. Abusive cannabis consumption can indeed induce atrial [23] or ventricular fibrillations [24] in predisposed patients and therefore represents a major risk for persons suffering from preexisting cardiac diseases. It is noteworthy that young cannabis consumers are also at risk in terms of cardiac consequences [25, 26].

Cannabis also has a strong impact on the respiratory system. The smoke of cannabis joints contains the same constituents as tobacco (nicotine, noxious mixtures of gases and particulates) and smoking cannabis chronically causes coughing, bronchitis, and emphysema. Even if the daily number of smoked cannabis joints is generally much lower than smoked conventional cigarettes, the differing manners in which cannabis is smoked may enhance the deposition of smoke particulates at the pulmonary level in cannabis smokers, and therefore explains specific respiratory consequences of cannabis [27]. It has been suggested that by increasing oxidative stress and inducing mitochondrial dysfunctions [27] Δ^9-THC may participate, in the long-term, to the development of chronic airway diseases, pulmonary infections, and even lung cancer in heavy smokers [13, 28, 29]. More attention should be given to these adverse respiratory effects as habitual smoking of cannabis has greatly increased in our modern society.

http://dx.doi.org/10.5772/63172

Among other adverse effects of cannabis use, immunosuppressive and endocrine properties have also been described as disturbing reproductive functions and fertility [18]. Depending on the individual, cannabis can also induce a reduction in salivary secretion (sensation of dry mouth) and an increase in appetite [30].

1.5. Current uses of medicinal cannabis

Medicinal or therapeutic cannabis refers to preparations using *Cannabis sativa* for a pure medicinal purpose. Intake of these phytocannabinoids can include smoking, inhaling, local application, or ingestion. Depending on the country, medicinal cannabis use is not allowed, permitted, or accepted. In France, any use of cannabis was removed from the French Pharmacopoeia in 1953 [31]. Its use, importation, sale, transportation, and production are strictly forbidden. On the other hand, medicinal cannabis use is authorized in several countries, including Canada, New-Zealand, Australia, Netherlands, Spain, United Kingdom, and more than 20 states in the United States of America. In Canada, for example, production and sale is allowed under the supervision of Health Canada [32]. In the United States of America, therapeutic cannabis is still classified as a "schedule I controlled substance" [33]. The American Medical Association recently proposed rescheduling it to become a "Schedule II controlled substance," meaning that it has potential abuse risk and is accepted for therapeutic use [34]. Some states have voted on an amendment to permit medicinal use in conditions under physician agreement for specific indications such as severe pain, cancer, cachexy, glaucoma, AIDS, multiple sclerosis (MS), severe nausea, or sleep disorders [33–37]. This creates a patchwork of state laws in the United States of America for legal use of medicinal cannabis, its indications and maximal amount tolerated.

International nonproprietary name	Brand name	Active ingredient(s)	Indications
Dronabinol	Marinol®	Δ^9-THC	Chemotherapy-induced nausea and vomiting AIDS-related loss of appetite and weight loss
Nabilone	Cesamet®	Synthetic analogue of Δ^9-THC	Chemotherapy-induced nausea and vomiting
Nabiximols	Sativex®	Δ^9-THC and CBD (ratio 1:1)	MS-related spasticity

Table 1. Marketed cannabinoid-based medicines.

Phytocannabinoids or derived compounds already exist on the market for some medicinal interventions (**Table 1**). Δ^9-THC is mostly used as a therapeutic compound for its antiemetic and orexigenic properties. It has been commercialized under Dronabinol (Marinol®) to suppress nausea produced by chemotherapy and anorexia symptoms associated with AIDS. A synthetic analogue of Δ^9-THC, Nabilone (Cesamet®), has also been produced to treat nausea and vomiting linked to chemotherapy. Nabiximols (Sativex®) contains an equal mixture of the phytocannabinoids Δ^9-THC and CBD and is usually prescribed to relieve pain in adult patients with MS or advanced cancer. It is administrated as a buccal spray in several countries, including Canada, Spain, Denmark, Germany, and United Kingdom [38]. Interestingly, these compounds are reported to only be used for recreational purposes and are therefore abused extremely rarely [39]. Indeed, the mode of consumption (oral) and their pharmacokinetic features delays a potential high effect for several hours and is therefore much less euphoric than cannabis. Recently, Sativex has been suggested as a potential substitutive medication for cannabis dependence and may help decrease withdrawal syndromes [40]. **Table 2** summarizes the current pathologies or symptoms treated with the approved phytocannabinoids derivatives.

Pathologies	Symptoms of the pathologies targeted by the cannabinoids	References
Acquired immune deficiency syndrome (AIDS)	Anorexia (loss of appetite and weight loss related)	[38]
Cancers and chemotherapies	Nausea and vomiting	[38]
Neuropathic/chronic/inflammatory pain	Pain intensity, inflammation, spasticity	[35, 39, 42, 48]
Gilles de la Tourette syndrome	Motor and verbal tics	[43, 44]
Multiple sclerosis (MS)	Spasticity	[36, 45]
Amyotrophic lateral sclerosis (ALS)	Tremors, motor deficiencies	[234, 235]
Huntington's chorea	Motor and cognitive disorders	[232]
Psychosis and schizophrenia	Anxiety, hallucinations, paranoia	[219, 220]
Depression	Sadness, demotivation, loss of interest, sleep disorders	[255, 257]
Heroin addiction	Craving	[221]
Cannabis addiction	Withdrawal syndrome	[189, 268]
Cocaine addiction	Hyperlocomotion, rewarding effects of cocaine	[66, 127]
Osteoporosis	Osteoclastogenesis, bone resorption, and bone fragility	[236]

Table 2. Pathologies and associated symptoms targeted by cannabinoids.

For example, clinical studies have investigated the analgesic properties of medicinal cannabis [35]. A comparison of cannabis's analgesic effect was performed between patients smoking cannabis and a placebo. A significant improvement in various types of pain including chronic, postoperative or neuropathic pain, as well as pain in patients suffering of AIDS was obtained [35]. A randomized clinical assay was conducted on patients with neuropathic pain who smoked high or low concentrated cannabis (Δ^9-THC) or a placebo. This study showed that cannabis is effective at ameliorating neuropathic pain [41]. Similar results were obtained in another randomized study including adults with AIDS-associated sensory neuropathy where the effect of smoking low concentrated cannabis three times per day over 5 days was compared with a placebo [42]. Other studies have suggested a potential role of smoking cannabis to alleviate some symptoms of Tourette's syndrome, a central nervous system (CNS) disorder characterized by motor or verbal tics [43, 44]. Also, orally administered cannabis (a mixture of Δ9-THC and CBD) has been tested in cohorts of patients with MS and lower spasm frequency and increase mobility has been observed [45]. Symptoms in patients who have MS with muscle spasticity were treated with oral Δ9-THC, cannabis extract, or placebo, and results have shown that the first compound is more efficient in alleviating some aspects of the disability [46]. These observations confirm the therapeutic interests of oral administration of drugs containing Δ9-THC such as Marinol® or Cesamet®.

1.6. Adverse effects of medicinal cannabis

It has been observed that the more Δ9-THC content in medicinal cannabis, the more efficient it is in alleviating pain [47]. But with high dose formulations, secondary effects such as headache, dizziness, sleepiness, dry mouth or eye sensation, sedative effects, hypotension, and impairments in memory and cognition can be observed by some patients [35, 47]. Also, the best equilibrium to have an analgesic effect with the minimum side effects is strongly dependent on the individual and the preparation of the drug (various content of phytocannabinoids), which renders the dosage regimen particularly difficult. Indeed, in certain cases it has also been shown that the benefit/risk ratio is not positive for chronic pain treatment as cannabis only moderately reduce pain [48]. Recently, dronabinol has been tested for treatment of opiate withdrawal in a clinical trial and some adverse effects, including increased heart rate, were observed at the examined dose [49]. These observations raise some concerns globally about the dosage of such compound for potential benefits. Besides these potential adverse effects, poor knowledge about the interaction of medicinal cannabis with other drugs and possible psychotic and cognitive effects on patients are high safety concerns. Altogether, these observations still limit current cannabis therapeutic use [35, 37].

It is noteworthy that current therapeutic use is directed to alleviate several symptoms of various pathologies rather than being a cure for the patient. Cannabis plants containing high level of CBD are associated with lower adverse effects [50] and therefore represent a major therapeutic line of research for further drug design together with some synthetic derivatives of cannabis (see below).

2. The endogenous cannabinoid system

In recent decades, the discovery and characterization of the endogenous cannabinoid system represents a great milestone for research in the field, with considerable efforts being given to create a better understanding of the mode of action of cannabinoids. The endocannabinoid system comprises two well-characterized receptors, cannabinoid receptors CB1 and CB2, and their lipid neuromodulators (endocannabinoids), enzymes for their synthesis and their degradation.

2.1. Cannabinoid receptors

Cannabinoid receptors are receptors that were discovered in the early 1990s with CB1 and CB2 cloned from rat brain in 1990 and rat spleen in 1993, respectively [51–53]. They both are membrane receptors coupled to G-protein (Gαi/o) (GPCR) and share common signaling properties (see below). They both bind Δ^9-THC, the main component of cannabis [54, 55].

CB1 and CB2 receptors share 48% peptidic sequence homology [10]. Radioligand binding studies revealed a rather different distribution of these two receptors [56]. CB1 receptors are mainly expressed in peripheral and central nervous systems as well as in the reproductive and neuroendocrine systems [55, 57]. This receptor is highly abundant in the brain in areas involved in memory and cognitive functions like the hippocampus, involved in reward processes such as the striatum, ventral tegmental area, and prefrontal cortex, as well as in motor coordination and psychomotor performances such as the cerebellum [58–62]. CB1 is also present in brain structures involved in the regulation of appetite and nociception. With this wide pattern of expression, CB1 receptors are therefore involved in various physiological functions and are responsible for most of the psychoactive and central effects of cannabis.

CB2 receptors are highly expressed in the immune system in spleen, tonsil, thymus, mastocytes, and blood cells. It has also been described in microglial cells [53, 55]. Several studies have reported significant mRNA expression of CB2 receptors in brain areas such as granular cells of the cerebellum [63, 64] in brain stem [65] as well as in dopaminergic neurons of the VTA [66] and in a subset of excitatory and inhibitory neurons in CA1, CA3, and dentate gyrus of the hippocampus [67]. Detection of CB2 proteins in brain structures is still controversial because of the low expression and/or low specificity of available antibodies. Very little data are available on the CB2 receptor's central function and a very recent study using a reporter mouse line may help better clarifying the potential role of this receptor in brain functions [68]. The authors generated BAC transgenic GFP reporter mice to trace CB2 expression and could detect, using fluorescence techniques, that the major sources for GFP-CB2 expression are in B-cells in the spleen, blood, and microglia in the brain.

Pharmacological studies have proposed that other non-CB1 and non-CB2 receptors interact with endocannabinoids such as channel vanilloid TRPV1 recognizing capsaicin [69] or the orphan GPCR GPR55 [70, 71]. These receptors are not yet classified among cannabinoid receptors, but interactions with cannabis could potentially explain some pharmacological effects of this drug that cannot be accounted for by CB1 and CB2 activation [72].

2.2. Endocannabinoid synthesis and degradation

Two main endogenous ligands were discovered in the early 1990s: *N*-arachidonoylethalonamine or anandamide (AEA) which was isolated from pig brain [51] and 2-arachidonoylglycerol (2-AG) which was isolated from rat brain and dog intestine [73, 74]. Other endocannabinoids have been identified, such as the *N*-arachidonoyl-dopamine (NADA), the *O*-arachidonoyl-ethanolamine (virhodamine), or the 2-arachidonoyl-glycerylether (2-AGE or noladin), but their specific physiologic role needs further clarification [72].The 2-AG is a full agonist at both CB1 and CB2 receptors, whereas AEA is a partial agonist [75]. Interestingly, it has recently been shown that 2-AG can be self-administered by rats and can stimulate dopamine (DA) transmission [76]. AEA also acts at TRPV1 receptors [11]. Both ligands show no strong selectivity for CB1 and CB2, with a ratio generally below 10 [73, 77, 78]. Endogenous cannabinoids are lipid neuromodulators synthesized from distinct phospholipid precursors. Several pathways have been described for their biosynthesis, noticeably for AEA (for a recent review, see [79]). The *N*-arachidonoyl phosphatidylethanolamine (NAPE) is one precursor for AEA, which can be generated through a two-step process involving a calcium-dependent transacylase and phospholipase D (NAPE-PLD) [80]. 2-AG synthesis mainly involves phospholipase C and diacylglycerol lipases (DAGL) [74, 81, 82]. It has recently been demonstrated using genetically modified mice that the DAGLα enzyme is directly responsible for 2-AG synthesis in the CNS [83]. Interestingly, 2-AG participates in the synthesis of arachidonic acid used for prostaglandin synthesis.

Postsynaptic neurons release endocannabinoid lipids. They cross the membrane by passive diffusion or using still not well characterized transporter systems, and then mainly act on presynaptic cannabinoid receptors. They are therefore retrograde synaptic messengers which regulate synaptic transmission. The decrease of neurotransmitter release will occur both at excitatory (glutamate) and inhibitory (gamma-aminobutyric acid or GABA) synapses (recently reviewed in [79, 84]). Endocannabinoids' local action is fast, as they are rapidly degraded through a recapture step through transporters, followed by enzymatic degradation with the fatty acid amide hydrolase (FAAH) for AEA [85, 86] and the monoacylglycerol lipase (MAGL) for 2-AG [87].

2.3. Signaling pathways

Several signaling pathways are activated by cannabinoid receptors and have been extensively reviewed [54, 55, 88]. Agonist activation induces inhibition of adenylate cyclase and a reduction of intracellular AMPc levels and therefore a decrease of protein kinase A activity [89]. On the other hand, beta and gamma subunits inhibit calcium voltage-gated channels and activate the opening of potassium channels. This effect results in membrane hyperpolarization and a reduction in neurons excitability and therefore a decrease in neurotransmitter release. At the presynaptic level this effect decreases the release of glutamate and GABA as well as acetylcholine, noradrenaline, cholecystokinin, or corticotrophin [10]. Activation of cannabinoid receptors also activates intracellular effectors stimulating MAPKinase signaling. This regulation induces phosphorylation of transcription factors and leads to gene expression modulation. CB1 signaling is well characterized and additional pathways have been described, including activation by CB1 receptors of sphingolipid metabolism by either direct synthesis of ceramide by serine-palmitoyltransferases or hydrolysis of sphingomyelin [90]. In astrocytes and glial cells, CB1 receptors are coupled to sphingomyelinase enzymes by chaperone molecules to produce ceramide that participate to apoptotic signaling [91, 92]. On the other hand, CB2 activation modulates a similar range of signaling pathways as the CB1 receptor, but clearly adenylate cyclase and MAPK pathways have been the most studied in regard to selective CB2 agonists (recently reviewed in [93]).

2.4. Physiological roles of the endocannabinoids

Endocannabinoids, by regulating the release of many neurotransmitters, act on various biological processes in the nervous, digestive, reproductive, pulmonary, and immune systems. Therefore, this system plays a critical role in a wide range of physiological functions, including energy balance, nociception and modulation of pain responses, and cognition and emotion as well as in reward. The central and peripheral roles of the endocannabinoid system have recently been extensively reviewed (see [94–101]) and the physiology and pathophysiology of this system have been largely studied using classical pharmacology and genetically modified animals [102]. Here, we provide just a few important specific points to illustrate these many roles.

The endocannabinoid system participates in several perception processes. Among them, nociception and modulation of pain responses have been particularly well studied and stimulation of the endocannabinoid system globally decreases pain sensitivity [98, 103]. CB1 receptors are a central player in these responses, but CB2 receptors also play a crucial role in the modulation of the immune response of the nervous system during neuropathic or joint pain [104, 105]. The endocannabinoid system has been shown to participate in different types of pain including acute, inflammatory, and neuropathic pain. Endocannabinoids like AEA also have strong antinociceptive properties [106] and can decrease pain perception in a situation of chemical skin damage, for example [107]. In terms of perception, this system also plays a role in retina physiology [108]. CB1 receptors have been shown to be expressed in the inner and outer plexiform layers of the retina of several species. Its activation in retinal bipolar cells decreases the amplitude of voltage-gated L-type calcium channel currents and therefore modulates photoreceptor activity. Also, CB2 expression has been demonstrated at RNA [109] and protein [110] levels and a specific role for this receptor in shaping retinal responses to light has been proposed [111]. These observations illustrate a modulatory role for the endocannabinoid system in visual processing. Agonists for these receptors significantly decrease intraocular pressure indicating a potential therapeutic effect for glaucoma treatment [112].

Noticeably, energy balance is an essential basic function where the endocannabinoid system has been revealed to play a major role. Indeed, cannabis is well known for hunger activation and specifically stimulating an appetite for sweet. Orexigenic properties of Δ^9-THC have been confirmed on rat studies [113] and food intake is increased by CB1 receptor activation in hypothalamic structures of the brain [114]. The endocannabinoid system is therefore clearly involved, mainly through central CB1 receptor activation, in food intake behaviors and energy balance [114–116]. It also plays a role in these processes by directly acting on peripheral organs like the gastrointestinal tract where both CB1 and CB2 receptors are expressed and participate in the regulation of motility and barrier function [117].

In the periphery, cannabinoid receptors are also expressed in cardiovascular tissues and their endogenous ligands have distinct effects. For example, it has been shown that AEA and 2-AG induce vasodilation which can trigger hypotension [118]. They can also induce depressor effects and bradycardia [119]. The endocannabinoid system clearly plays a role in cardiovascular-related diseases and opposing effects of activation of CB1 and CB2 have been suggested, highlighting potential therapeutic intervention [117].

In the brain, CB1 receptors are highly expressed throughout many structures including the hippocampus, cerebellum, and prefrontal cortex, suggesting a crucial role in cognitive functions such as learning and memory, motor coordination, and emotions like anxiety or depression and reward. Cannabis has been initially consumed to modify one's mood state and CB1 is proposed as a strong contributor for this effect. A rodent model for depressive-like behaviors has recently been proposed with genetically modified animals where this receptor is absent [120]. Dysfunction of many other processes is also produced by cannabis consumption and these events are thought to be mainly mediated through CB1 receptors. Interestingly, a possible implication in psychiatric disorders has been more recently proposed for CB2 receptors. A link between CB2 activation and schizophrenia has been considered [121, 122]. In addition, recent evidence suggests a neuromodulator role of CB2 receptors in addictive processes, with an implication in cocaine, nicotine, or ethanol effects [122–127]. Whether these central effects are due to CB2 expression in neurons, microglia, or inflammatory cells is still under investigation (see in [79]).

The endocannabinoid system also plays a neuroprotective role in some pathological conditions as it has been shown that CB1 receptors expressed specifically in glutamatergic hippocampal neurons are both necessary and sufficient to provide substantial endogenous protection against kainic-acid-induced seizures [128]. This system also modulates adult neurogenesis in the hippocampus with a pivotal role in some steps of this process, probably through activation of both CB1 and CB2 receptors (reviewed in [129].

Altogether pharmacological studies and preclinical models have allowed substantial progress in understanding the cellular and molecular mechanisms of the prolonged use of cannabinoids [130, 131]. In particular, genetically modified animal models, using knockout and conditional knockout methodologies together with viral approaches (inactivation or re-expression of components of the endocannabinoid system), have greatly improved our knowledge on the physiological and pathophysiological relevance of endocannabinoid signaling (see [102]). The use of animal models is also greatly evolving with rapid genome engineering technologies being developed using CRISPR-Cas9 and will surely improve our knowledge of the cannabinoid system [132, 133].

In conclusion, endocannabinoids are neuromodulators of important homeostatic mechanisms, including nociception and control of pain, vision, digestive and reproductive systems, energy balance, mood regulation, cognitive functions, and immune system and reward processing. Dysfunction of the system may induce pathologies and we particularly explore the role of this system in the development of addiction.

3. Cannabis misuse and dependence

3.1. Cannabis misuse

Besides its medicinal use, cannabis has been used for its psychotropic effects and the addictive potential of its components, including Δ^9-THC, has been well described since the discovery of the endogenous system. Indeed, cannabis and its derivatives represent the most consumed illicit drug in modern countries worldwide. More popular than cocaine, amphetamines, ecstasy, or opiate in Europe, about 21.7% of citizens (15–64 years old) have taken cannabis at least once in their life. This represents an estimated 14 million Europeans aged 15–34 using the drug in the last year and about 3 millions using it daily. Among intensive cannabis users, close to 7% of individuals have become dependent [134] and are now seeking treatment for cannabis-induced disorders. Even if this represents a minority of consumers, it globally represents a large number of people that may develop a cannabis-related health problem and is therefore a growing recognized public health threat [4]. Prevalence among young people is greater and corresponds to recreational use. Moreover, it has been reported that more men use cannabis, which may correspond to increased risk-taking behavior, but one cannot exclude a further increase of this behavior toward cannabis in women, as it has been observed for other drugs of abuse such as tobacco or alcohol in recent years. Also, global intake of cannabis is rather stable in Europe (Norway, Germany, France, and United Kingdom). Nevertheless, some European countries where prevalence used to be low now show a noticeable increase in cannabis use (Italy and Bulgaria). Internationally, cannabis use is still controversial, as a strong disparity for its use and legal state is observed [4]. In the United States of America, about 3 million adults and adolescents tried cannabis for the first time and about 10% of the population (32 million citizens) have used this drug in 2012 [135]. It is noteworthy that cannabis consumption is easier in the United States of America as it is more and more accessible due to its legalization in some state for either therapeutic intervention (20 states in March 2014: Alaska, Arizona, California, Colorado, Connecticut, Delaware, Hawaï, Maine, Massachusetts, Michigan, Montana, Nevada, New Jersey, New-Mexico, Oregon, Rhode Island, Vermont, Virginia, Washington DC, and Washington state) [33, 34, 136] or even more recently for recreational use (Alaska, Colorado, and Washington state, [137, 138]).

In conclusion, misuse or repeated use of cannabis may lead to societal and health issues. Cannabis abuse is correlated with poor academic performance, legal problems, risky behaviors, unemployment, road accidents, and a higher risk of developing psychological disorders, respiratory diseases, and cardiovascular problems [6, 19, 139–141]. In addition, its consumption is often associated with other psychostimulants to potentiate their effects, which makes this polyconsumption more dangerous for the individual. For example, alcohol taken together with cannabis may increase the risk of death car accident of about 15 times [142].

3.2. Cannabis and adolescents

The popularity of cannabis has grown substantially in recent years among young people. In Europe, a survey performed in 2011 (European School Project on Alcohol and other Drugs) showed that about 24% of the young population has taken cannabis at least once, 20% in the year 2011, and 12% within the last month [4, 142]. Similar to patterns of adult use, more boys are consumers of cannabis (1.5 times more than girls), probably because risk-taking behavior is more pronounced in boys. Consumption is recreational for most young users, but about 2% of them become intensive users. Even though cannabis is still illegal in most places, it is largely perceived as harmless. Thus, there is a normalization of usage among the young population which has spread among many countries and is therefore a growing health concern. Indeed, the most striking observations related to consumption during adolescence are a predisposition to develop psychiatric and cardiovascular pathologies [6, 134]. In the latter case, a recent study was performed on data collected by the French Addictovigilance Network from 2006 to 2010, a nationwide network of regional addictovigilance centers focused on achieving reliable surveillance of abuse and pharmacodependence cases. They analyzed spontaneous reports of cardiovascular complications related to cannabis use and showed some death cases from coronary syndromes, juvenile arteriopathies, and acute cerebral angiopathy [143]. Association with an increased risk of myocardial infarction has also been reported, with aggravation of coronary ischemia and even triggering of myocardial infarction [144]. Also, myocardial infarction, sudden cardiac death, cardiomyopathy, stroke, transient ischemic attack, and arteritis have been described [136]. Complications can occur in young users without preexisting cardiovascular problems [136] and at a greater frequency [143]. Therefore, potential for marijuana-associated adverse cardiovascular effects is of extreme seriousness as it may even have been underestimated if the analysis were based on spontaneous reports [143].

Recreational consumption by adolescents may lead to subsequent drug abuse. Cannabis has been proposed as a gateway drug [145, 146]. This hypothesis is still debated and neurobiological mechanisms are still not fully understood. Preclinical studies suggest nevertheless that cannabis may facilitate the sampling of other drugs of abuse such as alcohol, cocaine, and heroin. Indeed, rat exposure to Δ^9-THC during adolescence increases voluntary heroin intake in adulthood [147]. Furthermore, data analysis of transcriptomic and DNA methylation modifications has revealed a generational transmission of adaptations both at the neurobiological and behavioral levels in animals with parental exposure to Δ^9-THC [148, 149]. These observations suggest long-term adaptations and germinal transmission which may involve epigenetic events with gene expression modulations such as DNA methylation or histone post-translational modification [150, 151].

Academic difficulties have also been observed among occasional cannabis users during adolescence [139]. Regular consumption is predictive of a person having a higher risk of problems with other drugs in adulthood, along with psychological and societal issues [139]. It has been shown that consumption during adolescence may increase chronic psychosis and this phenomenon is reinforced when there is a genetic predisposition to the problem [19].

3.3. Dependence on cannabis

As opposed to cocaine or heroin, cannabis has often been considered a less harmful drug with low dependence properties and minimal negative effects, but its addictive potential has long been questioned [152]. Recent research has made strong progress in the knowledge of the mechanisms of action of cannabis and no doubt has subsisted that cannabis is an addictive drug. Moreover, an increasing number of cannabis consumers are seeking efficient treatments indicating that a growing fraction of the population is being dependent on cannabis.

Chronic consumption of a drug may lead to addiction and this brain disease can be characterized by specific behavioral consequences: compulsive drug seeking, uncontrolled-drug intake, craving for the drug, and strong potential for relapse. This addictive behavior evolves despite its adverse consequences on everyday life. This phenomenon has been well documented by several reviews which propose a model for this spiral of addiction [62, 153–156]. It develops in a small proportion of casual users and relies on psychological, genetic and environmental factors participating to the individual vulnerability [157–160]. To precisely evaluate this pathological process, the American Psychiatric Association has proposed the DSM-V (Diagnostic and Statistical Manual of Mental Disorders) as a reference for diagnosing addiction as a mental disorder [161]. Several criterions are documented for this evaluation and allow classifying the severity of the individual addiction depending on the numbers of criterions identified.

When cannabis plant is taken, Δ^9-THC enters the body through the lungs and circulating blood, which causes it to quickly reach the brain. When cannabis is eaten (space-cake for example), absorption is slower [35]. Δ^9-THC targets the cannabinoid receptors and therefore heavily activates the endocannabinoid system, which triggers the psychological and physical effects of the drug. Among the criterion listed for cannabis, the development of tolerance [162] and withdrawal syndromes caused by the interruption of consumption [152] are well recognized. Tolerance is characterized by a decrease of the effects following repeated drug consumption or by a need to increase the amount taken to reach similar effects [163]. Nevertheless, development of tolerance can vary between individuals in terms of physiological responses or behavior [164]. Withdrawal syndromes appear when the individual is under abstinence following chronic intake of the drug or when the individual seeks for the same drug or another one to alleviate these symptoms [15, 163]. Spontaneous withdrawal is observed in humans to cause increased agitation and excitability, insomnia, anxiety, aggressiveness, depression state, anorexia, and tremors [13, 152]. Interestingly, the criterion of craving cannabis has been added for the first time to the DSM-V.

Specific animal models have been developed to study drug rewarding effects mediated by specific brain structures in preclinical research. In order to characterize cannabis effects observed in humans, rodent models using repeated administration of cannabinoid agonists have been elaborated to evaluate consequences of such a chronic exposure as well as the addictive power of these cannabinoids [165]. This allowed a better understanding of motivational and reinforcing properties of these drugs [15]. The self-administration paradigm (SA) is recognized as the most powerful model for measuring both the rewarding and motivational effects of a drug [166]. It is an operant system based on a voluntary procedure to obtain the drug, coupled with the association of a signal [167]. Intravenous (iv) SA has been rather difficult to establish for Δ^9-THC (probably due to its partial agonistic nature) and several adaptations were necessary to obtain a reliable model. Indeed drug priming, low doses, food restriction, and animal restraint were useful to measure cannabinoid agonists properties in this task [96, 165, 168]. Both Δ^9-THC and the synthetic cannabinoid WIN55,212-2 have been successfully described to promote self-administration in rats and mice, and extended to the study of mice deficient for cannabinoid receptors [169–172]. Other synthetic compounds were also successful, such as CP 55,940 and HU-210 [173]. Moreover, the selective antagonist of CB1 receptor (rimonabant or SR141716A) was able to reverse cannabinoid-induced iv SA, illustrating the major role of this receptor in reinforcing properties of the drugs [171]. Interestingly, stable iv

SA of Δ^9-THC was obtained in squirrel monkeys, with much lower doses than for rodent studies [174, 175], illustrating potential differences in the pharmacodynamic and kinetic properties of this drug across species.

A task evaluating the conditioned place preference (CPP) has been developed to study reinforcing properties of drugs associated with an environmental cue like the context in which the drug is administered [176]. Interestingly, conflicting evidence exist about either positive (CPP) or negative (CPA) properties of cannabinoids, depending on experimental conditions used [96]. Agonists such as Δ^9-THC and CP 55,940 used at high doses produce aversion, therefore animals will avoid the compartment where the drug was injected [177–180]. Also, the antagonist SR141716A induced CPP at low and high doses in rats, revealing reinforcing properties [180]. Nevertheless, reinforcing properties can be observed with low doses of Δ^9-THC, longer conditioning periods or priming injections of the drug in the home cage prior to conditioning [181]. This nonoperant paradigm with specific experimental conditions has been used to study cannabinoid effects in genetically modified mice (for review see [182]). Finally, withdrawal signs following repeated exposure to Δ^9-THC can be measured in rodents. They may be either spontaneous or precipitated by a selective CB1 antagonist, and somatic signs can be scored for providing an index of dependence [152, 183]. For example, mice exhibited several signs including tremor, ataxia, piloerection, ptosis, and decreased motor activity [177, 184].

3.4. Medications for cannabis dependence

Besides preclinical evidence of cannabis-induced dependence in rodent studies, demand for treatment of cannabis use disorders is increasing. This illustrates the fact that an increasing number of people are dependent on cannabis. In the United States of America, more people are dependent on cannabis than cocaine (4.5 and 1 million in 2010, respectively) and therefore more people are seeking treatment for the first, rather than second, drug [185]. In 2013, about 845,000 people aged more than 12 years old received treatment because of their cannabis consumption [5]. In general, adults seeking treatment have been regular users for more than 10 years and have already tried to reduce or stop their behavior [134, 152].

There are currently no approved medications for the treatment of cannabis dependence and cannabinoid antagonists could be a potential pharmacotherapy [186]. The use of selective CB1 antagonists for the treatment of drug dependence has been investigated in preclinical studies as CB1 receptors are highly expressed in brain structures related to reward (see Section 2.1) [187, 188]. In a study using squirrel monkeys, rimonabant, a selective CB1 antagonist with some inverse agonistic properties, blocked cue-induced drug seeking, Δ^9-THC-induced drug seeking, and the direct reinforcing effects of Δ^9-THC suggesting that this compound may help to maintain abstinent behavior [189]. Such medications might be effective treatments for cannabinoid dependence, but they have not been tested on humans' cannabis reinforcing effects.

Cognitive behavioral therapy associated with contingency management is quite efficient for treating cannabis dependence [4, 134]. Moreover, family-based interventions may help adolescents dealing with cannabis withdrawal and craving and social help for employment is also crucial for limiting relapse [4]. Proposed therapeutic approaches are based on existing ones known to be effective in the treatment of other drug use disorders like baclofen for alcoholic withdrawal. Some clinical studies suggest that existing medications for other indications may be promising target for cannabis use disorder. Among them, buspirone, bupropion (Zyban®), sodium divalproate (Depakote®), and lithium may have therapeutic benefits [190]. Bupropion (Zyban®) is an inhibitor of noradrenalin and dopamine recapture, and an antagonist of nicotinic receptors. It is used to treat nicotinic withdrawal, and is an antidepressant. Sodium divalproate (Depakote®) is an antiepileptic drug used to treat bipolar symptoms. Buspirone is used as an anxiolytic and lithium as a thymoregulator. Finally, novel approaches have focused on cannabinoid replacement therapy (CRT) and showed that Sativex®(Nabiximols), a buccal spray containing Δ^9-THC and CBD used to treat spasticity associated with MS, may be a useful substitutive medication for cannabis dependence [40]. Nevertheless, controlled clinical trials are needed to confirm potential therapeutic efficacy of these molecules in cannabis-dependent treatment [190].

3.5. Synthetic cannabinoids

A more recent problem that has strongly increased the risks of drug use is the proliferation worldwide of new derivatives of synthetic cannabinoids. These drugs, also known as synthetic marijuana, "Spice," or "K2," are often less controlled and are being sold on the Internet which greatly facilitates their access [2, 191, 192]. Spices usually look like a mixture of dry herb plants where a multitude of compounds have been sprayed. More recently, these molecules have been sold for liquid preparation used in e-cigarettes [193]. These synthetic compounds are analogs of cannabinoids, but the exact content of the mixtures is not fully known and many chemical types of compounds are now being produced. They induce similar euphoric and relaxing effects as classical cannabis derivatives but they present a much higher potency. It is not even clear that they all contain Δ^9-THC [194]. Also, they do not contain CBD, which is suggested to balance the antipsychotic effects of Δ^9-THC in cannabis [195]. There may be specific risks associated with these new drugs compared to those known for cannabis. Indeed, they produce increased or even additional adverse effects, such as tachycardia, hypertension, chest pain, cardiac palpitation, intense sweating, convulsions, drowsiness, and agitation [192, 193, 196]. In adolescents, hallucinations, paranoia, and myocardial infarction have been reported [197]. More toxicology studies are needed to better characterize the adverse effects of these substances [198]. Altogether, synthetic cannabinoids represent a significant public health issue with an evolving legal market place that specifically target young populations and is difficult to control.

3.6. Cannabinoid-opioid interactions

Mechanisms of action are yet more complex as the endocannabinoid system interacts with other neuromodulatory systems such as the hypocretin, dopaminergic, adenosinergic, and opioid systems. The latter is of particular interest as the endocannabinoid and the opioid systems share neuroanatomical, neurochemical, and pharmacological characteristics [199–202]. The opioid system consists of three GPCR named mu, delta, and kappa receptors which interact with endogenous ligands (enkephalins, dynorphins, and endorphins) as well as exogenous ligands, including morphine or heroin. A hypothesis of cross-modulation includes the release of opioid peptides induced by cannabinoids (or reversely of endocannabinoids by opioids), and possible direct interaction at the level of receptors or signaling pathways. Evidence for specific interactions in the modulation of nociception has been provided both with *in vitro* and *in vivo* approaches [203, 204]. In the context of responses associated with reward and relapse, specific mechanisms have been highlighted, in particular with the use of knockout approaches [182]. Noticeably the mu opioid receptor has been proposed as a convergent molecular target mediating rewarding properties of opioid compounds but also of other drugs of abuse, including cannabinoids [205, 206]. The participation of the enkephalinergic system, with a joint action of mu and delta receptors, in behavioral responses associated with cannabinoid dependence has been clearly demonstrated. Moreover, chronic exposure to cannabinoid agonists induced a modification in both the density of mu opioid receptors and their activity in structures related to reward, which may contribute to the development of cannabinoid dependence [207]. Interestingly, studies using cannabinoid iv SA experiments have shown that opioid antagonists can block cannabinoid intake in mice and rats [169] and in squirrel monkeys [175]. Moreover, iv SA of morphine is abolished in animals deficient for the CB1 receptor [208], confirming a role for CB1 receptor in the modulation of opioid reward [182, 209]. Additionally, the antagonist rimonabant can precipitate withdrawal signs in morphine dependent animals and reciprocally, the opioid antagonist naloxone can precipitate these effects in cannabinoid dependent rats [210]. Another cross-interaction occurs at the cellular levels with colocalization of CB1 and opioid receptors observed in several brain structures including limbic areas, mid-brain, brain stem, or spinal cord [182, 211, 212]. Also, heterodimerization processes between cannabinoid and opioid receptors have been reported in both *in vitro* and more recently *in vivo*, in neuronal populations [213, 214]. This physical proximity is suggested mainly for CB1 receptors and delta or mu receptors and may impact on signaling properties of these receptors in specific brain structures, therefore possibly influencing analgesic or addictive responses involving these receptors. More research remains to be done to decipher the physiological role of such heteromers [214, 215].

4. Therapeutic perspectives

Even though cannabinoids are considered a drug of abuse and can induce dependence, they are used to treat several pathologies, including drug dependence. As developed earlier in this chapter, there are several risks associated with cannabis use, including altered short-term memory and decision making, increased anxiety and psychosis, and an increased risk of cardiovascular and lung diseases. On the other hand, the beneficial effects of cannabinoids in specific pathologies are worth trying to develop for medical use and therefore represent a main therapeutic challenge for health science. Several therapeutic strategies are currently being developed with some limitations. **Figure 1** and **Table 3** summarize some of these approaches.

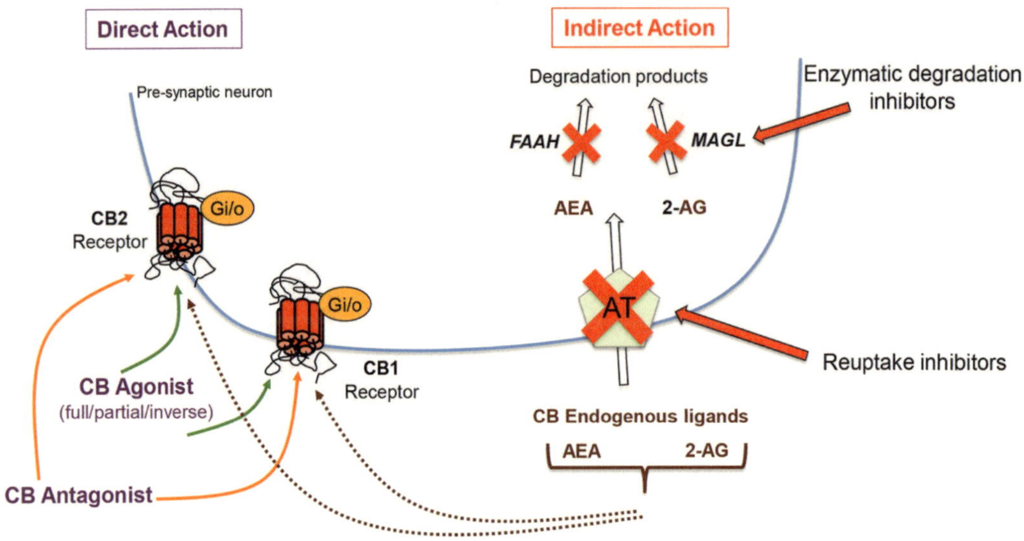

Figure 1. Therapeutic interventions targeting the endocannabinoid system. Commercialized compounds or molecules under study for targeting the endocannabinoid system are acting on different processes. Two main strategies are being developed to target the endocannabinoid system. A **direct** process will focus on compounds that bind to the cannabinoid receptors CB1 and/or CB2 receptors, with full, partial, or inverse agonists or antagonists (see text for details). An **indirect** process will aim at increasing endocannabinoid levels *in situ* and, therefore, target either the reuptake of anandamide and 2-AG or their degradation by their specific enzymes, FAAH and MAGL, respectively. Only the presynaptic neuron is represented here. Thin arrows represent the action of endogenous (hatched) or exogenous (plain) ligands on cannabinoid receptors. For detailed references, see the text. Abbreviations: AEA, anandamide; 2-AG, 2-arachidonoylglycerol; AT, anandamide transporter; CB, cannabinoid; FAAH, fatty acid amide hydrolase; MAGL, monoacylglycerol lipase.

4.1. Cannabidiol as a promising therapeutic medication

Cannabidiol (CBD) is a phytocannabinoid that has a low affinity for both receptors CB1 and CB2 with inverse agonistic properties [96, 216] and antagonistic effects, with CB2 receptors in particular [216] (see Section 1). This action explains the opposite effects of CBD toward Δ^9-THC and illustrates the interest to associate both compounds for developing a new medication. As mentioned earlier, CBD is commercialized in association with Δ^9-THC as Sativex®. Other properties such as anxiolytic, antidepressor, and antipsychotic effects have been observed with CBD [217]. Recent studies have revealed that CBD can decrease the cognitive and memory impairments induced by Δ^9-THC in male rhesus monkeys [218]. Evidence from several research domains suggests that CBD can be used for antipsychotic treatment (for reviews, see [219, 220]). A clinical study shows that anxiety and psychotic effects produced by a high concentration of Δ^9-THC can be reversed by CBD administration. Animal studies investigated the pharmacological profile of this phytocannabinoid and revealed a similar pattern to atypical antipsychotic drugs (clozapine or risperidone). Also, clinical studies on schizophrenic patients using CBD demonstrated a potential for this drug to be used as an alternative treatment for schizophrenia [220]. More investigations are still needed to better demonstrate the potential of this phytocannabinoid as a medication.

http://dx.doi.org/10.5772/63172

Strategy	Therapeutic potential	Limitation
Medicinal cannabis (phytocannabinoid including: Δ^9-THC, CBD, Δ^8-THC, CBN, etc.)	Severe pain (neuropathic, AIDS-associated, postsurgery, chronic) Muscle spasticity; cancer; cachexia, glaucoma, nausea	Adverse effects (psychosis) Safety issues (drug interaction unknown) Therapeutic benefit not fully proved Various pharmacodynamic and pharmacologic profiles Difficult dosage regimen
Cannabidiol	Anxiety; depression; psychosis(schizophrenia, bipolar disorders) Opiate dependence Pain Neurodegenerative diseases (AD, PD) Inflammatory diseases (rheumatoid arthritis) Brain ischemia Diabetes; nausea ; cancer	Clinical trials needed
CB2 receptor agonist	Chronic inflammatory and neuropathic pain Neurodegenerative and neuroinflammatory diseases (AD, MS, HD, ALS, brain ischemia) Osteoporosis Peripheric inflammatory disorders (atherosclerosis, nephropathy, liver disease) Cocaine dependence	Poor results in clinical trials compare with preclinical data
CB1 receptor antagonist	Drugs of abuse dependence(cannabinoids, nicotine, alcohol, opiates) Obesity; metabolic disorders	Adverse effects (anxiety, depression, suicides) Clinical trials needed
Peripheric CB1 receptor antagonist	Weight gain Atherosclerosis Gastrointestinal, liver, pancreatic or coronary artery diseases Arthritis	Preclinical studies to complete Clinical trials needed
Inhibitors of endocannabinoids degradation or inhibitors of recapture transporter	Anxiety; depression Opiate dependence	Clinical trials needed

This table lists examples of strategies targeting directly or indirectly the endocannabinoid system being developed or in progress for treating several pathologies. Most of trials were perform in preclinical studies. For most of candidate medications clinical trials must be perform or completed to confirm the efficiency in human and the safety of the various compounds. For detailed references, see the text.

Table 3. Examples of therapeutic strategies targeting the endocannabinoid system.

Interestingly, a rodent study using iv SA of heroin has revealed a potential for CBD as a medication for heroin dependence [221]. Indeed, the authors show in their model that CBD does not alter the intake of heroin, but specifically impairs the seeking behavior reinstated by a conditioned stimulus cue. This CBD effect is associated with the normalization of neurobiological changes observed in this model, noticeably in the CB1 receptor expression in structures related to reward like Nucleus Accumbens. In humans, opiate dependence is mostly treated with substitutive therapy like methadone but this molecule does not affect heroin craving. Therefore, CBD represents a potential alternative to treat heroin craving and relapse [221].

CBD has been shown to have analgesic properties. Paclitaxel is an anticancer drug that induces neuropathic pain. In a rodent model with chemotherapy-induced neuropathic pain and this medication, CBD was able to decrease mechanical sensitivity [222]. It had no conditioned rewarding effects and did not affect conditioned learning and memory. The precise mechanism of action is still not clear and may partly involve the serotonin system [222]. An interaction of CBD with CB2 receptor has also been suggested in heterologous system [216]. CBD may be an efficient treatment to reduce the neuropathic pain induced by chemotherapy without any of the potential side effects of cannabinoids.

Finally, other pathological situations, such as neurodegenerative diseases (Parkinson and Alzheimer), cerebral ischemia, diabetes, nausea, rheumatoid arthritis, or other inflammatory problems could be treated with CBD [223, 224]. Additionally, the potential for CBD as a medical intervention in psychotic disorder has been reviewed recently [219]. CBD represents a therapeutic approach for several disorders, but more clinical studies are needed. Also, plants with higher content in CBD or a low ratio Δ^9-THC/CBD are being produced for medical application and may not be of interest for euphoric purposes.

4.2. CB2 receptors as targets for medication

Pharmacology has provided many synthetic cannabinoid ligands that specifically interact with cannabinoid receptors and therefore represent great tools for research and clinical applications. The limitation for the use of these compounds as therapeutic drugs so far is that most of them target CB1 receptors and therefore may lead to adverse psychotic effects [225]. Indeed, CB1 receptor activation induces most of the central and psychotic effects of cannabis (see Section 2.1). Even though CB2 receptors are expressed in the CNS (see Section 2.1), they are mostly involved in inflammatory processes and are therefore less implicated in adverse central effects. Noteworthy activation of CB2 is not associated with tolerance or withdrawal syndrome in animal models of neuropathic pain [226]. In addition, no CPP or CPA could be measured using the CB2 agonist JWH-133 at the doses tested in mice, neither SA with this same agonist in mice able to self-administer cocaine, revealing no direct role of the CB2 receptor associated with reinforcing properties of cannabinoids [127]. Targeting these receptors for therapeutic purposes is therefore of strong interest [93].

As CB2 is highly expressed in immune cells, a potential role in treating several diseases including inflammation, cancer, osteoporosis, and liver diseases has been proposed (for a recent review, see [227]). Thus, CB2 agonists represent promising medication strategies in

http://dx.doi.org/10.5772/63172

several therapeutic applications with modulation of inflammatory processes without triggering psychotic effect [228, 229]. For example, selective activation of CB2 receptors by the synthetic cannabinoid JWH-015 suppresses CD40 expression in a model of cultured microglial cells activated by IFN-gamma, suggesting a beneficial role of CB2 activation in pathological activation of microglial cells [230]. This effect may be of interest in the context of neurodegenerative and neuroinflammatory diseases such as Alzheimer disease (AD), MS, or Huntington's disease [230–233]. Interestingly, another selective agonist of CB2, AM1241, was effective at slowing signs of disease progression in an amyotrophic lateral sclerosis (ALS) mouse model (G93A-SOD1 transgenic mice) when administered at the onset of tremor signs [234]. Daily injections of this CB2 agonist also increased the survival interval after disease onset by 56%, with reduction of motor neuron degeneration and preservation of motor function. Interestingly, a strong increase of CB2 mRNA expression is observed in the spinal cord of this mouse model [235]. These observations highlight the therapeutic potential of CB2 agonists for the treatment of these chronic pathologies.

A study using genetically modified mice deficient for CB2 receptors has revealed a low bone mass phenotype, suggesting that endocannabinoids play an essential role in the maintenance of bone mass by signaling through CB2. The authors showed that CB2 receptors are expressed in cells of both the osteoblast and osteoclast lineages and that exposure of these cells to a CB2-specific agonist (HU-308) results in direct stimulation of osteoblasts and inhibition of osteoclasts, suggesting that CB2 signaling contributes to the maintenance of normal bone mass [236]. Thus CB2 selective agonists could play a protector role in osteoporosis and represent a treatment strategy. In addition, selective agonists for CB2 receptors have been proposed for the treatment of inflammatory disorders in periphery, including atherosclerosis [237], nephropathy [238] or chronic liver disease [239].

Finally, CB2 receptor expression has been detected in neurons and a modulator role of this receptor has been proposed in drug addiction (see Section 2.4). Chronic administration of JWH-133 CB2 agonist inhibits iv SA of cocaine, cocaine-induced hyperlocomotion, and cocaine-induced levels of dopamine in the Nucleus Accumbens, in wild-type and mice deficient for CB1 receptors, but not in knockout mice for CB2 [127]. A similar effect is observed in the ventral tegmental area with inhibition of dopaminergic activity both *in vivo* and *in vitro* [66]. Therefore, the development of CB2 agonists for the treatment of cocaine dependence may be a future strategy.

In conclusion, preclinical studies are encouraging for CB2 agonist use in therapeutic approaches, but clinical results are rather poor and more studies are still needed. These limited results may be due to low *in vivo* selectivity of the tested compounds (which may also interact with CB1 receptors), individual (gender, age) or interspecies differences in CB2 receptors and associated signaling pathways [93].

4.3. Cannabinoid antagonists to treat several disorders

Other therapeutic strategies have explored the use of specific antagonists to block cannabinoid effects [188]. Rimonabant was the first CB1 antagonist introduced into clinical practice [240]. In 2006 in Europe, it was initially developed as a medication (Acomplia®) to treat obesity disorders and associated risks such as dyslipidemia, diabetes, and metabolic syndromes [241–243]. The anorexigenic properties of rimonabant were also encouraging to evaluate the potential of this compound to avoid weight gain when stopping nicotine consumption. A random double-blind clinical study has revealed that the addition of a nicotinic patch with rimonabant was more efficient than a placebo patch associated with rimonabant to prolonged abstinence following 6–9 weeks of treatment, but weight gain was similar in both groups [244]. Besides promising effects of this compound, it was withdrawn from the market in 2008 as strong psychiatric adverse effects have been observed during clinical trials (increased anxiety, deep depression, and suicide) [38, 240, 245] and was therefore not authorized by the Food and Drug Administration in the United States of America.

Knowing the adverse effects of rimonabant in human, development of any new selective cannabinoid antagonists with different pharmacodynamics properties (more neutral antagonist) that would possess the same activity both in animals and humans is greatly needed. In addition, such compound would have to yield a positive benefit/risk ratio to be considered for a therapeutic use and be tested in clinical research under strictly controlled circumstances that maximize safety [240]. Alternative perspectives for specific medical conditions are oriented toward cannabinoid antagonists that will only act on the periphery without CNS related adverse effects. Such compounds are being developed to treat pain (see [246]) and may also be useful for obesity and metabolic disorder, as preclinical studies have demonstrated decreased food intake using LH-21, an antagonist with a poor penetration rate into the central nervous system [247]. Likewise, peripheral antagonism may be beneficial for other pathologies with noticeable peripheral pathophysiologic mechanisms including gastrointestinal, liver, pancreatic, or coronary artery diseases ([240] and references therein).

Cannabinoid antagonists have also been evaluated for their potential in opiate-dependence therapy. Indeed, bidirectional interactions between cannabinoid and opioid systems on reward processes revealed by both pharmacological and genetic approaches (see Section 3.6) suggest a possible therapeutic intervention with cannabinoid antagonist for opiate dependence. For example, rimonabant administration suppresses morphine-induced CPP and morphine SA in mice, and heroin SA in rats [173], with the latter effect appearing only in opiate-dependent rats but not in nondependent animals [248]. Another therapeutic use for cannabinoid antagonists would be for treatment of nicotine abuse. Preclinical studies have revealed that CB1 selective antagonists, including rimonabant and AM251, reduced nicotinic SA, as well as nicotinic-induced CPP behaviors (see [249]). Besides, clinical studies have shown that rimonabant was efficient for tobacco smoking cessation, but the therapeutic effects were not better than other substitutive medications and results for abstinence were not fully convincing [250].

Moreover, CB1 antagonists have been evaluated for their use in alcohol dependence (recently reviewed in [251]). In preclinical studies, evidence accumulates for the good efficiency of cannabinoid antagonists to significantly reduce alcohol consumption and attenuate alcohol withdrawal symptoms. For example, a preclinical study demonstrated that rimonabant may be effective in reduction of alcohol consumption, most probably by indirect modulation of dopaminergic transmission [252]. On the other hand, results obtained in animals do not

http://dx.doi.org/10.5772/63172

necessary translate to human studies. Indeed, a double blind clinical trial with placebo has been conducted to examine the effect of a 12-week rimonabant treatment on alcohol-dependent patients under detoxification and only a mild effect was observed for efficiency against relapse [253]. Globally, results on cannabinoid efficiency for alcohol dependence are highly inconsistent and more clinical studies are needed to confirm an effect in human for this major health concern worldwide.

4.4. Inhibition of endocannabinoid degradation as a therapeutic strategy

An indirect strategy that is currently developed to target the endocannabinoid system is to limit the endocannabinoid degradation in order to increase their natural concentration *in situ* and amplify their effects. The most targeted enzyme is the FAAH enzyme (see Section 2.2) which hydrolyses AEA and therefore, by developing potent and selective inhibitors AEA actions may be prolonged. For example, the URB597 is a selective inhibitor of this enzyme [254, 255]. In both rats and mice it elicits antidepressive and antianxiolytic like effects, likely via CB1 receptor mediated modulation of serotonin and norepinephrine neurotransmission [255–258]. These observations highlight FAAH as an interesting pharmacological target to directly modulate endocannabinoid levels in the brain and therefore offer a potential treatment for depression and anxiety phenotype.

In addition, several preclinical studies have shown that the inhibitors of catabolic enzymes (FAAH and MAGL) may be useful against opiate abuse. Indeed, URB597 protects against tolerance and memory deficits in chronic morphine treatment and does not interfere with drug-induced reinstatement of either conditioned floor preference or avoidance [259]. Moreover, these inhibitors reduce somatic morphine withdrawal signs but not aversive aspects (CPA paradigm) [260]. The MAGL inhibitor JZL184 attenuates spontaneous withdrawal signs in morphine dependent mice. Morphine-dependent mice challenged with the opiate antagonist, naloxone, display a profound withdrawal syndrome. In these conditions, both PF-3845 (FAAH inhibitor) and JZL184 reduce these withdrawal signs, a process that is reversed by a CB1 antagonist SR141716A [261]. Interestingly, the FAAH inhibitors do not show any adverse effects such as hypothermia, hypomotility, or catalepsia [81, 262]. In addition, they do not show reinforcing properties and therefore are a promising therapeutic strategy to treat opiate dependence with the minimal risk of abuse that is classically observed with cannabinoid agonists [257, 260]. Interestingly, other authors have evaluated the effects of structurally different FAAH inhibitors in an animal model of working memory known to be sensitive to impairment by Δ^9-THC and showed that one FAAH inhibitor (AM3506) decreased accuracy in the memory task via a CB1-dependent mechanism, whereas the others had no effect [263].

Another target for increasing endogenous levels of the cannabinoid-receptor agonist would be to block the AEA transporter. The endocannabinoid uptake inhibitor AM404 can have antidepressant effects in the forced swim test in rat (decreased immobility), suggesting a potential therapeutic effect as for the FAAH inhibitors [264]. On the other hand, a very recent study demonstrated that AM404 was able to effectively reinforce SA behavior and induce reinstatement of drug-seeking behavior in abstinent squirrel monkeys, indicating that such a compound that promotes increased endocannabinoids may have a potential for abuse [265].

All these indirect strategies are of particular interest as they amplify cannabinoid receptor activation specifically where the endocannabinoids are produced, therefore increase signaling in defined brain structures [255]. Nevertheless, clinical studies are needed to confirm the therapeutic potential of these molecules in human and it will be crucial to evaluate the effects of such inhibitors with respect to their potential for memory impairment, abuse liability, and probably other cannabis-like effects in clinical trials before any specific therapeutic application.

5. Conclusion

The growing consumption of cannabis and its derivatives in the population and particularly in the adolescent population represents a real public health challenge. A growing interest has been developed in cannabis and related compounds in research. Furthermore, considerable debates involving its legalization are still being conducted and this may have political consequences. Risk should not be neglected and it seems crucial to widely disseminate more scientific knowledge about this family of compounds before legalization becomes a normalization. Cannabis exposure produces a range of behavioral and neurobiological adaptations and the general public should be more aware of the clinical implications of the long-term impact of this drug. Among adaptations, long-term exposure to drugs of abuse or specific exposure during a critical period of development may elicit gene expression changes through epigenetic mechanisms. Recent research using genomic technology has investigated plasticity mechanisms taking place in brain structures involved in reward circuitry and highlighted epigenetic control of gene transcription (see Section 3.2). An expected increase of scientific data in this field will help clarify the molecular mechanisms of drug abuse vulnerability. This research will also be a new avenue for proposing novel therapeutic interventions for long-term cannabis exposure or spreading abuse of synthetic cannabinoids.

Cannabinoid derivatives have positive effects on several other pathologies besides drug dependence. These applications need further rigorous clinical trials to ensure efficiency and safety in human and additional cannabinoid-related compounds need to be developed. In conjunction, a combination of strategies may be foreseen, as this is the case in other pharmacological fields, with specific care to the dose and duration of treatments. Inventive therapeutic approaches for treating pain or dependence may also consider targeting heterodimers of cannabinoid and opioid receptors using antibodies or bivalent ligands or indirectly acting on both systems using dual enkephalinase and cannabinoid catabolic enzyme inhibitors [266, 267]. Intensive research is now oriented toward such perspectives.

To conclude, and as for the opiate compounds that are used as medication, in particular, to treat pain (e.g., morphine) or abused for euphoric effects (e.g., heroin), cannabinoids by targeting a complex endogenous system also constitute a powerful pharmacological tool with both drug and medication properties. Therefore, future investigations are necessary in order to propose optimal therapeutic approaches for managing complex diseases and promising strategies for reducing dependence. The ultimate goal is to propose innovative strategies to current treatments with increased safety usage.

http://dx.doi.org/10.5772/63172

Acknowledgements

We would like to thank Dominique Massotte for constant support and fruitful discussions and Emma Stephens for English proof reading of the manuscript. We would also like to thank funding sources including the Centre National de la Recherche Scientifique, the Université de Strasbourg, and Investissements d'Avenir PEPS2015.

Author details

Léa Giron[1,2,3] and Katia Befort[2,3*]

*Address all correspondence to: katia.befort@unistra.fr

1 Laboratory of Cognitive and Adaptative Neuroscience (LNCA), UMR University of Strasbourg -CNRS, Neuropole of Strasbourg, Faculty of Psychology, 12, rue Goethe, Strasbourg (France)

2 Laboratory of Cognitive and Adaptative Neuroscience (LNCA), UMR University of Strasbourg -CNRS, Neuropole of Strasbourg, Faculty of Psychology, 12, rue Goethe, Strasbourg (France)

3 LNCA UMR, CNRS, 12 rue Goethe, Strasbourg

References

[1] Zuardi AW. History of cannabis as a medicine: a review. Rev Bras Psiquiatr. 2006;28(2): 153–157.

[2] Leung L. Cannabis and its derivatives: review of medical use. J Am Board Fam Med. 2011;24(4):452–462.

[3] AIHW. National Drug Strategy Household Survey 2013 [accessed April 16, 2015]. Available from: http://www.aihw.gov.au/alcohol-and-other-drugs/ndshs-2013/.

[4] OFDT. European survey on drugs 2014 [accessed December 7, 2014]. Available from: www.ofdt.fr/BDD/publications/docs/OEDT2014EDRrap.pdf.

[5] SAMHSA. Results from the 2013 National Survey on Drug Use and Health: Summary of National Findings [accessed April 16, 2015]. Available from: http://www.samhsa.gov/data/sites/default/files/NSDUHresultsPDFWHTML2013/Web/NSDUHresults2013.htm.

[6] Hall W, Degenhardt L. Adverse health effects of non-medical cannabis use. Lancet. 2009;374(9698):1383–1391.

[7] Adams IB, Martin BR. Cannabis: pharmacology and toxicology in animals and humans. Addiction. 1996;91(11):1585–1614.

[8] Mechoulam R, Gaoni Y. Hashish. IV. The isolation and structure of cannabinolic cannabidiolic and cannabigerolic acids. Tetrahedron. 1965;21(5):1223–1229.

[9] Mechoulam R. Marihuana chemistry. Science. 1970;168(3936):1159–1166.

[10] Howlett AC, Barth F, Bonner TI, Cabral G, Casellas P, Devane WA, et al. International Union of Pharmacology. XXVII. Classification of cannabinoid receptors. Pharmacol Rev. 2002;54(2):161–202.

[11] Pertwee RG. Pharmacological actions of cannabinoids. Handb Exp Pharmacol. 2005(168):1–51.

[12] Mechoulam R, Parker L. Towards a better cannabis drug. Br J Pharmacol. 2013;170(7): 1363–1364.

[13] Ashton CH. Pharmacology and effects of cannabis: a brief review. Br J Psychiatry. 2001;178:101–106.

[14] Hillig KW, Mahlberg PG. A chemotaxonomic analysis of cannabinoid variation in Cannabis (Cannabaceae). Am J Bot. 2004;91(6):966–975.

[15] Maldonado R, Berrendero F, Ozaita A, Robledo P. Neurochemical basis of cannabis addiction. Neuroscience. 2011;181:1–17.

[16] Johns A. Psychiatric effects of cannabis. Br J Psychiatry. 2001;178:116–122.

[17] Hall W, Solowij N. Adverse effects of cannabis. Lancet. 1998;352(9140):1611–1616.

[18] Maykut MO. Health consequences of acute and chronic marihuana use. Prog Neuropsychopharmacol Biol Psychiatry. 1985;9(3):209–238.

[19] Henquet C, Krabbendam L, Spauwen J, Kaplan C, Lieb R, Wittchen HU, et al. Prospective cohort study of cannabis use, predisposition for psychosis, and psychotic symptoms in young people. BMJ. 2005;330(7481):11.

[20] Le Bec PY, Fatseas M, Denis C, Lavie E, Auriacombe M. Cannabis and psychosis: search of a causal link through a critical and systematic review. Encephale. 2009;35(4):377–385.

[21] Shapiro GK, Buckley-Hunter L. What every adolescent needs to know: cannabis can cause psychosis. J Psychosom Res. 2010;69(6):533–539.

[22] Kocabay G, Yildiz M, Duran NE, Ozkan M. Acute inferior myocardial infarction due to cannabis smoking in a young man. J Cardiovasc Med (Hagerstown). 2009;10(9):669–670.

[23] Lehavi A, Shay M, Gilony C, Even L. Marijuana smoking and paroxysmal atrial fibrillation. Harefuah. 2005;144(1):2–3, 72.

[24] Baranchuk A, Johri AM, Simpson CS, Methot M, Redfearn DP. Ventricular fibrillation triggered by marijuana use in a patient with ischemic cardiomyopathy: a case report. Cases J. 2008;1(1):373.

[25] Bailly C, Merceron O, Hammoudi N, Dorent R, Michel PL. Cannabis induced acute coronary syndrome in a young female. Int J Cardiol. 2010;143(1):e4–e6.

[26] Basnet S, Mander G, Nicolas R. Coronary vasospasm in an adolescent resulting from marijuana use. Pediatr Cardiol. 2009;30(4):543–545.

[27] Tashkin DP. Smoked marijuana as a cause of lung injury. Monaldi Arch Chest Dis. 2005;63(2):93–100.

[28] Moir D, Rickert WS, Levasseur G, Larose Y, Maertens R, White P, et al. A comparison of mainstream and sidestream marijuana and tobacco cigarette smoke produced under two machine smoking conditions. Chem Res Toxicol. 2008;21(2):494–502.

[29] Reid PT, Macleod J, Robertson JR. Cannabis and the lung. J R Coll Physicians Edinb. 2010;40(4):328–323; quiz 33–34.

[30] Mazidi M, Baghban Taraghdari S, Rezaee P, Kamgar M, Jomezadeh MR, Akbarieh Hasani O, et al. The effect of hydroalcoholic extract of *Cannabis sativa* on appetite hormone in rat. J Complement Integr Med. 2014;11(4):253–257.

[31] Cabut S, Santi P. Cannabis: la fin d'un interdit Le Monde [accessed February 7, 2015]. Available from: http://www.lemonde.fr/sciences/article/2013/09/09/cannabis-la-fin-d-un-interdit_3473572_1650684.html.

[32] Health_Canada. Medical use of Marijuana [Accessed January 17, 2015]. Available from: http://www.hc-sc.gc.ca/dhp-mps/marihuana/index-eng.php.

[33] MacDonald J. Medical marijuana: informational resources for family physicians. Am Fam Physician. 2009;80(8):779.

[34] Hoffmann DE, Weber E. Medical marijuana and the law. N Engl J Med. 2010;362(16): 1453–1457.

[35] Borgelt LM, Franson KL, Nussbaum AM, Wang GS. The pharmacologic and clinical effects of medical cannabis. Pharmacotherapy. 2013;33(2):195–209.

[36] Clark AJ, Ware MA, Yazer E, Murray TJ, Lynch ME. Patterns of cannabis use among patients with multiple sclerosis. Neurology. 2004;62(11):2098–2100.

[37] Seamon MJ, Fass JA, Maniscalco-Feichtl M, Abu-Shraie NA. Medical marijuana and the developing role of the pharmacist. Am J Health Syst Pharm. 2007;64(10):1037–1044.

[38] Pertwee RG. Emerging strategies for exploiting cannabinoid receptor agonists as medicines. Br J Pharmacol. 2009;156(3):397–411.

[39] Ware MA, St Arnaud-Trempe E. The abuse potential of the synthetic cannabinoid nabilone. Addiction. 2010;105(3):494–503.

[40] Allsop DJ, Lintzeris N, Copeland J, Dunlop A, McGregor IS. Cannabinoid replacement therapy (CRT): nabiximols (Sativex) as a novel treatment for cannabis withdrawal. Clin Pharmacol Ther. 2015; 97(6): 571-574.

[41] Wilsey B, Marcotte T, Tsodikov A, Millman J, Bentley H, Gouaux B, et al. A randomized, placebo-controlled, crossover trial of cannabis cigarettes in neuropathic pain. J Pain. 2008;9(6):506–521.

[42] Abrams DI, Jay CA, Shade SB, Vizoso H, Reda H, Press S, et al. Cannabis in painful HIV-associated sensory neuropathy: a randomized placebo-controlled trial. Neurology. 2007;68(7):515–521.

[43] Hemming M, Yellowlees PM. Effective treatment of Tourette's syndrome with marijuana. J Psychopharmacol. 1993;7(4):389–391.

[44] Sandyk R, Awerbuch G. Marijuana and Tourette's syndrome. J Clin Psychopharmacol. 1988;8(6):444–445.

[45] Vaney C, Heinzel-Gutenbrunner M, Jobin P, Tschopp F, Gattlen B, Hagen U, et al. Efficacy, safety and tolerability of an orally administered cannabis extract in the treatment of spasticity in patients with multiple sclerosis: a randomized, double-blind, placebo-controlled, crossover study. Mult Scler. 2004;10(4):417–424.

[46] Zajicek JP, Sanders HP, Wright DE, Vickery PJ, Ingram WM, Reilly SM, et al. Cannabinoids in multiple sclerosis (CAMS) study: safety and efficacy data for 12 months follow up. J Neurol Neurosurg Psychiatry. 2005;76(12):1664–1669.

[47] Ware MA, Wang T, Shapiro S, Robinson A, Ducruet T, Huynh T, et al. Smoked cannabis for chronic neuropathic pain: a randomized controlled trial. CMAJ. 2010;182(14):E694–E701.

[48] Martin-Sanchez E, Furukawa TA, Taylor J, Martin JL. Systematic review and meta-analysis of cannabis treatment for chronic pain. Pain Med. 2009;10(8):1353–1368.

[49] Jicha CJ, Lofwall MR, Nuzzo PA, Babalonis S, Elayi SC, Walsh SL. Safety of oral dronabinol during opioid withdrawal in humans. Drug Alcohol Depend. 2015;157:179–183.

[50] Schubart CD, Sommer IE, van Gastel WA, Goetgebuer RL, Kahn RS, Boks MP. Cannabis with high cannabidiol content is associated with fewer psychotic experiences. Schizophr Res. 2011;130(1–3):216–221.

[51] Devane WA, Hanus L, Breuer A, Pertwee RG, Stevenson LA, Griffin G, et al. Isolation and structure of a brain constituent that binds to the cannabinoid receptor. Science. 1992;258(5090):1946–1949.

[52] Matsuda LA, Lolait SJ, Brownstein MJ, Young AC, Bonner TI. Structure of a cannabinoid receptor and functional expression of the cloned cDNA. Nature. 1990;346(6284): 561–564.

[53] Munro S, Thomas KL, Abu-Shaar M. Molecular characterization of a peripheral receptor for cannabinoids. Nature. 1993;365(6441):61–65.

[54] Howlett AC. Cannabinoid receptor signaling. Handb Exp Pharmacol. 2005(168):53–79.

[55] Rodriguez de Fonseca F, Del Arco I, Bermudez-Silva FJ, Bilbao A, Cippitelli A, Navarro M. The endocannabinoid system: physiology and pharmacology. Alcohol Alcohol. 2005;40(1):2–14.

[56] Matsuda LA. Molecular aspects of cannabinoid receptors. Crit Rev Neurobiol. 1997;11(2–3):143–166.

[57] Fasano S, Meccariello R, Cobellis G, Chianese R, Cacciola G, Chioccarelli T, et al. The endocannabinoid system: an ancient signaling involved in the control of male fertility. Ann NY Acad Sci. 2009;1163:112–124.

[58] Fride E. Endocannabinoids in the central nervous system– an overview. Prostaglandins Leukot Essent Fatty Acids. 2002;66(2–3):221–233.

[59] Herkenham M, Lynn AB, Little MD, Johnson MR, Melvin LS, de Costa BR, et al. Cannabinoid receptor localization in brain. Proc Natl Acad Sci U S A. 1990;87(5):1932–1936.

[60] Tsou K, Brown S, Sanudo-Pena MC, Mackie K, Walker JM. Immunohistochemical distribution of cannabinoid CB1 receptors in the rat central nervous system. Neuroscience. 1998;83(2):393–411.

[61] Di Chiara G, Bassareo V, Fenu S, De Luca MA, Spina L, Cadoni C, et al. Dopamine and drug addiction: the nucleus accumbens shell connection. Neuropharmacology. 2004;47(Suppl 1):227–241.

[62] Everitt BJ, Robbins TW. Neural systems of reinforcement for drug addiction: from actions to habits to compulsion. Nat Neurosci. 2005;8(11):1481–1489.

[63] Gong JP, Onaivi ES, Ishiguro H, Liu QR, Tagliaferro PA, Brusco A, et al. Cannabinoid CB2 receptors: immunohistochemical localization in rat brain. Brain Res. 2006;1071(1): 10–23.

[64] Skaper SD, Buriani A, Dal Toso R, Petrelli L, Romanello S, Facci L, et al. The ALIAmide palmitoylethanolamide and cannabinoids, but not anandamide, are protective in a delayed postglutamate paradigm of excitotoxic death in cerebellar granule neurons. Proc Natl Acad Sci U S A. 1996;93(9):3984–3989.

[65] Van Sickle MD, Duncan M, Kingsley PJ, Mouihate A, Urbani P, Mackie K, et al. Identification and functional characterization of brainstem cannabinoid CB2 receptors. Science. 2005;310(5746):329–332.

[66] Zhang HY, Gao M, Liu QR, Bi GH, Li X, Yang HJ, et al. Cannabinoid CB2 receptors modulate midbrain dopamine neuronal activity and dopamine-related behavior in mice. Proc Natl Acad Sci U S A. 2014;111(46):E5007–E5015.

[67] Li Y, Kim J. Neuronal expression of CB2 cannabinoid receptor mRNAs in the mouse hippocampus. Neuroscience. 2015;311:253–267.

[68] Schmole AC, Lundt R, Gennequin B, Schrage H, Beins E, Kramer A, et al. Expression analysis of CB2-GFP BAC transgenic mice. PLoS One. 2015;10(9):e0138986.

[69] Zygmunt PM, Petersson J, Andersson DA, Chuang H, Sorgard M, Di Marzo V, et al. Vanilloid receptors on sensory nerves mediate the vasodilator action of anandamide. Nature. 1999;400(6743):452–457.

[70] Baker D, Pryce G, Davies WL, Hiley CR. In silico patent searching reveals a new cannabinoid receptor. Trends Pharmacol Sci. 2006;27(1):1–4.

[71] Brown AJ. Novel cannabinoid receptors. Br J Pharmacol. 2007;152(5):567–575.

[72] De Petrocellis L, Di Marzo V. Non-CB1, non-CB2 receptors for endocannabinoids, plant cannabinoids, and synthetic cannabimimetics: focus on G-protein-coupled receptors and transient receptor potential channels. J Neuroimmun Pharmacol. 2010;5(1):103–1021.

[73] Mechoulam R, Ben-Shabat S, Hanus L, Ligumsky M, Kaminski NE, Schatz AR, et al. Identification of an endogenous 2-monoglyceride, present in canine gut, that binds to cannabinoid receptors. Biochem Pharmacol. 1995;50(1):83–90.

[74] Sugiura T, Kondo S, Sukagawa A, Nakane S, Shinoda A, Itoh K, et al. 2-Arachidonoylglycerol: a possible endogenous cannabinoid receptor ligand in brain. Biochem Biophys Res Commun. 1995;215(1):89–97.

[75] Sugiura T, Kishimoto S, Oka S, Gokoh M. Biochemistry, pharmacology and physiology of 2-arachidonoylglycerol, an endogenous cannabinoid receptor ligand. Prog Lipid Res. 2006;45(5):405–446.

[76] De Luca MA, Valentini V, Bimpisidis Z, Cacciapaglia F, Caboni P, Di Chiara G. Endocannabinoid 2-arachidonoylglycerol self-administration by Sprague–Dawley rats and stimulation of in vivo dopamine transmission in the nucleus accumbens shell. Front Psychiatry. 2014;5:140.

[77] Lin S, Khanolkar AD, Fan P, Goutopoulos A, Qin C, Papahadjis D, et al. Novel analogues of arachidonylethanolamide (anandamide): affinities for the CB1 and CB2 cannabinoid receptors and metabolic stability. J Med Chem. 1998;41(27):5353–5361.

[78] Pertwee RG, Howlett AC, Abood ME, Alexander SP, Di Marzo V, Elphick MR, et al. International Union of Basic and Clinical Pharmacology. LXXIX. Cannabinoid receptors and their ligands: beyond CB(1) and CB(2). Pharmacol Rev. 2010;62(4):588–631.

[79] Lu HC, Mackie K. An introduction to the endogenous cannabinoid system. Biol Psychiatry.2015; 79(7):516-525.

[80] Liu J, Wang L, Harvey-White J, Huang BX, Kim HY, Luquet S, et al. Multiple pathways involved in the biosynthesis of anandamide. Neuropharmacology. 2008;54(1):1–7.

[81] Ahn K, McKinney MK, Cravatt BF. Enzymatic pathways that regulate endocannabinoid signaling in the nervous system. Chem Rev. 2008;108(5):1687–1707.

[82] Piomelli D. The molecular logic of endocannabinoid signalling. Nat Rev Neurosci. 2003;4(11):873–884.

[83] Tanimura A, Yamazaki M, Hashimotodani Y, Uchigashima M, Kawata S, Abe M, et al. The endocannabinoid 2-arachidonoylglycerol produced by diacylglycerol lipase alpha mediates retrograde suppression of synaptic transmission. Neuron. 2010;65(3):320–327.

[84] Ohno-Shosaku T, Kano M. Endocannabinoid-mediated retrograde modulation of synaptic transmission. Curr Opin Neurobiol. 2014;29C:1–8.

[85] Desarnaud F, Cadas H, Piomelli D. Anandamide amidohydrolase activity in rat brain microsomes. Identification and partial characterization. J Biol Chem. 1995;270(11): 6030–6035.

[86] Cravatt BF, Giang DK, Mayfield SP, Boger DL, Lerner RA, Gilula NB. Molecular characterization of an enzyme that degrades neuromodulatory fatty-acid amides. Nature. 1996;384(6604):83–87.

[87] Dinh TP, Carpenter D, Leslie FM, Freund TF, Katona I, Sensi SL, et al. Brain monoglyceride lipase participating in endocannabinoid inactivation. Proc Natl Acad Sci U S A. 2002;99(16):10819–10824.

[88] Schlicker E, Kathmann M. Modulation of transmitter release via presynaptic cannabinoid receptors. Trends Pharmacol Sci. 2001;22(11):565–572.

[89] Wade MR, Tzavara ET, Nomikos GG. Cannabinoids reduce cAMP levels in the striatum of freely moving rats: an in vivo microdialysis study. Brain Res. 2004;1005(1–2):117–123.

[90] Velasco G, Galve-Roperh I, Sanchez C, Blazquez C, Haro A, Guzman M. Cannabinoids and ceramide: two lipids acting hand-by-hand. Life Sci. 2005;77(14):1723–1731.

[91] Galve-Roperh I, Sanchez C, Cortes ML, Gomez del Pulgar T, Izquierdo M, Guzman M. Anti-tumoral action of cannabinoids: involvement of sustained ceramide accumulation and extracellular signal-regulated kinase activation. Nat Med. 2000;6(3):313–319.

[92] Sanchez C, Galve-Roperh I, Rueda D, Guzman M. Involvement of sphingomyelin hydrolysis and the mitogen-activated protein kinase cascade in the Delta9-tetrahydrocannabinol-induced stimulation of glucose metabolism in primary astrocytes. Molecular pharmacology. 1998;54(5):834–843.

[93] Dhopeshwarkar A, Mackie K. CB2 Cannabinoid receptors as a therapeutic target-what does the future hold? MolPharmacol. 2014;86(4):430–437.

[94] Flores A, Maldonado R, Berrendero F. Cannabinoid-hypocretin cross-talk in the central nervous system: what we know so far. Frontiers in neuroscience. 2013;7:256.

[95] Gatta-Cherifi B, Cota D. Endocannabinoids and metabolic disorders. Handb Exp Pharmacol. 2015;231:367–391.

[96] Panagis G, Mackey B, Vlachou S. Cannabinoid regulation of brain reward processing with an emphasis on the role of CB1 receptors: a step back into the future. Front Psychiatry. 2014;5:92.

[97] Solinas M, Goldberg SR, Piomelli D. The endocannabinoid system in brain reward processes. Br J Pharmacol. 2008;154(2):369–383.

[98] Woodhams SG, Sagar DR, Burston JJ, Chapman V. The role of the endocannabinoid system in pain. Handb Exp Pharmacol. 2015;227:119–143.

[99] Zanettini C, Panlilio LV, Alicki M, Goldberg SR, Haller J, Yasar S. Effects of endocannabinoid system modulation on cognitive and emotional behavior. Frontiers in behavioral neuroscience. 2011;5:57.

[100] Moreira FA, Jupp B, Belin D, Dalley JW. Endocannabinoids and striatal function: implications for addiction-related behaviours. Behav Pharmacol. 2015;26(1–2):59–72.

[101] Meccariello R, Battista N, Bradshaw HB, Wang H. Updates in reproduction coming from the endocannabinoid system. Int JEndocrinol. 2014;2014:412354.

[102] Zimmer A. Genetic manipulation of the endocannabinoid system. Handb Exp Pharmacol. 2015;231:129–183.

[103] Walker JM, Hohmann AG. Cannabinoid mechanisms of pain suppression. Handb Exp Pharmacol. 2005(168):509–554.

[104] Racz I, Nadal X, Alferink J, Banos JE, Rehnelt J, Martin M, et al. Crucial role of CB(2) cannabinoid receptor in the regulation of central immune responses during neuropathic pain. J Neurosci. 2008;28(46):12125–12135.

[105] La Porta C, Bura SA, Aracil-Fernandez A, Manzanares J, Maldonado R. Role of CB1 and CB2 cannabinoid receptors in the development of joint pain induced by monosodium iodoacetate. Pain. 2013;154(1):160–174.

[106] Martin BR, Lichtman AH. Cannabinoid transmission and pain perception. Neurobiol Dis. 1998;5(6 Pt B):447–461.

[107] Calignano A, La Rana G, Giuffrida A, Piomelli D. Control of pain initiation by endogenous cannabinoids. Nature. 1998;394(6690):277–281.

[108] Straiker A, Stella N, Piomelli D, Mackie K, Karten HJ, Maguire G. Cannabinoid CB1 receptors and ligands in vertebrate retina: localization and function of an endogenous signaling system. Proc Natl Acad Sci U S A. 1999;96(25):14565–14570.

[109] Lu Q, Straiker A, Lu Q, Maguire G. Expression of CB2 cannabinoid receptor mRNA in adult rat retina. VisNeurosci. 2000;17(1):91–95.

[110] Lopez EM, Tagliaferro P, Onaivi ES, Lopez-Costa JJ. Distribution of CB2 cannabinoid receptor in adult rat retina. Synapse. 2011;65(5):388–392.

[111] Cecyre B, Zabouri N, Huppe-Gourgues F, Bouchard JF, Casanova C. Roles of cannabinoid receptors type 1 and 2 on the retinal function of adult mice. Invest Ophthalmol Vis Sci. 2013;54(13):8079–8090.

[112] Mainolfi N, Powers J, Amin J, Long D, Lee W, McLaughlin ME, et al. An effective prodrug strategy to selectively enhance ocular exposure of a cannabinoid receptor (CB1/2) agonist. J Med Chem. 2013;56(13):5464–5472.

[113] Williams CM, Rogers PJ, Kirkham TC. Hyperphagia in pre-fed rats following oral delta9-THC. Physiol Behav. 1998;65(2):343–346.

[114] Di Marzo V, Matias I. Endocannabinoid control of food intake and energy balance. Nat Neurosci. 2005;8(5):585–589.

[115] Pagotto U, Marsicano G, Cota D, Lutz B, Pasquali R. The emerging role of the endocannabinoid system in endocrine regulation and energy balance. Endocr Rev. 2006;27(1):73–100.

[116] Mazier W, Saucisse N, Gatta-Cherifi B, Cota D. The endocannabinoid system: pivotal orchestrator of obesity and metabolic disease. Trends Endocrinol Metab. 2015;26(10): 524–537.

[117] Maccarrone M, Bab I, Biro T, Cabral GA, Dey SK, Di Marzo V, et al. Endocannabinoid signaling at the periphery: 50 years after THC. Trends Pharmacol Sci. 2015;36(5): 277–296.

[118] Kunos G, Batkai S, Offertaler L, Mo F, Liu J, Karcher J, et al. The quest for a vascular endothelial cannabinoid receptor. Chem Phys Lipids. 2002;121(1–2):45–56.

[119] Randall MD, Harris D, Kendall DA, Ralevic V. Cardiovascular effects of cannabinoids. Pharmacol Ther. 2002;95(2):191–202.

[120] Valverde O, Torrens M. CB1 receptor-deficient mice as a model for depression. Neuroscience. 2012;204:193–206.

[121] Ishiguro H, Horiuchi Y, Ishikawa M, Koga M, Imai K, Suzuki Y, et al. Brain cannabinoid CB2 receptor in schizophrenia. Biol Psychiatry. 2010;67(10):974–982.

[122] Ortega-Alvaro A, Aracil-Fernandez A, Garcia-Gutierrez MS, Navarrete F, Manzanares J. Deletion of CB2 cannabinoid receptor induces schizophrenia-related behaviors in mice. Neuropsychopharmacology. 2011;36(7):1489–1504.

[123] Aracil-Fernandez A, Trigo JM, Garcia-Gutierrez MS, Ortega-Alvaro A, Ternianov A, Navarro D, et al. Decreased cocaine motor sensitization and self-administration in mice overexpressing cannabinoid CB(2) receptors. Neuropsychopharmacology. 2012;37(7): 1749–1763.

[124] Ignatowska-Jankowska BM, Muldoon PP, Lichtman AH, Damaj MI. The cannabinoid CB2 receptor is necessary for nicotine-conditioned place preference, but not other behavioral effects of nicotine in mice. Psychopharmacology (Berl). 2013;229(4):591–601.

[125] Navarrete F, Rodriguez-Arias M, Martin-Garcia E, Navarro D, Garcia-Gutierrez MS, Aguilar MA, et al. Role of CB2 cannabinoid receptors in the rewarding, reinforcing, and physical effects of nicotine. Neuropsychopharmacology. 2013;38(12):2515–2524.

[126] Ortega-Alvaro A, Ternianov A, Aracil-Fernandez A, Navarrete F, Garcia-Gutierrez MS, Manzanares J. Role of cannabinoid CB2 receptor in the reinforcing actions of ethanol. Addict Biol. 2015;20(1):43–55.

[127] Xi ZX, Peng XQ, Li X, Song R, Zhang HY, Liu QR, et al. Brain cannabinoid CB(2) receptors modulate cocaine's actions in mice. Nat Neurosci. 2011;14(9):1160–1166.

[128] Monory K, Massa F, Egertova M, Eder M, Blaudzun H, Westenbroek R, et al. The endocannabinoid system controls key epileptogenic circuits in the hippocampus. Neuron. 2006;51(4):455–466.

[129] Prenderville JA, Kelly AM, Downer EJ. The role of cannabinoids in adult neurogenesis. Br J Pharmacol. 2015;172(16):3950–3963.

[130] Fratta W, Fattore L. Molecular mechanisms of cannabinoid addiction. Curr Opin Neurobiol. 2013;23(4):487–492.

[131] Maldonado R, Valverde O, Berrendero F. Involvement of the endocannabinoid system in drug addiction. Trends Neurosci. 2006;29(4):225–232.

[132] Doudna JA, Charpentier E. Genome editing. The new frontier of genome engineering with CRISPR-Cas9. Science. 2014;346(6213):1258096.

[133] Hsu PD, Lander ES, Zhang F. Development and applications of CRISPR-Cas9 for genome engineering. Cell. 2014;157(6):1262–1278.

[134] Copeland J, Swift W. Cannabis use disorder: epidemiology and management. Int Rev Psychiatry. 2009;21(2):96–103.

[135] Time. What is America high on right now? [accessed December 22, 2014]. Available from: http://time.com/american-drug-use/.

[136] Rezkalla S, Kloner RA. Recreational marijuana use: is it safe for your patient? J Am Heart Assoc. 2014;3(2):e000904.

[137] Pardo B. Cannabis policy reforms in the Americas: a comparative analysis of Colorado, Washington, and Uruguay. Int J Drug Policy. 2014;25(4):727–735.

[138] Thomas G, Kloner RA, Rezkalla S. Adverse cardiovascular, cerebrovascular, and peripheral vascular effects of marijuana inhalation: what cardiologists need to know. Am J Cardiol. 2014;113(1):187–190.

[139] Degenhardt L, Coffey C, Carlin JB, Swift W, Moore E, Patton GC. Outcomes of occasional cannabis use in adolescence: 10-year follow-up study in Victoria, Australia. Br J Psychiatry. 2010;196(4):290–295.

[140] Ferdinand RF, Sondeijker F, van der Ende J, Selten JP, Huizink A, Verhulst FC. Cannabis use predicts future psychotic symptoms, and vice versa. Addiction. 2005;100(5):612–618.

[141] Friedman AS, Glassman K, Terras BA. Violent behavior as related to use of marijuana and other drugs. J Addict Dis. 2001;20(1):49–72.

[142] MILDECA. Cannabis [accessed December 22, 2014]. Available from: http://www.drogues.gouv.fr/drogues-illicites/cannabis/index.html.

[143] Jouanjus E, Lapeyre-Mestre M, Micallef J. Cannabis use: signal of increasing risk of serious cardiovascular disorders. J Am Heart Assoc. 2014;3(2):e000638.

[144] Lindsay AC, Foale RA, Warren O, Henry JA. Cannabis as a precipitant of cardiovascular emergencies. Int J Cardiol. 2005;104(2):230–232.

[145] Hall WD, Lynskey M. Is cannabis a gateway drug? Testing hypotheses about the relationship between cannabis use and the use of other illicit drugs. Drug Alcohol Rev. 2005;24(1):39–48.

[146] Spano MS, Fadda P, Fratta W, Fattore L. Cannabinoid-opioid interactions in drug discrimination and self-administration: effect of maternal, postnatal, adolescent and adult exposure to the drugs. Curr Drug Targets. 2010;11(4):450–461.

[147] Ellgren M, Spano SM, Hurd YL. Adolescent cannabis exposure alters opiate intake and opioid limbic neuronal populations in adult rats. Neuropsychopharmacology. 2007;32(3):607–615.

[148] Szutorisz H, DiNieri JA, Sweet E, Egervari G, Michaelides M, Carter JM, et al. Parental THC exposure leads to compulsive heroin-seeking and altered striatal synaptic plasticity in the subsequent generation. Neuropsychopharmacology. 2014;39(6):1315–1323.

[149] Watson CT, Szutorisz H, Garg P, Martin Q, Landry JA, Sharp AJ, et al. Genome-wide DNA methylation profiling reveals epigenetic changes in the rat nucleus accumbens

associated with cross-generational effects of adolescent THC Exposure. Neuropsychopharmacology. 2015;40(13):2993–3005.

[150] Nestler EJ. Epigenetic mechanisms of drug addiction. Neuropharmacology. 2014;76(Pt B):259–268.

[151] Szutorisz H, Hurd YL. Epigenetic effects of cannabis exposure. Biol Psychiatry.2015; 79(7):586-594.

[152] Budney AJ, Hughes JR. The cannabis withdrawal syndrome. Curr Opin Psychiatry. 2006;19(3):233–238.

[153] Winstanley CA, Olausson P, Taylor JR, Jentsch JD. Insight into the relationship between impulsivity and substance abuse from studies using animal models. Alcohol Clin Exp Res. 2010;34(8):1306–1318.

[154] Koob GF. Neurobiological substrates for the dark side of compulsivity in addiction. Neuropharmacology. 2009;56(Suppl 1):18–31.

[155] Leshner AI. Addiction is a brain disease, and it matters. Science. 1997;278(5335):45–47.

[156] Robinson TE, Berridge KC. Review. The incentive sensitization theory of addiction: some current issues. Philos Trans R Soc Lond B Biol Sci. 2008;363(1507):3137–3146.

[157] Belin D, Deroche-Gamonet V. Responses to novelty and vulnerability to cocaine addiction: contribution of a multi-symptomatic animal model. Cold Spring Harbor Perspect Med. 2012; 2 :a011940

[158] Pattij T, De Vries TJ. The role of impulsivity in relapse vulnerability. CurrOpinNeurobiol. 2013;23(4):700–705.

[159] Saunders BT, Robinson TE. Individual variation in resisting temptation: implications for addiction. NeurosciBiobehav Rev. 2013;37(9 Pt A):1955–1975.

[160] Swendsen J, Le Moal M. Individual vulnerability to addiction. Ann N Y Acad Sci. 2011;1216:73–85.

[161] APA. In: Edition F, editor. The diagnostic and statistical manual of mental disorders, 5th edition (DSM-V). Washington, DC: American Psychiatric Association; 2013.

[162] Lichtman AH, Martin BR. Cannabinoid tolerance and dependence. Handb Exp Pharmacol. 2005(168):691–717.

[163] APA. In: Edition F, editor. The diagnostic and statistical manual of mental disorders, 4th edition (DSM-IV). Washington, DC: American Psychiatric Association; 2000.

[164] Pope HG, Jr., Gruber AJ, Hudson JI, Huestis MA, Yurgelun-Todd D. Neuropsychological performance in long-term cannabis users. Arch Gen Psychiatry. 2001;58(10):909–915.

[165] Maldonado R. Study of cannabinoid dependence in animals. Pharmacol Ther. 2002;95(2):153–164.

[166] Sanchis-Segura C, Spanagel R. Behavioural assessment of drug reinforcement and addictive features in rodents: an overview. Addict Biol. 2006;11(1):2–38.

[167] Panlilio LV, Goldberg SR. Self-administration of drugs in animals and humans as a model and an investigative tool. Addiction. 2007;102(12):1863–1870.

[168] Panlilio LV, Justinova Z, Goldberg SR. Animal models of cannabinoid reward. Br J Pharmacol. 2010;160(3):499–510.

[169] Fattore L, Cossu G, Martellotta CM, Fratta W. Intravenous self-administration of the cannabinoid CB1 receptor agonist WIN 55,212-2 in rats. Psychopharmacology (Berl). 2001;156(4):410–416.

[170] Flores A, Maldonado R, Berrendero F. The hypocretin/orexin receptor-1 as a novel target to modulate cannabinoid reward. Biol Psychiatry. 2014;75(6):499–507.

[171] Martellotta MC, Cossu G, Fattore L, Gessa GL, Fratta W. Self-administration of the cannabinoid receptor agonist WIN 55,212-2 in drug-naive mice. Neuroscience. 1998;85(2):327–330.

[172] Mendizabal V, Zimmer A, Maldonado R. Involvement of kappa/dynorphin system in WIN 55,212-2 self-administration in mice. Neuropsychopharmacology. 2006;31(9): 1957–1966.

[173] Navarro M, Carrera MR, Fratta W, Valverde O, Cossu G, Fattore L, et al. Functional interaction between opioid and cannabinoid receptors in drug self-administration. J Neurosci. 2001;21(14):5344–5350.

[174] Justinova Z, Tanda G, Redhi GH, Goldberg SR. Self-administration of delta9-tetrahydrocannabinol (THC) by drug naive squirrel monkeys. Psychopharmacology (Berl). 2003;169(2):135–140.

[175] Tanda G, Munzar P, Goldberg SR. Self-administration behavior is maintained by the psychoactive ingredient of marijuana in squirrel monkeys. Nat Neurosci. 2000;3(11): 1073–1074.

[176] Tzschentke TM. Measuring reward with the conditioned place preference (CPP) paradigm: update of the last decade. Addict Biol. 2007;12(3–4):227–462.

[177] Hutcheson DM, Tzavara ET, Smadja C, Valjent E, Roques BP, Hanoune J, et al. Behavioural and biochemical evidence for signs of abstinence in mice chronically treated with delta-9-tetrahydrocannabinol. Br J Pharmacol. 1998;125(7):1567–1577.

[178] McGregor IS, Issakidis CN, Prior G. Aversive effects of the synthetic cannabinoid CP 55,940 in rats. Pharmacol Biochem Behav. 1996;53(3):657–664.

[179] Parker LA, Gillies T. THC-induced place and taste aversions in Lewis and Sprague–Dawley rats. Behav Neurosci. 1995;109(1):71–78.

[180] Sanudo-Pena MC, Tsou K, Delay ER, Hohman AG, Force M, Walker JM. Endogenous cannabinoids as an aversive or counter-rewarding system in the rat. Neurosci Lett. 1997;223(2):125–128.

[181] Valjent E, Maldonado R. A behavioural model to reveal place preference to delta 9-tetrahydrocannabinol in mice. Psychopharmacology (Berl). 2000;147(4):436–438.

[182] Befort K. Interactions of the opioid and cannabinoid systems in reward: insights from knockout studies. Front Pharmacol. 2015;6:6.

[183] Maldonado R, Blendy JA, Tzavara E, Gass P, Roques BP, Hanoune J, et al. Reduction of morphine abstinence in mice with a mutation in the gene encoding CREB. Science. 1996;273(5275):657–659.

[184] Maldonado R, Rodriguez de Fonseca F. Cannabinoid addiction: behavioral models and neural correlates. J Neurosci. 2002;22(9):3326–3331.

[185] SAMHSA. Results from the 2010 National Survey on Drug Use and Health: Summary of National Findings [accessed April 16, 2015]. Available from: http://www.samhsa.gov/data/sites/default/files/NSDUHresults2010/NSDUHresults2010.pdf.

[186] Marshall K, Gowing L, Ali R, Le Foll B. Pharmacotherapies for cannabis dependence. Cochrane Database Syst Rev. 2014;12:CD008940.

[187] De Vries TJ, Schoffelmeer AN. Cannabinoid CB1 receptors control conditioned drug seeking. Trends Pharmacol Sci. 2005;26(8):420–426.

[188] Le Foll B, Goldberg SR. Cannabinoid CB1 receptor antagonists as promising new medications for drug dependence. J Pharmacol Exp Ther. 2005;312(3):875–883.

[189] Justinova Z, Munzar P, Panlilio LV, Yasar S, Redhi GH, Tanda G, et al. Blockade of THC-seeking behavior and relapse in monkeys by the cannabinoid CB(1)-receptor antagonist rimonabant. Neuropsychopharmacology. 2008;33(12):2870–2877.

[190] Vandrey R, Haney M. Pharmacotherapy for cannabis dependence: how close are we? CNS Drugs. 2009;23(7):543–553.

[191] Fattore L, Fratta W. Beyond THC: The New Generation of cannabinoid designer drugs. Front Behav Neurosci. 2011;5:60.

[192] Vandrey R, Johnson MW, Johnson PS, Khalil MA. Novel drugs of abuse: a snapshot of an evolving marketplace. Adolesc Psychiatry (Hilversum). 2013;3(2):123–134.

[193] Debruyne D, Le Boisselier R. Emerging drugs of abuse: current perspectives on synthetic cannabinoids. Subst Abuse Rehabil. 2015;6:113–129.

[194] Lindigkeit R, Boehme A, Eiserloh I, Luebbecke M, Wiggermann M, Ernst L, et al. Spice: a never ending story? Forensic Sci Int. 2009;191(1–3):58–63.

[195] Cohen J, Morrison S, Greenberg J, Saidinejad M. Clinical presentation of intoxication due to synthetic cannabinoids. Pediatrics. 2012;129(4):e1064–e1067.

[196] Wells DL, Ott CA. The "new" marijuana. Ann Pharmacother. 2011;45(3):414–417.

[197] Mir A, Obafemi A, Young A, Kane C. Myocardial infarction associated with use of the synthetic cannabinoid K2. Pediatrics. 2011;128(6):e1622–e1627.

[198] Rech MA, Donahey E, Cappiello Dziedzic JM, Oh L, Greenhalgh E. New drugs of abuse. Pharmacotherapy. 2015;35(2):189–197.

[199] Fattore L, Deiana S, Spano SM, Cossu G, Fadda P, Scherma M, et al. Endocannabinoid system and opioid addiction: behavioural aspects. Pharmacol Biochem Behav. 2005;81(2):343–359.

[200] Robledo P, Berrendero F, Ozaita A, Maldonado R. Advances in the field of cannabinoid–opioid cross-talk. Addict Biol. 2008;13(2):213–224.

[201] Trigo JM, Martin-Garcia E, Berrendero F, Robledo P, Maldonado R. The endogenous opioid system: acommon substrate in drug addiction. Drug Alcohol Depend. 2010; 108(3):183-194.

[202] Vigano D, Rubino T, Parolaro D. Molecular and cellular basis of cannabinoid and opioid interactions. Pharmacol Biochem Behav. 2005;81(2):360–368.

[203] Nadal X, La Porta C, Andreea Bura S, Maldonado R. Involvement of the opioid and cannabinoid systems in pain control: new insights from knockout studies. Eur J Pharmacol. 2013;716(1–3):142–157.

[204] Welch SP. Interaction of the cannabinoid and opioid systems in the modulation of nociception. Int Rev Psychiatry. 2009;21(2):143–151.

[205] Charbogne P, Kieffer BL, Befort K. 15 years of genetic approaches in vivo for addiction research: opioid receptor and peptide gene knockout in mouse models of drug abuse. Neuropharmacology. 2014;76(Pt B):204–217.

[206] Contet C, Kieffer BL, Befort K. Mu opioid receptor: a gateway to drug addiction. Curr Opin Neurobiol. 2004;14(3):370–378.

[207] Fattore L, Vigano D, Fadda P, Rubino T, Fratta W, Parolaro D. Bidirectional regulation of mu-opioid and CB1-cannabinoid receptor in rats self-administering heroin or WIN 55,212-2. Eur J Neurosci. 2007;25(7):2191–2200.

[208] Ledent C, Valverde O, Cossu G, Petitet F, Aubert JF, Beslot F, et al. Unresponsiveness to cannabinoids and reduced addictive effects of opiates in CB1 receptor knockout mice. Science. 1999;283(5400):401–404.

[209] Maldonado R, Robledo P, Berrendero F. Endocannabinoid system and drug addiction: new insights from mutant mice approaches. Curr Opin Neurobiol. 2013;23(4):480–486.

[210] Navarro M, Chowen J, Rocio ACM, del Arco I, Villanua MA, Martin Y, et al. CB1 cannabinoid receptor antagonist-induced opiate withdrawal in morphine-dependent rats. Neuroreport. 1998;9(15):3397–3402.

[211] Rodriguez JJ, Mackie K, Pickel VM. Ultrastructural localization of the CB1 cannabinoid receptor in mu-opioid receptor patches of the rat *Caudate putamen* nucleus. J Neurosci. 2001;21(3):823–833.

[212] Salio C, Fischer J, Franzoni MF, Mackie K, Kaneko T, Conrath M. CB1-cannabinoid and mu-opioid receptor co-localization on postsynaptic target in the rat dorsal horn. Neuroreport. 2001;12(17):3689–3692.

[213] Fujita W, Gomes I, Devi LA. Revolution in GPCR signalling: opioid receptor heteromers as novel therapeutic targets: IUPHAR review 10. Br J Pharmacol. 2014;171(18): 4155–4176.

[214] Massotte D. In vivo opioid receptor heteromerization: where do we stand? Br J Pharmacol. 2015;172(2):420–434.

[215] Scavone JL, Sterling RC, Van Bockstaele EJ. Cannabinoid and opioid interactions: implications for opiate dependence and withdrawal. Neuroscience. 2013;248:637–654.

[216] Thomas A, Baillie GL, Phillips AM, Razdan RK, Ross RA, Pertwee RG. Cannabidiol displays unexpectedly high potency as an antagonist of CB1 and CB2 receptor agonists in vitro. Br J Pharmacol. 2007;150(5):613–623.

[217] Campos AC, Moreira FA, Gomes FV, Del Bel EA, Guimaraes FS. Multiple mechanisms involved in the large-spectrum therapeutic potential of cannabidiol in psychiatric disorders. Philos Trans R Soc Lond B Biol Sci. 2012;367(1607):3364–3378.

[218] Wright MJ, Jr., Vandewater SA, Taffe MA. Cannabidiol attenuates deficits of visuospatial associative memory induced by Delta(9) tetrahydrocannabinol. Br J Pharmacol. 2013;170(7):1365–1373.

[219] Schubart CD, Sommer IE, Fusar-Poli P, de Witte L, Kahn RS, Boks MP. Cannabidiol as a potential treatment for psychosis. Eur Neuropsychopharmacol. 2014;24(1):51–64.

[220] Zuardi AW, Crippa JA, Hallak JE, Moreira FA, Guimaraes FS. Cannabidiol, a *Cannabis sativa* constituent, as an antipsychotic drug. Braz J Med Biol Res. 2006;39(4):421–429.

[221] Ren Y, Whittard J, Higuera-Matas A, Morris CV, Hurd YL. Cannabidiol, a nonpsychotropic component of cannabis, inhibits cue-induced heroin seeking and normalizes discrete mesolimbic neuronal disturbances. J Neurosci. 2009;29(47):14764–14769.

[222] Ward SJ, McAllister SD, Kawamura R, Murase R, Neelakantan H, Walker EA. Cannabidiol inhibits paclitaxel-induced neuropathic pain through 5-HT(1A) receptors without diminishing nervous system function or chemotherapy efficacy. Br J Pharmacol. 2014;171(3):636–645.

[223] Izzo AA, Borrelli F, Capasso R, Di Marzo V, Mechoulam R. Non-psychotropic plant cannabinoids: new therapeutic opportunities from an ancient herb. Trends Pharmacol Sci. 2009;30(10):515–527.

[224] Zuardi AW. Cannabidiol: from an inactive cannabinoid to a drug with wide spectrum of action. Rev Bras Psiquiatr. 2008;30(3):271–280.

[225] Volkow ND, Baler RD, Compton WM, Weiss SR. Adverse health effects of marijuana use. N Engl J Med. 2014;370(23):2219–2227.

[226] Deng L, Guindon J, Cornett BL, Makriyannis A, Mackie K, Hohmann AG. Chronic cannabinoid receptor 2 activation reverses paclitaxel neuropathy without tolerance or cannabinoid receptor 1-dependent withdrawal. Biol Psychiatry. 2014;77(5):475–487.

[227] Leleu-Chavain N, Desreumaux P, Chavatte P, Millet R. Therapeutical potential of CB(2) receptors in immune-related diseases. Curr Mol Pharmacol. 2013;6(3):183–203.

[228] Han S, Chen JJ, Chen JZ. Latest progress in the identification of novel synthetic ligands for the cannabinoid CB2 receptor. Mini Rev Med Chem. 2014;14(5):426–443.

[229] Leleu-Chavain N, Body-Malapel M, Spencer J, Chavatte P, Desreumaux P, Millet R. Recent advances in the development of selective CB(2) agonists as promising anti-inflammatory agents. Curr Med Chem. 2012;19(21):3457–3474.

[230] Ehrhart J, Obregon D, Mori T, Hou H, Sun N, Bai Y, et al. Stimulation of cannabinoid receptor 2 (CB2) suppresses microglial activation. J Neuroinflammation. 2005;2:29.

[231] Dittel BN. Direct suppression of autoreactive lymphocytes in the central nervous system via the CB2 receptor. Br J Pharmacol. 2008;153(2):271–276.

[232] Sagredo O, Pazos MR, Valdeolivas S, Fernandez-Ruiz J. Cannabinoids: novel medicines for the treatment of Huntington's disease. Recent Pat CNS Drug Discov. 2012;7(1): 41–48.

[233] Zhang M, Martin BR, Adler MW, Razdan RK, Jallo JI, Tuma RF. Cannabinoid CB(2) receptor activation decreases cerebral infarction in a mouse focal ischemia/reperfusion model. J Cereb Blood Flow Metab. 2007;27(7):1387–1396.

[234] Kim K, Moore DH, Makriyannis A, Abood ME. AM1241, a cannabinoid CB2 receptor selective compound, delays disease progression in a mouse model of amyotrophic lateral sclerosis. Eur J Pharmacol. 2006;542(1–3):100–105.

[235] Shoemaker JL, Seely KA, Reed RL, Crow JP, Prather PL. The CB2 cannabinoid agonist AM-1241 prolongs survival in a transgenic mouse model of amyotrophic lateral sclerosis when initiated at symptom onset. J Neurochem. 2007;101(1):87–98.

[236] Ofek O, Karsak M, Leclerc N, Fogel M, Frenkel B, Wright K, et al. Peripheral cannabinoid receptor, CB2, regulates bone mass. Proc Natl Acad Sci U S A. 2006;103(3):696–701.

[237] Mach F, Montecucco F, Steffens S. Cannabinoid receptors in acute and chronic complications of atherosclerosis. Br J Pharmacol. 2008;153(2):290–298.

[238] Barutta F, Piscitelli F, Pinach S, Bruno G, Gambino R, Rastaldi MP, et al. Protective role of cannabinoid receptor type 2 in a mouse model of diabetic nephropathy. Diabetes. 2011;60(9):2386–2396.

[239] Mallat A, Teixeira-Clerc F, Deveaux V, Lotersztajn S. Cannabinoid receptors as new targets of antifibrosing strategies during chronic liver diseases. Expert Opin Ther Targets. 2007;11(3):403–409.

[240] Le Foll B, Gorelick DA, Goldberg SR. The future of endocannabinoid-oriented clinical research after CB1 antagonists. Psychopharmacology (Berl). 2009;205(1):171–174.

[241] Despres JP, Ross R, Boka G, Almeras N, Lemieux I. Effect of rimonabant on the high-triglyceride/ low-HDL-cholesterol dyslipidemia, intraabdominal adiposity, and liver fat: the ADAGIO-Lipids trial. Arterioscler Thromb Vasc Biol. 2009;29(3):416–423.

[242] Hampp C, Hartzema AG, Kauf TL. Cost-utility analysis of rimonabant in the treatment of obesity. Value Health. 2008;11(3):389–399.

[243] Despres JP, Golay A, Sjostrom L. Effects of rimonabant on metabolic risk factors in overweight patients with dyslipidemia. N Engl J Med. 2005;353(20):2121–2134.

[244] Rigotti NA, Gonzales D, Dale LC, Lawrence D, Chang Y. A randomized controlled trial of adding the nicotine patch to rimonabant for smoking cessation: efficacy, safety and weight gain. Addiction. 2009;104(2):266–276.

[245] Christensen R, Kristensen PK, Bartels EM, Bliddal H, Astrup A. Efficacy and safety of the weight-loss drug rimonabant: a meta-analysis of randomised trials. Lancet. 2007;370(9600):1706–1713.

[246] Romero-Sandoval EA, Asbill S, Paige CA, Byrd-Glover K. Peripherally Restricted cannabinoids for the treatment of pain. Pharmacotherapy. 2015;35(10):917–925.

[247] Pavon FJ, Serrano A, Perez-Valero V, Jagerovic N, Hernandez-Folgado L, Bermudez-Silva FJ, et al. Central versus peripheral antagonism of cannabinoid CB1 receptor in obesity: effects of LH-21, a peripherally acting neutral cannabinoid receptor antagonist, in Zucker rats. J Neuroendocrinol. 2008;20 Suppl 1:116–123.

[248] Navarro M, Carrera MR, Del Arco I, Trigo JM, Koob GF, Rodriguez de Fonseca F. Cannabinoid receptor antagonist reduces heroin self-administration only in dependent rats. Eur J Pharmacol. 2004;501(1–3):235–237.

[249] Le Foll B, Forget B, Aubin HJ, Goldberg SR. Blocking cannabinoid CB1 receptors for the treatment of nicotine dependence: insights from pre-clinical and clinical studies. Addict Biol. 2008;13(2):239–252.

[250] Cahill K, Ussher M. Cannabinoid type 1 receptor antagonists (rimonabant) for smoking cessation. Cochrane Database Syst Rev. 2007(3):CD005353.

[251] Kleczkowska P, Smaga I, Filip M, Bujalska-Zadrozny M. Cannabinoid ligands and alcohol addiction: a promising therapeutic tool or a humbug? Neurotox Res. 2016;29(1): 173–196.

[252] Cohen C, Perrault G, Voltz C, Steinberg R, Soubrie P. SR141716, a central cannabinoid (CB(1)) receptor antagonist, blocks the motivational and dopamine-releasing effects of nicotine in rats. Behav Pharmacol. 2002;13(5–6):451–463.

[253] Soyka M, Koller G, Schmidt P, Lesch OM, Leweke M, Fehr C, et al. Cannabinoid receptor 1 blocker rimonabant (SR 141716) for treatment of alcohol dependence: results from a placebo-controlled, double-blind trial. J Clin Psychopharmacol. 2008;28(3):317–324.

[254] Piomelli D, Tarzia G, Duranti A, Tontini A, Mor M, Compton TR, et al. Pharmacological profile of the selective FAAH inhibitor KDS-4103 (URB597). CNS Drug Rev. 2006;12(1):21–38.

[255] Gaetani S, Dipasquale P, Romano A, Righetti L, Cassano T, Piomelli D, et al. The endocannabinoid system as a target for novel anxiolytic and antidepressant drugs. Int Rev Neurobiol. 2009;85:57–72.

[256] Kathuria S, Gaetani S, Fegley D, Valino F, Duranti A, Tontini A, et al. Modulation of anxiety through blockade of anandamide hydrolysis. Nat Med. 2003;9(1):76–81.

[257] Gobbi G, Bambico FR, Mangieri R, Bortolato M, Campolongo P, Solinas M, et al. Antidepressant-like activity and modulation of brain monoaminergic transmission by blockade of anandamide hydrolysis. Proc Natl Acad Sci U S A. 2005;102(51):18620–18625.

[258] Bambico FR, Duranti A, Nobrega JN, Gobbi G. The fatty acid amide hydrolase inhibitor URB597 modulates serotonin-dependent emotional behaviour, and serotonin and serotonin activity in the hippocampus. Eur Neuropsychopharmacol. 2015; 26(3): 578-590.

[259] Hasanein P, Ghafari-Vahed M. Fatty acid amide hydrolase inhibitor URB597 prevented tolerance and cognitive deficits induced by chronic morphine administration in rats. Behav Pharmacol. 2016;27(1):37–43.

[260] Gamage TF, Ignatowska-Jankowska BM, Muldoon PP, Cravatt BF, Damaj MI, Lichtman AH. Differential effects of endocannabinoid catabolic inhibitors on morphine withdrawal in mice. Drug Alcohol Depend. 2015;146:7–16.

[261] Ramesh D, Ross GR, Schlosburg JE, Owens RA, Abdullah RA, Kinsey SG, et al. Blockade of endocannabinoid hydrolytic enzymes attenuates precipitated opioid withdrawal symptoms in mice. J Pharmacol Exp Ther. 2011;339(1):173–185.

[262] Clapper JR, Mangieri RA, Piomelli D. The endocannabinoid system as a target for the treatment of cannabis dependence. Neuropharmacology. 2009;56(Suppl 1):235–243.

[263] Panlilio LV, Thorndike EB, Nikas SP, Alapafuja SO, Bandiera T, Cravatt BF, et al. Effects of fatty acid amide hydrolase (FAAH) inhibitors on working memory in rats. Pharmacol (Berl). 2016; 233(10):1879-1888.

[264] Hill MN, Gorzalka BB. Pharmacological enhancement of cannabinoid CB1 receptor activity elicits an antidepressant-like response in the rat forced swim test. Eur Neuropsychopharmacol. 2005;15(6):593–599.

[265] Schindler CW, Scherma M, Redhi GH, Vadivel SK, Makriyannis A, Goldberg SR, et al. Self-administration of the anandamide transport inhibitor AM404 by squirrel monkeys. psychopharmacol (Berl). 2016; 233(10):1867-1877.

[266] Le Naour M, Akgun E, Yekkirala A, Lunzer MM, Powers MD, Kalyuzhny AE, et al. Bivalent ligands that target mu opioid (MOP) and cannabinoid1 (CB1) receptors are potent analgesics devoid of tolerance. J Med Chem. 2013;56(13):5505–5513.

[267] Roques BP, Fournie-Zaluski MC, Wurm M. Inhibiting the breakdown of endogenous opioids and cannabinoids to alleviate pain. Nat Rev Drug Discov. 2012;11(4):292–310.

[268] Hart CL. Increasing treatment options for cannabis dependence: a review of potential pharmacotherapies. Drug Alcohol Depend. 2005;80(2):147–159.